Barbara Sehsering

CLINICS IN DEVELOPMENTAL MEDICINE NO. 104/105
THE DEVELOPMENT OF MATURE WALKING

Clinics in Developmental Medicine No. 104/105

THE DEVELOPMENT OF MATURE WALKING

DAVID H. SUTHERLAND
RICHARD A. OLSHEN
EDMUND N. BIDEN
MARILYNN P. WYATT

Motion Analysis Laboratory
Children's Hospital and Health Center
San Diego

1988
Mac Keith Press
OXFORD: Blackwell Scientific Publications Ltd.
PHILADELPHIA: J. B. Lippincott Co.

©1988 Mac Keith Press
5a Netherhall Gardens, London NW3 5RN

All rights reserved. No part of this publication may be reproduced, stored in a retrieval system, or transmitted in any form or by any means, electronic, mechanical, photocopying, recording or otherwise, without the prior permission of the publishers (Mac Keith Press, 5a Netherhall Gardens, London NW3 5RN)

First published 1988

British Library Cataloguing in Publication Data

The development of mature walking.—
  (Clinics in developmental medicine, ISSN 0069-4835; no. 104/105).
  1. Children. Motor skills. Development
  I. Sutherland, David H. II. Series
  155.4'12

ISBN (UK) 0 632-01902 6
      (USA) 0 397 44622 5

Printed in Great Britain at The Lavenham Press Ltd., Lavenham, Suffolk
Mac Keith Press is supported by **The Spastics Society, London, England**

This book is dedicated to:

Anne, David, Tom, Paul, Jeff and Kathy

Susan

Bernadette and Emily

Frank and Taylor

AUTHORS' APPOINTMENTS

DAVID H. SUTHERLAND, M.D.
Professor of Surgery, Division of Orthopaedics and Rehabilitation, University of California, San Diego.

Chief of Orthopaedic Surgery; Medical Director, Motion Analysis Laboratory, Children's Hospital, San Diego.

RICHARD A. OLSHEN, Ph.D.
Professor, Department of Mathematics; Director, Laboratory for Mathematics and Statistics, University of California, San Diego.

EDMUND N. BIDEN, D.Phil.
Associate Professor, Mechanical Engineering, University of New Brunswick, Fredericton, New Brunswick, Canada.

MARILYNN P. WYATT, M.A., R.P.T.
Supervisor, Motion Analysis Laboratory, Children's Hospital, San Diego.

CONTENTS

FOREWORD — Martin Bax — page ix

1. INTRODUCTION — 1
2. METHODS — 3
3. MODELING AND PREDICTION REGIONS FOR MOTION DATA — 24
4. STUDY PLAN — 30
5. ANTHROPOMETRIC MEASUREMENTS AND DEVELOPMENTAL SCREENING — 33
6. TIME/DISTANCE PARAMETERS BY AGE — 55
7. JOINT ANGLES AND FILM TRACINGS — 65
8. DYNAMIC ELECTROMYOGRAPHY BY AGE — 154
9. FORCE-PLATE VALUES BY AGE — 163
10. AGE AND GAIT — 178
11. RELATIONSHIP BETWEEN NEURAL DEVELOPMENT AND WALKING — 183
12. RELEVANCE TO CLINICAL PRACTICE — 188
13. FUTURE DIRECTIONS — 206

APPENDICES — 210

REFERENCES — 215

ACKNOWLEDGEMENTS — 219

INDEX — 222

FOREWORD

Upright gait has always been seen as one of the most distinctive of human characteristics. 'Man', wrote Aristotle, 'alone among all living beings walks erect, because his nature and his being are divine.' And the anthropomorphic Greek gods surely walked erect.

This recognition of the importance of upright gait as a unique characteristic has long led to an interest in its development. Peiper, in his classic work on the development of cerebral function[1], remarked on the young child's drive towards motility: 'Progress is made possible by the strong urge for movement and activity, which continuously drives the child to new experiments and which is not inhibited by many failures.' (Interestingly he added, 'To further this development by special aides who are trained in "infant gymnastics" seems to me needless, at least for the healthy child.')

Peiper himself provided us with excellent descriptions of the gait patterns of young children, as did a number of other early authors. However, to take the analysis of the development of gait in man beyond a descriptive stage is not a simple matter. Those early workers made numerous films of walking infants and toddlers, but the great problem in analysing such work is the time needed to view the material and later to compress it into any sensible form.

Yet over recent years the development of new ideas about therapy for children with movement problems has become widespread throughout the developed world. The objective measurement of movement in the young child has become vitally important in order to assess the effectiveness of the wide range of treatments offered to children with motor disabilities.

In order to make such assessments it is essential to have clear data on the normative gait of young children. For some time we have been able to carry out objective measurements using cinematography, dynamic EMG and force plates; however, the problem has been to analyse the resultant data in an understandable way. Today, the advent of computer analysis has led to the modern gait laboratory.

In this book Sutherland and his colleagues provide us for the first time with norms of gait development through the first seven years of life. At every age from one year up detailed measurements of hip, knee and ankle joints across the gait cycle are clearly described and displayed in a way that is readily accessible to all.

There are many different groups of people who should find this material fascinating, and I fancy that some parents will enjoy looking more knowingly at the progress of their young child's walking. But for all of us professionally engaged in the observation of child development, whether we be doctors, nurses, psychologists or therapists, it will add a new depth to our clinical work by providing a thorough understanding of the development of this most basic human attribute.

The authors have not only mastered the techniques of analysis but, equally, have developed ways of presenting them to other researchers and clinicians.

Readers who do not have access to such expensively equipped laboratories will find that the display of information will make their own clinical observations much more meaningful and, as the authors state, much of the analysis can be conducted using much simpler methods than the highly sophisticated techniques used here.

On the basis of this monumental and classic study we can move forward with more confidence to describe the abnormal gait patterns we see in our patients with disabilities, and hopefully begin at last to provide them with treatments which have been properly assessed.

MARTIN BAX

REFERENCE

1. Peiper, A. (1961) *Cerebral Function in Infancy and Childhood.* London: Pitman Medical. *[Translated from the German original (1942).]*

1
INTRODUCTION

The current development of gait analysis and its increasing application to the study of pathological gait has created an urgent need for normative data. This is most evident in the study of children. The walking patterns of small children differ substantially from those of adults, so measurements at various ages are required for critical comparisons. If objective gait measurements—including averages and population variability around them—are available, the process of identifying departures from normal patterns has at least the beginnings of a scientific foundation.

To meet the need for measurements from onset of walking to 7 years of age, 449 studies of 309 normal children were performed in the Motion Analysis Laboratory at the Children's Hospital, San Diego. The objectives of this study were: (1) to outline changes in gait from the age of first walking to 7 years; (2) to define mature gait in terms of specific gait parameters; and (3) to provide a substantial data base for comparing children with possible gait problems against normal children of the same age.

The study is now sufficiently detailed that it seems worthwhile to present this monograph on its most cogent findings to date. A summary has already been published of many aspects of 186 of our subjects (Sutherland *et al.* 1980a). The current material covers the entire study sample and includes anthropometric measurements not discussed in the previous publication. Normal data have been helpful in the studies of pathological gait done at this laboratory, providing means and prediction regions essential to the recognition of abnormality, as well as giving insights into the normal maturation process.

These data are useful even to those who have no access to a sophisticated gait laboratory. Many of the measurements can be made in simpler ways—for example, chalk dust or ink can be placed on the soles of the subject's feet, allowing measurement of the width of the base, step length, stride length, and foot rotation with respect to the line of progression. With a stopwatch and a measured distance, walking velocity can be calculated and cadence counted.

Tracings from cine film of the walking cycle of a representative child in each of the 10 age-groups studied have been included to provide visual representation of gait. The reader is encouraged to correlate joint angles displayed graphically with limb-segment positions as they are observed by the human eye. The emergence of gait analysis as a scientific tool does not substitute for skills in visual gait observation. Gait analysis can, however, correct errors in visual observation, reinforce accurate observation, and measure subtleties that are beyond the scope of the human eye to discern.

Advanced statistical techniques have been used in the study, and appropriate attention is focused on them in order to establish the credibility of our methods of data handling. We have examined sex, laterality and the determinants of mature gait. Particular attention has been given to providing gait parameters by age. This information will be useful to many disciplines dealing with the growth and development of children. Chapters have been organized so as to allow ready reference to gait parameters and anthropometric measurements by age. A pediatrician wishing to assess the walking function of a 2-year-old can readily locate normal gait measurements. S/he can also see front- and side-view film tracings of the walk cycle of a representative 2-year-old normal subject.

An accurate description of walking, with measurements of gait parameters, is only the first step in understanding the complex function of walking, and many areas are yet to be explored. The struggle to understand the subject fully is in its infancy, and much growth and development in our comprehension lie ahead.

2
METHODS

Description of the laboratory
The Motion Analysis Laboratory at the Children's Hospital, San Diego, was built first and foremost as a gait analysis facility. The testing area forms the core of the laboratory, with office space and computer rooms arranged around it. Equipment used in gait analysis is permanently set up and available for use. Every attempt is made to put subjects at ease and to gain their confidence. The staff avoid the 'white coat' hospital uniform where possible and toys are provided for younger subjects to play with. Parents and other family members are encouraged to stay during the testing and often play an active part in encouraging reluctant children to perform.

In this chapter we describe the facility, and provide definitions and descriptions of the measurements we make. The descriptions are divided into four sections: (1) movement measurements; (2) force measurements; (3) electromyographic measurements; and (4) computer systems. Each section describes the sort of equipment used and the procedures followed. Tables 2.I and 2.II at the end of the chapter provide a detailed equipment list and other technical data.

Movement measurements
For this study, and for all clinical gait analysis from the time the lab opened until 1987, when we began using a VICON* system (see Chapter 13, p. 207), movement data were collected photographically (Fig. 2.1). Four 16mm motion picture cameras were used. The front camera, equipped with a telephoto lens, was placed about 17 meters from the center of the lab and tipped on its side to take advantage of the aspect ratio of the film to get a more complete view of the patient. Cameras to the subject's right and left were placed between 5 and 6 meters from the walkway, providing a sagittal field of view which for most subjects was sufficient to record two or three complete gait cycles during each pass down the walkway. The fourth camera was placed beneath a clear force plate (see below) to photograph the bottom of the subject's foot as s/he stepped over it. The right, front and left cameras all ran at 50 frames per second (fps) and the pit camera at 24fps. The cameras ran independently, each with its own speed control, although they were started and stopped by remote control. To provide synchronization between cameras, a digital time display was placed in each camera's field of view. The four displays, all controlled by a master clock, counted in tenths of seconds while the cameras were running. Thus, frames for two views could be synchronized by matching the time displays.

Subjects walked several times down the walkway while data were collected. The exposed film was processed off-site by a commercial laboratory, and on return

---
*VICON is a registered trademark of Oxford Medllog Inc.

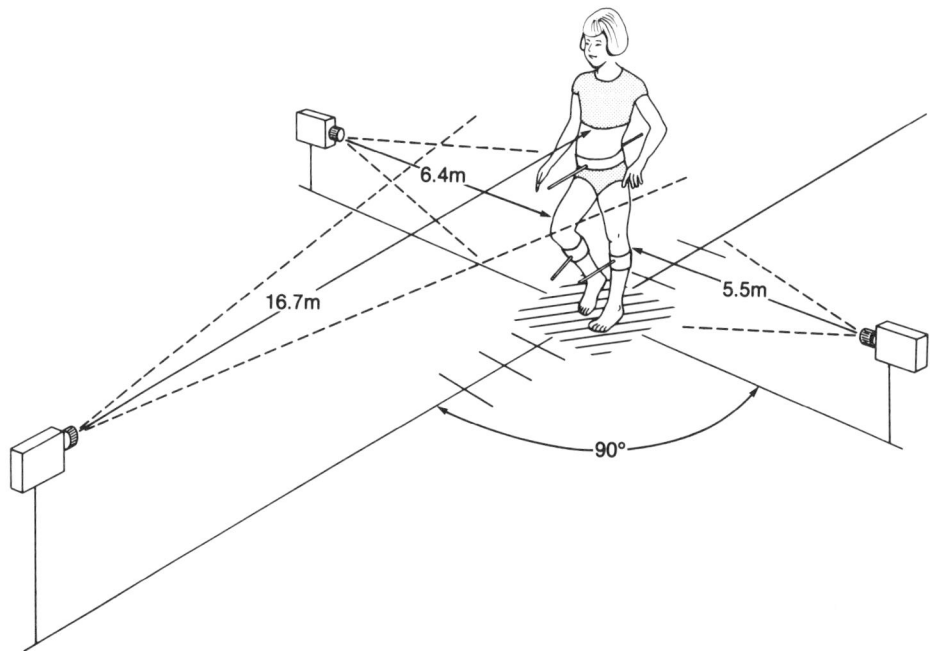

Fig. 2.1. Arrangement of cameras and force plate in the gait laboratory. (A fourth camera is situated below the force plate.)

was edited so that the film for each subject was all together. The usual sequence was to edit right-side views first, followed by front and left views, with the view from the pit placed last in the sequence. Each subject's completed film was placed in its own container, which was filed to allow easy retrieval.

Once edited, the subject's film was studied using a motion analyzer. The film was projected on a rear-projection screen and analyzed frame by frame. The first stage of analysis was to measure the time/distance parameters for six to 10 individual gait cycles for each side of the body. The most representative cycle was selected on the basis of these parameters, and the joint angles in that cycle were measured. As each frame was projected, a Graf-Pen sonic digitizer attached to the motion analyzer was used to measure the x,y positions of various 'landmarks' on the subject (Fig. 2.2). The Graf-Pen is an acoustic device consisting of a sound source and two transducers (one placed along the top and the other along the left-hand side of the viewing screen). The observer places the sound source over the point to be digitized, then activates it by pressing a button. The x,y coordinates are computed from the time taken by the sound pulse to travel from the source to each of the transducers. For this study the x,y data were recorded on magnetic tape using a dedicated tape-drive and then transferred to the lab computer for analysis.

Basic computer analysis included the calculation of 12 different 'joint angles' for each side of the body. Sagittal angles (see pp. 65–67) were derived from the side-view film. Frontal and transverse rotations were calculated from the front

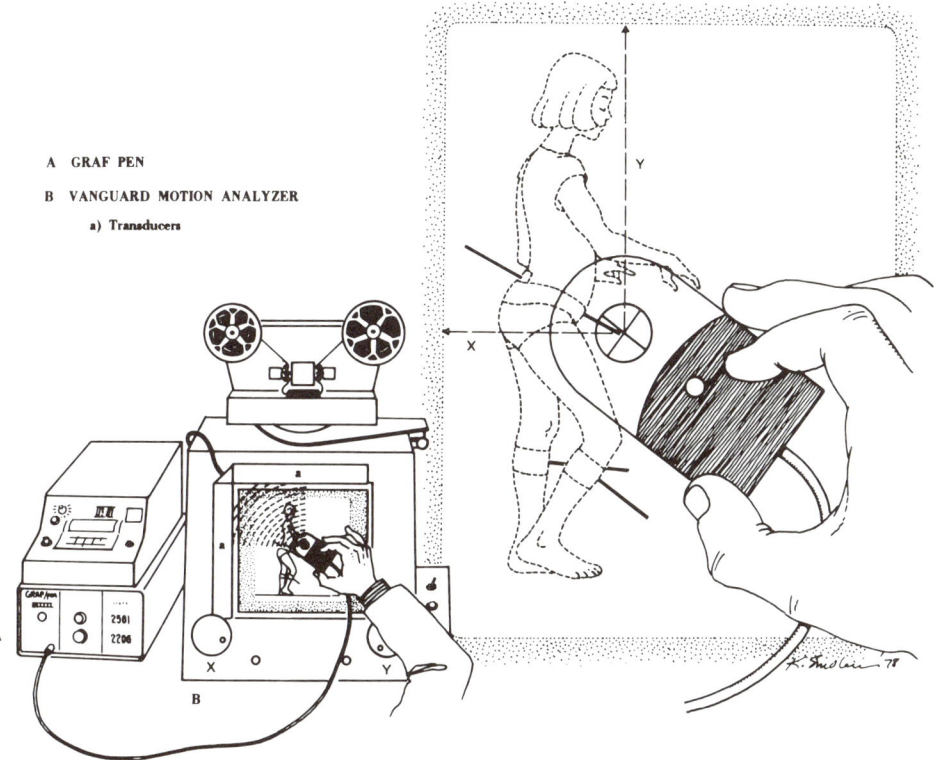

Fig. 2.2. Vanguard motion analyzer and Graf-Pen sonic digitizer used to determine the x,y coordinates of the markers shown on the viewing screen. (Sutherland *et al.* 1980*a*; reproduced by permission.)

camera view, correcting for parallax bias by means of a prepared table which listed these corrections as a function of the subject's position on the walkway. Position on the walkway was determined from the corresponding side view. For subjective analysis the joint-angle data were plotted in 'raw' form. For statistical analysis, Fourier series were found for each rotation for each subject (see Chapter 3).

Force measurements
Force data were collected using a single, custom-made, clear-topped force platform (see Fig. 2.6). This consisted of a square plexiglas panel, seven piezoelectric transducers, and six charge amplifiers (one of which was wired to collect two signals simultaneously, the combined signal being 'decoded' on later analysis). The panel, supported on the transducers, allowed for measurement of the three force components: vertical force, fore/aft shear and medial/lateral shear (see p. 16–17 for definitions). Torque in the plane of the force plate and the 'center of pressure' were calculated later. Signals were measured by the transducers, converted from charge to voltage and amplified by the charge amplifiers. A 32-channel, instrument-quality tape recorder was used to record the voltages from the charge amplifiers.

These voltage readings were later transferred to the laboratory computer using an analog-to-digital converter.

Force data were collected as the subjects were filmed. Since the motion analysis was performed using the 'most representative' gait cycle, often the force data and motion data were not derived from the same pass down the walkway.

A single foot-strike on the force platform was desired, with the opposite foot striking the floor beyond. In this manner a complete record of the force on the foot during single-limb stance was produced. Older subjects succeeded in this better than younger (smaller) ones, who would often strike the force plate with both feet. In those instances data were not recorded after the second foot hit.

As the subject's foot struck the force plate, it was photographed from below by the pit camera. Tracings from these films were matched to the 'center of pressure' plots to show the location of the ground-reaction force on the foot.

Electromyographic measurements
Measurements of the electrical activity of muscles were made after the motion and force data had been collected. The electromyographic (EMG) system comprised four channels for surface electrodes and a channel for footswitches. Commercially packaged electrodes with integral pre-amplifiers were used. These were connected via a lightweight cable to the EMG recording system. The cable included power lines to provide electrode and footswitch power and signal lines for the output signals. EMG signals were passed through a second amplifier with three gain settings and were bandpass filtered. The output was then directed to an oscillograph which recorded the EMG and footswitch signals on light-sensitive paper, and to a four-channel oscilloscope which displayed the EMG signals in view of one lens of a twin-lens camera, set up to superimpose these signals over a cine-film record of the subject walking.

'On' and 'off' times for the muscles relative to the gait cycle were determined by analyzing the oscillograph recordings or, when these had not been made, by examining the oscilloscope trace on the cine film. The beginning and end frames of a gait cycle were determined, and the frame numbers marking the start and end of activity were noted. This was repeated for between six and 10 cycles and the results were averaged. For subjects who had oscillograph recordings made, cycles were identified using the footswitch signals. The 'on' and 'off' times were then expressed as a percentage of the cycle by relating them to the distance on the chart between successive foot-strikes.

Computer systems
Two computer systems were used during this project. The first, which was used for all the data collection and for the initial analysis of motion and force, was an EPI 118, a small mini-computer running BASIC as its language. It was equipped with two 1.5 megabyte disk-drives, an analog-to-digital converter system, a plotter and a cassette tape drive. The motion data were loaded on this system using the motion analyzer and the cassette drive, and the force data were loaded from the magnetic tape drive via the analog-to-digital converter. Joint-angle and force calculations were made using this computer.

Shortly after the end of the data-collection phase of the project, the EPI 118 was replaced as the lab computer by a Digital Equipment Corp. PDP 11/44. This system has extensive real-time data collection facilities and considerably greater computing power than the EPI. Joint-angle and force data were transferred from the EPI to the new system for statistical processing. All software for the PDP 11/44 was developed in FORTRAN 77.

Test procedure
Contact was made with the parents of potential subjects, and children who met the study criteria (see p. 30) were scheduled for a session of around 1½ to 2 hours in the lab. Developmental milestones were gathered from a questionnaire filled out by the parents (Appendix A). On arrival at the lab, the subject changed into brief underclothing or a swimsuit-style outfit, and was then tested by a physical therapist for range of motion and for the anthropometric variables included in the study. When these tests were complete, markers were positioned over various bony landmarks to facilitate the digitization process. A set of four 'sticks', to measure the tilt and rotation of the pelvis and the rotations of the tibias, was also attached to the subject (Fig. 2.3). They were placed as the child was standing, one on the Michael's rhomboid of the sacrum, one on each anterior tibial crest, and one on the mid-anterior pelvis. The first three were attached by means of molded thermoplastic bases and tape or Velcro straps, and the latter by means of a pelvic belt. The actual points that were digitized are illustrated in Figure 2.4. Motion and force data were gathered as described above.

Usually subjects were asked to walk up and down the lab a number of times before the actual data collection, so as to accustom them to the markers and to allow the staff to assess the best place from which to start them walking in order to obtain clean foot-strikes on the force plate. When the subject was ready, s/he was told to stand still at the end of the walkway and then, on command from the staff member running the cameras, was told to walk.

In order to minimize the likelihood that subjects would 'target' the force plate, they were not told its real purpose. It is our experience that once children become aware that clean foot-strikes are the desired outcome, they will modify their step length accordingly, thereby altering their normal pattern of walking. Thus subjects were simply told that a number of walks were needed. The usual practice was to try to obtain two 'good' left and two 'good' right foot-strikes. Often it took six to 10 trips down the walkway to achieve this.

As soon as the motion and force data had been gathered, the markers were removed and the EMG portion of the study begun. Usually this involved two sets of four surface electrodes with footswitches. The electrodes were first coated with a special gel to improve conductivity, then placed over the muscle belly and secured with adhesive tape and with a rubber strap around the limb. Footswitches were placed under the heels to indicate foot-strike.

Once the footswitches and electrodes were in place they were connected by cable to the recording system. Tests were then made on the muscles to ensure proper placement and function of the electrodes. Levels for the oscillograph and oscilloscope were set to provide clear differentiation of when the muscles were 'on'

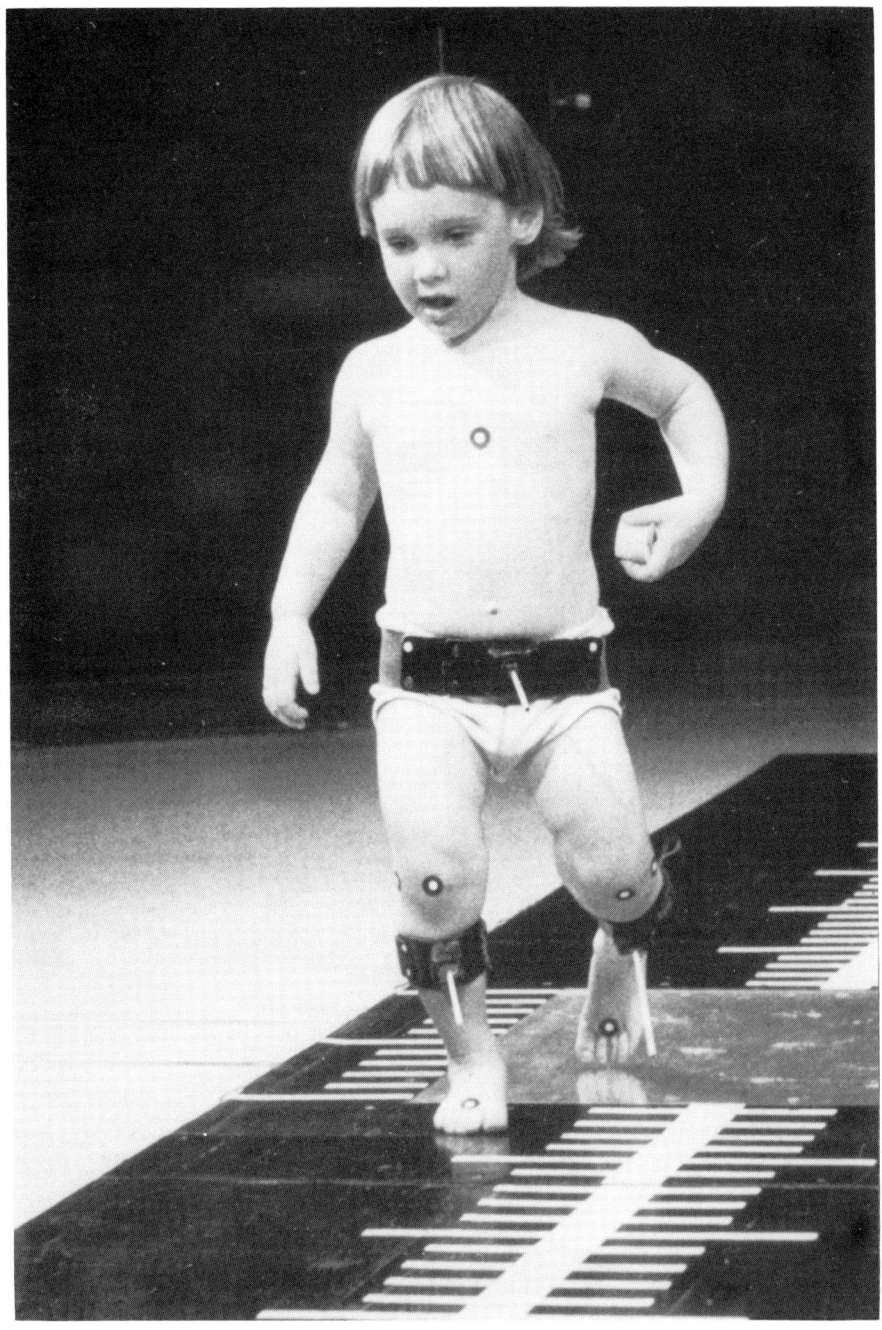

Fig. 2.3. Subject on the walkway. Note positioning of markers and marker 'sticks', from which joint rotations will be measured (see Fig. 2.4). As the photograph is taken the right foot is in contact with the ground just beyond the force plate; thus, a 'good' left foot-strike has been registered and the force data generated may be included in later analysis.

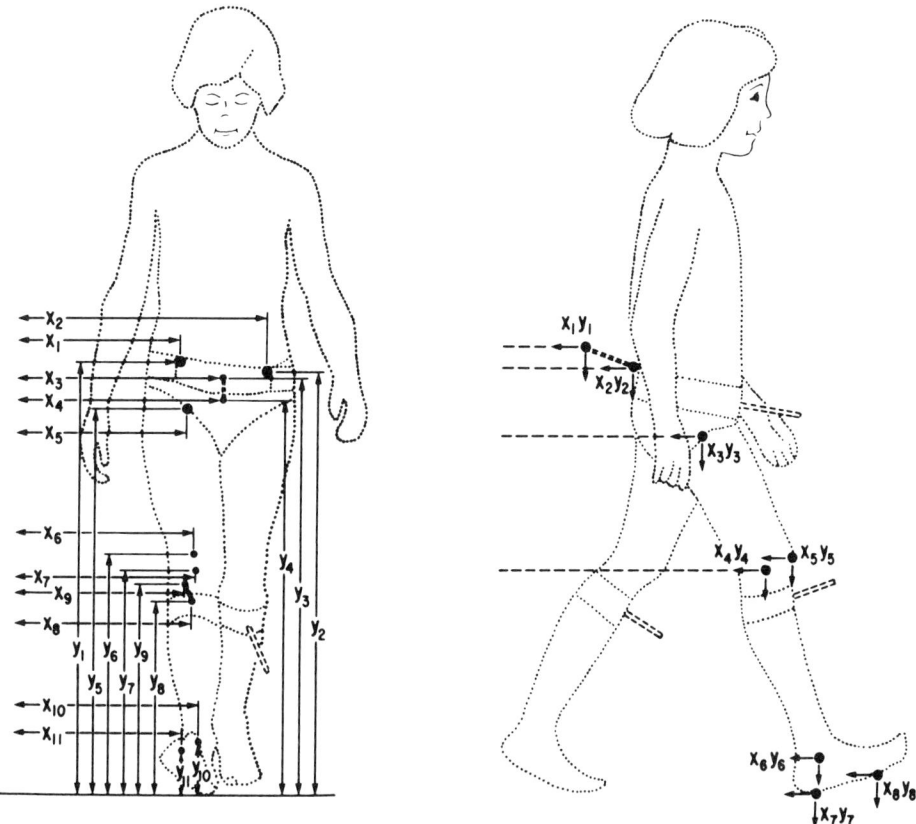

Fig. 2.4. Summary figure showing placement of the 12 markers and four sticks whose coordinates are digitized. Coordinates of both base and tip of each stick are digitized. (Specific details are illustrated in Figure 2.5.) Subscripts indicate the order in which data points are taken and later identified in computer calculations. The zero reference lines for the x,y coordinates are established by the Graf-Pen sonic digitizer. (Sutherland *et al.* 1980*a*; reproduced by permission.)

or 'off'. Absolute gain was not recorded because only timing information was required. When the electrodes were in their correct position the child was helped down from the examining table and asked to walk up and down the lab. Once s/he had become accustomed to the electrodes, data were recorded for two trips up the length of the walkway and back. This usually involved 30 to 40 complete steps.

When the first set of EMG data had been gathered the subject was returned to the examining table, a second set of electrodes was applied, and data were gathered as before. Data were analyzed, as described above, after the subject had left the lab.

As one might expect, this procedure works well with children who are old enough to understand and obey directions. With very young children, the physical examination was often done on a mat or blanket on the floor, and perhaps from the child's point of view seemed more like a game than a visit to the doctor. Often the younger children were encouraged to walk by asking them to carry toys or other objects to their parents or by offering them cereal or other food as a 'reward'. The inclusion in this study of such large numbers of young subjects is an indication of the dedication and creativity of the laboratory staff in encouraging or cajoling the children into co-operation.

Parameters measured
Joint angles
Angular rotations were measured throughout the left and right walking cycles of each subject. Methods of measurement are described below and illustrated in Figure 2.5 overleaf. The following four measurements were made using only the views obtained with the side cameras.

PELVIC TILT

Measured by means of the sacral stick. From the side view, the positions of the base and tip of the stick are noted (Fig. 2.5A). Neutral pelvic tilt (0°) is indicated when the stick is parallel to the floor. Increased pelvic tilt is recorded when the tip of the stick rises above the base and decreased tilt when the tip moves in the opposite direction.

HIP FLEXION/EXTENSION

Measured as the angle between a line segment joining the hip and knee centers and a line perpendicular to the sacral stick (Fig. 2.5B). The hip center is obtained by estimating the center of the soft-tissue outline of the upper thigh at the level of the greater trochanter. The knee center is obtained by estimating the center of the soft-tissue outline at the level of the marker on the lateral condyle of the femur.

KNEE FLEXION/EXTENSION

Measured as the angle formed by the line segments between the hip and knee centers and between the knee and ankle centers (Fig. 2.5C). The hip and knee centers are obtained as described above. The ankle center is obtained by estimating the center of the soft-tissue outline at the level of the marker on the lateral malleolus of the fibula. When the two line segments form a straight line, knee flexion/extension is 0°.

ANKLE DORSIFLEXION/PLANTAR FLEXION

Measured as the angle formed by a perpendicular to the line segment joining the knee and ankle centers and a line along the bottom of the foot (Fig. 2.5D). Negative angles indicate plantar flexion and positive ones indicate dorsiflexion.

The remaining measurements were all made using the film from the front-view camera, with the exception of femoral rotation which requires both front and side views. Even though the side view is not needed to measure pelvic, tibial or foot rotation, it must still be studied to establish the subject's position on the walkway for parallax correction.

PELVIC OBLIQUITY

Measured by means of a line of spots on the front of the pelvic belt (Fig. 2.5E). Pelvic obliquity is 0° when this line is parallel to the floor. If the marker on the right is higher than that on the left, pelvic obliquity is recorded as either 'up' for the right side or 'down' for the left, and vice-versa.

PELVIC ROTATION

Measured using the stick projecting from the front of the pelvic belt (Fig. 2.5F). When the tip and base of the stick are in line as seen from the front, the rotation is recorded as 0°. Internal pelvic rotation for the right side and external rotation for the left are indicated when the tip of the stick moves to the right of center as seen from the front (*i.e.* to the subject's left) and vice-versa.

FEMORAL ROTATION

To make this measurement it is necessary to take simultaneous readings from the front and side views. From the side view, a line segment is defined which intersects the center of the front of the patella and is perpendicular to the line between the hip and ankle centers (see above). From the corresponding front view, a second line segment is defined, intersecting the center of the front of the patella and perpendicular to the line between the hip and ankle centers. Because these two line segments (front view and side view) establish two sides of a right-angled triangle, the angle of rotation can then be calculated by trigonometry. In general, the angle of rotation is 0° if the markers for the hip, patella and ankle centers are in a straight line as seen from the front (Fig. 2.5G). Internal rotation is indicated if the patella is turned toward the midline of the body with respect to the hip/ankle line and external rotation when the patella is turned in the opposite direction.

TIBIAL ROTATION

Measured by means of the tibial stick. If the tip and base of the stick are in line as seen from the front, the rotation is 0°. Internal rotation is indicated when the tip of the stick is nearer the midline of the body and external rotation by the reverse (Fig. 2.5H).

FOOT ROTATION

Measured from the markers at the center of the ankle and between the second and third metatarsal heads. When the two points are in line as seen from the front, the rotation is 0°. The rotation is internal when the front of the foot moves toward the midline of the body, and external when it moves in the opposite direction (Fig. 2.5I).

HIP ABDUCTION/ADDUCTION

Measured in terms of the angle formed between the line segment joining the marker spots on the pelvic belt and that joining the hip and knee centers (see above). When this angle is 90°, the joint angle is 0°. Positive joint angles indicate adduction and negative ones indicate abduction (Fig. 2.5J).

A. PELVIC TILT

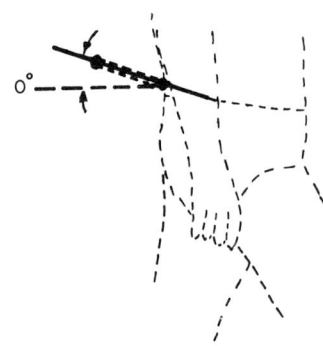

B. HIP FLEXION/EXTENSION

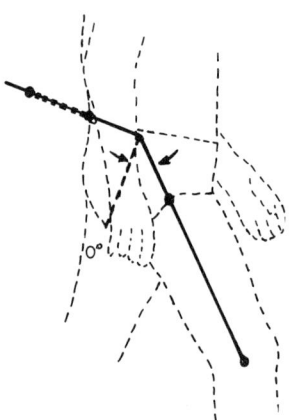

C. KNEE FLEXION/EXTENSION

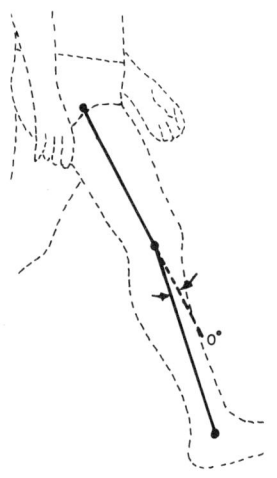

D. ANKLE DORSI-/PLANTAR FLEXION

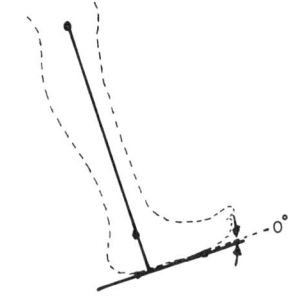

E. PELVIC OBLIQUITY

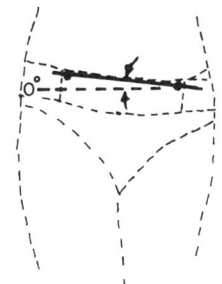

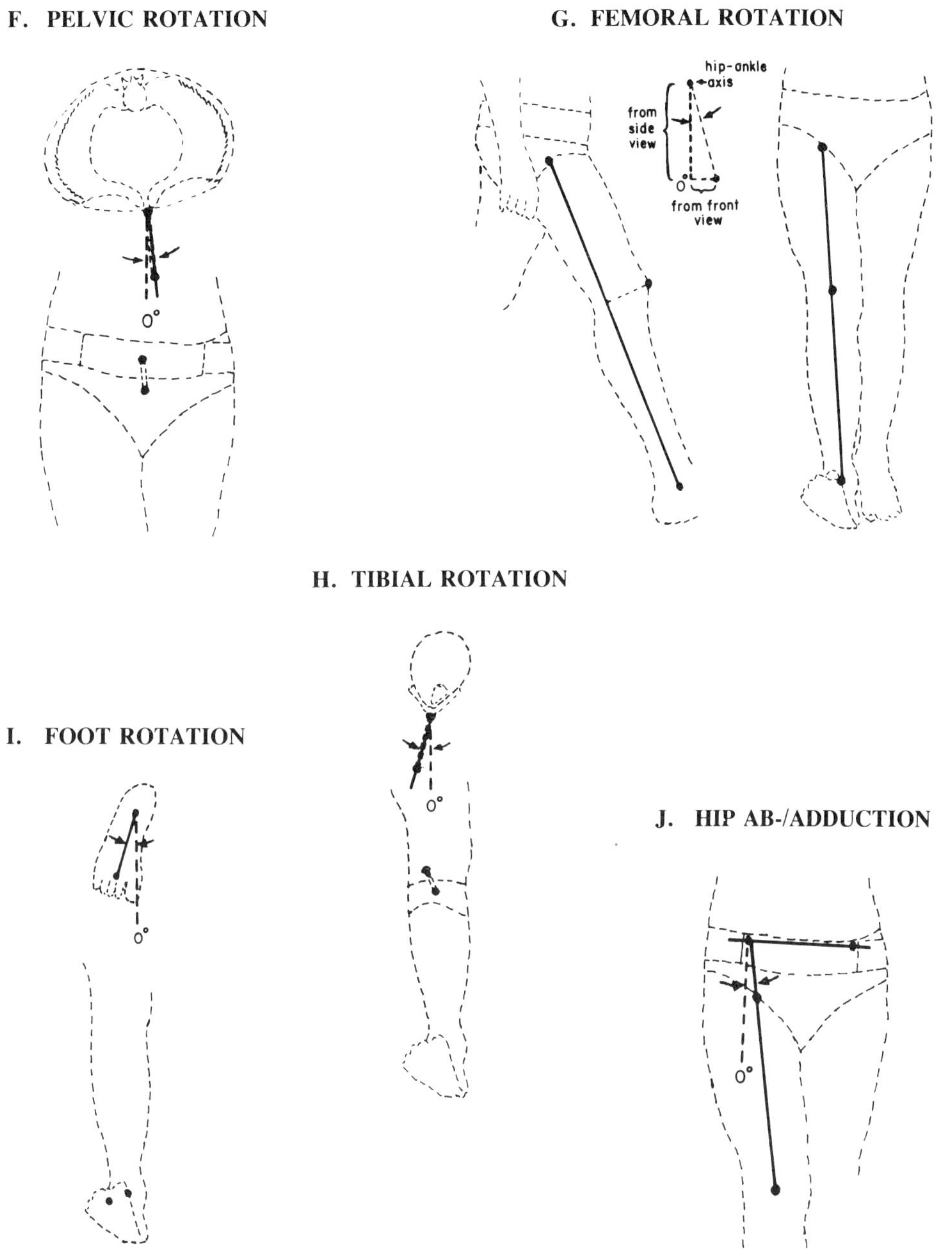

F. PELVIC ROTATION

G. FEMORAL ROTATION

H. TIBIAL ROTATION

I. FOOT ROTATION

J. HIP AB-/ADDUCTION

Figs. 2.5A–J. Measurement of joint-rotation angles. The large dots indicate the actual measurement points and the broken lines show 0° reference. (Sutherland *et al.* 1980*a*; reproduced by permission.)

HIP ROTATION
Calculated as the difference between pelvic rotation and femoral rotation.

KNEE ROTATION
Calculated as the difference between femoral rotation and tibial rotation.

Force data
The force data for each foot are reduced to six components (see pp. 16–17 for definitions): vertical force, fore/aft shear, medial/lateral shear, the x and y coordinates of center of pressure, and torque (Fig. 2.6). To allow inter-subject comparisons, forces have been expressed as percentage of body weight (with the exception of torque, measured in newton-meters).

Electromyography
To determine muscle phasic activity, surface EMGs were obtained of the following muscles: gluteus medius, vastus medialis, gluteus maximus, gastrocnemius-soleus, tibialis anterior, and medial and lateral hamstrings. The 'on' and 'off' times, expressed as a percentage of the gait cycle, were obtained for each muscle of each subject by averaging readings for six or more cycles. This was because a moderate variation in muscle phasic activity was observed from cycle to cycle. 'On' and 'off' times were usually within a range of ± 3 per cent of the gait cycle in comparison to the mean.

Time/distance parameters
The following data were also determined: time of opposite toe-off, time of opposite foot-strike and duration of single-limb stance (all expressed as a percentage of the walking cycle); walking velocity (in cm/sec.); cadence (steps/min.); step length and stride length (cm); cycle time (secs.); and ratio of pelvic span to ankle spread (measured during the double-limb support phase).

Anthropometric measurements and developmental screening
The following measurements were recorded and will be discussed fully in Chapter 6: standing height; length from crown to pubis and from pubis to toe; sitting height; arm span; body weight; hip, knee and ankle ranges of motion; tibial torsion; femoral/tibial angle; gross manual muscle test; and joint laxity (screening for excess, normal and tight laxity). Developmental screening and testing for motor control involved walking on toes and heels, standing and hopping on one leg, squatting, rising from the floor, walking on a balance beam, and running. Subjects were also tested for retained neonatal reflexes and upper-extremity protective extension, and for hand and foot preference or dominance.

Data handling (collection and reduction)
At least three passes down the walkway were observed on the motion analyzer. Each pass included about three full walking cycles. Data from linear measurements of the three passes were averaged and the walking cycle closest to the average was

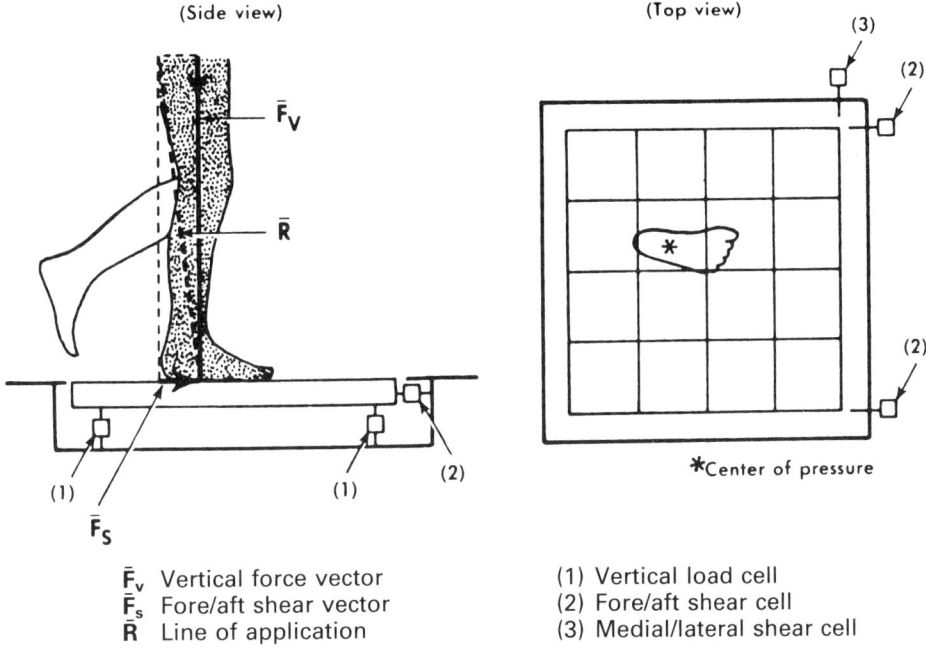

Fig. 2.6. Sketch of force plate with location of load cells. (Sutherland *et al.* 1980*a*; reproduced by permission.)

selected for analysis. The measurements used to determine a representative cycle were: cadence, cycle time, step length, duration of single-limb stance, and the points in the cycle at which toe-off, opposite toe-off and opposite foot-strike occurred.

The observer began reducing the data by projecting on the motion analyzer the right-side view film-frame showing heel-strike. 11 points were digitized (see Fig. 2.4): the tip and base of the sacral stick; the tip of the pelvic stick; the centers of the hip, knee and ankle joints (see p. 10); the patellar marker, the tip of the tibial stick, the bottom of the foot beneath the heel and near the fifth metatarsal head, and the center of the force plate. Because of limitations in the data collection and processing system, a maximum of 34 frames could be used to represent each gait cycle. Where there were more than 34 frames from foot-strike to foot-strike, the film was advanced two or three frames as required to give evenly spaced measurement increments throughout the cycle (for example, if a walk cycle consisted of 54 film frames, the first frame and every third frame up to the 25th were digitized; the 26th was skipped, and, starting with the 27th, every third frame up to the 54th were digitized, for a total of 19 measurements). When digitizing of the right-side view had been completed for the full gait cycle, the process was repeated for the corresponding front view. Here, 12 points were digitized (see

Fig. 2.4): the right and left pelvic-belt spots; the base and tip of the pelvic and tibial sticks; the hip, knee and ankle centers; the patellar marker; the marker between the second and third metatarsals on the dorsum of the foot; and the center of the force plate. Finally, when digitizing for the front view was complete, the process was repeated for the left side.

The digitized data were recorded on cassette and subsequently transferred to the computer, which was programmed to convert the coordinate points to joint angles and then plot them graphically.

Definitions

The *gait cycle* is defined as the movements and events that occur between successive footsteps of the same foot. In normal subjects the gait cycle begins with heel-strike, continues through stance and swing phases, and ends with heel-strike of the same foot. In pathological gait the forefoot may make the initial floor contact to begin the gait cycle. Figure 2.7 illustrates the gait cycle of a normal 7-year-old. Stance phase ends with toe-off which initiates swing phase. Swing phase ends with foot-strike. Opposite toe-off and opposite foot-strike are the other significant gait events; these separate the stance phase into periods of initial double-limb support, single-limb stance and second double support. In addition, reversal of fore/aft shear separates single-limb support into mid- and terminal stance. (This last separation cannot be determined accurately without a force plate.) Swing phase is separated into three periods—initial swing, mid-swing and terminal swing—by two events. The first is movement of the swinging ankle beyond the opposite standing tibia, and the second is vertical alignment of the swinging tibia. It is important for the reader to be familiar with these subdivisions of gait.

In order to allow comparisons between subjects, all events, phases and periods of the gait cycle have been expressed as percentages of the total cycle. This conversion to percentages normalizes individual cycles. All gait measurements are based on free-speed walking.

Duration of single-limb stance is the duration of single-limb support during the walking cycle.

Step length is the distance between the same point on each foot during double-limb support.

Stride length is the distance traveled by the same point on the same foot during two successive steps. Thus, each stride length comprises one right and one left step length.

Cadence is the number of steps per minute.

Walking velocity is the average distance traveled per second, calculated by dividing stride length by cycle time.

Vertical force is the vertical ground-reaction force.

Fore/aft shear is the horizontal ground-reaction force, directed along the line of progression.

Medial/lateral shear is the horizontal ground-reaction force, directed perpendicular to the line of progression.

The *line of application of the ground-reaction force* in the sagittal plane (R) is the resultant of the vertical force vector (F_v) and the fore/aft shear vector (F_s). The

TYPICAL NORMAL WALK CYCLE

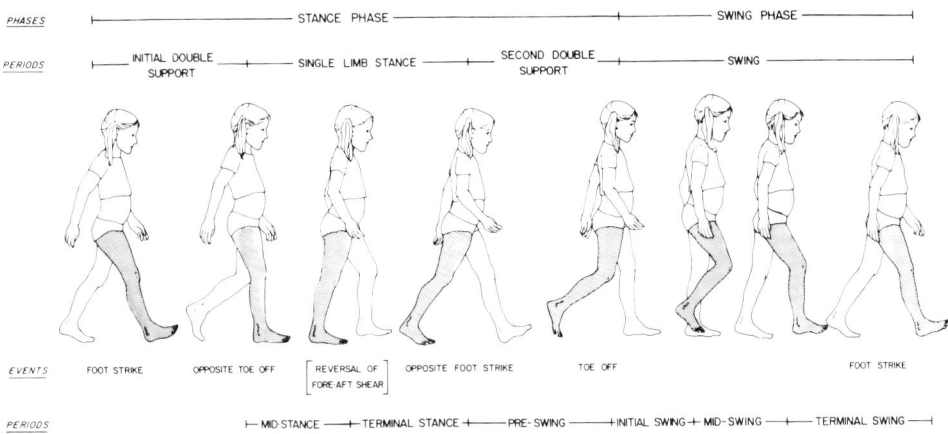

Fig. 2.7. Representative walk cycle of a normal 7-year-old girl, showing events, phases and periods of gait. (Sutherland 1981a; reproduced by permission.)

point of application of the ground-reaction force is at the *center of pressure* (see Fig. 2.6).

Torque is the moment applied about the center of pressure in the plane of the force plate.

Phasic muscle activity during the walking cycle occurs when there is electromyographic activity of a muscle.

Statistical methods
The motion data were subjected to Fourier analysis to determine mean rotations across the cycle and the 'harmonics' which describe the pattern of motion. Prediction regions—defining boundaries within which 95 per cent of normal children should lie throughout the gait cycle—were calculated using the resultant Fourier coefficients. To adjust for biases inherent in this process, we adapted a statistical technique known as the 'bootstrap'. These analytical methods are described in detail in Chapter 3.

Reproducibility of data
The clinical applicability of our studies depends on the extent to which the data gathered are reproducible. One must consider how much variation there is from step to step for an individual as well as how much variability is introduced by the digitizing process. The variation due to digitizing is affected not only by the operator's ability to reproduce his/her own work, but also by the ability to reproduce the work of others. We will discuss two aspects of the reproducibility question: first, the digitizing process itself; and second, the results of an experiment designed to measure the variability of data observed for a single subject.

The digitizing process, which has been described to some extent earlier in this chapter, comprises several stages. In the first, the film from the left-side camera is analyzed to produce 'linear measurements' or 'time/distance parameters' for several gait cycles (foot-strike to foot-strike). These measures of step length, walking velocity, cycle percentages and so on are then averaged, and the cycle nearest the mean is selected for subsequent digitizing. At this stage the films are checked to ensure that recordings are available from all three views (right, left and front) for the selected cycle. The film is then played through on the digitizer to determine the frame count for the selected cycle for each camera view. Remembering that the cameras all run independently and are synchronized by digital counters in the field of view, it can be seen that even if they all run at exactly the same speed, they can still be up to one half of the between-frames time out of synchronization. In practice it is not atypical to have frame counts among the three cameras varying by one or two frames even in near-ideal conditions.

Due to limitations of the computer system when the lab was built, and also to save time, the person doing the digitizing divides the gait cycle into between 16 and 34 intervals of approximately equal length. For example, if the cycle contains 42 frames, dividing it into 21 intervals would involve choosing frames 1, 3, 5 . . . 41. However, to ensure that the actual frames corresponding to foot-strike are digitized, often an additional frame is included near the middle so that the count might become: 1, 3, 5 . . . 21, then 24, 26, 28 . . . 42, with the extra frame added between frames 21 and 24.

A further discrepancy can be introduced when an event such as foot-strike occurs *between* two frames, in which case it is not necessarily clear which frame should be designated as the start or end of the cycle. One may well ask, what difference do single-frame errors make? Taking a typical gait cycle of something between 0.7 and 1.0 seconds, one has between 35 and 50 frames of data; thus, an 'error' of one frame corresponds to about 2 to 3 per cent of the total gait cycle.

The film is projected one frame at a time, and the person doing the digitizing identifies the various body points noted above. The scale factor from lab to screen is approximately 1:12, and the digitizing instrument has a resolution of about 0.1mm, corresponding to about 1mm on the subject in the lab. However, the person using the digitizer has a much lower resolving capability than the instrument. Tests on the lab staff indicated that multiple digitizations of the same point tend to fall within a circle of about 1.5mm diameter, which translates to a 15mm uncertainty on the subject. Considering a typical limb segment to be about 200 to 300mm in length, the error would be expected to lie in a range of approximately ±5°. In fact, the errors are not completely random, and the range is somewhat less in practice. It is also important to note that often the person digitizing is not identifying marked points but is using the body markers to identify joint levels and then estimating the 'center' of the joint. Thus, an element of personal judgment also enters the process.

Another effect is the influence of marker position. For many of the identified points, the marker is used only as a guide to the level of the joint. For other measures, such as tibial rotation, the measurement is made by looking at the orientation of the tibial stick. Here marker position is very important. For example, if a subject is tested, and the tibial stick is then removed and replaced so as to be internally rotated relative to the limb, subsequent measurements will have the same pattern as before but will be offset. This can also occur if the subject walks at an angle to the center of the lab, in which case transverse rotations will appear as though one limb is rotated internally and the other externally. It is important, when interpreting the data, that such 'artifacts' are recognized. In clinical gait analysis such marker repositioning often takes place when subjects are tested in and out of braces, or indeed if they are tested on more than one occasion to assess progress. We feel that at least some of the variability in the mean across the gait cycle (see Chapter 7) is due to these marker positioning errors.

In summary, the digitizing process introduces timing errors due to uncertainty about frame counts and frame synchronization, and therefore introduces errors into the measured joint angles. Figures 2.8, 2.9 and 2.10 show some results that illustrate these effects. In each of the graphs three curves are presented, all of which were measured from the same cycle for one subject. Curves D1 and D2 represent two different attempts by the same individual, and P is an attempt by another person. Both were experts at digitizing. In each case the 'A' portion of the figure shows the joint angles as calculated from the 'raw' digitized data, and the 'B' portion shows the curves produced by Fourier coefficients fitted using least squares (see Chapter 3).

In all three cases the D1 and D2 curves are nearer one another than the results for P. This is at least partly due to the fact that when individuals attempt to reproduce their own values they tend to be very careful about the actual frames digitized, thus eliminating timing or frame-count errors. As can be seen, the errors in the angles at a specific point tend to be less than 5°, and the mean error considerably less.

The differences between the D1/D2 curves and the P curve appear to be related more to a shift on the time base than to digitizing inconsistencies. The most likely cause of these differences is that the two individuals chose different frames to process.

The most dramatic differences are in hip flexion in the 60 to 80 per cent range and in foot rotation between 80 and 90 per cent. Neither of these can be explained easily by frame-counting errors; they are undoubtedly the result of differences in personal judgment as to where the digitized points defining the hip and the orientation of the foot should lie.

Perhaps the most important message is that any system of measurement requires interpretation which includes a critical assessment of the 'correctness' of the data. In our facility, when a subject's motion data are used for clinical purposes, they are checked at three levels. First the person doing the digitizing checks his/her own work to see if the curves produced 'make sense' when compared to what was actually observed in the lab and on film. Next the data are double-checked by some other member of the lab staff, again to make sure that they are a sensible reflection of the subject under study. Finally the data are reviewed by one of the physicians who consults on gait cases and an opinion is rendered. Inconsistencies observed at any level are investigated to ensure that the final data are as valid as possible

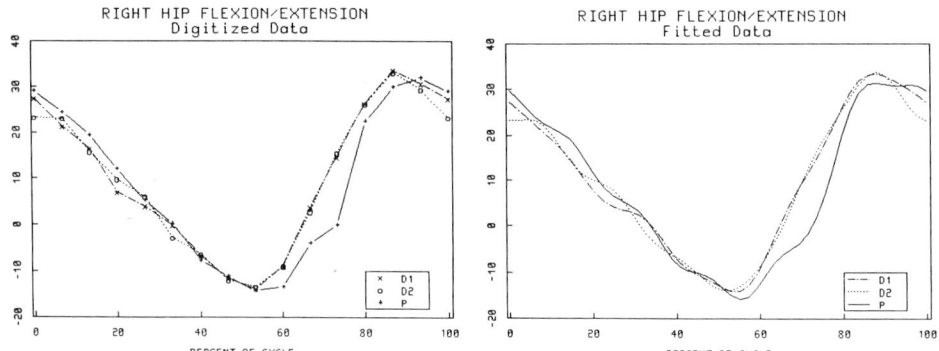

Fig. 2.8. Right hip flexion/extension. Repeated digitization of same cycle by one observer (D1, D2) and digitization of same cycle by a different observer (P).

In each of the three figures on this page, the left-hand graphs illustrate data prior to Fourier fitting, while the right-hand curves were produced by Fourier coefficients, fitted using least squares.

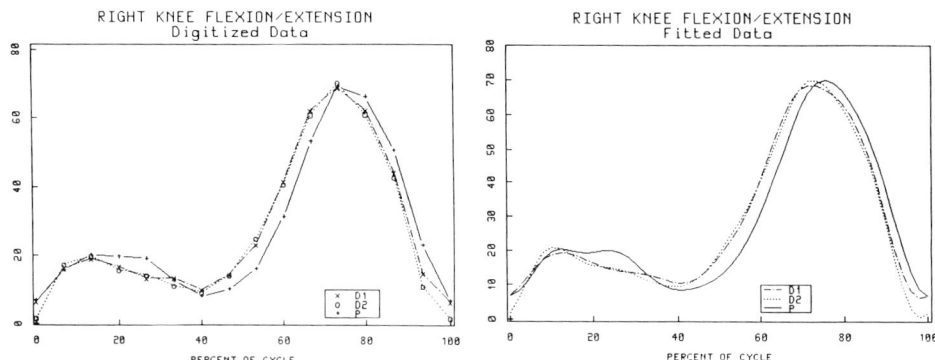

Fig. 2.9. Right knee flexion/extension. Repeated digitization of same cycle by one observer (D1, D2) and digitization of same cycle by a different observer (P).

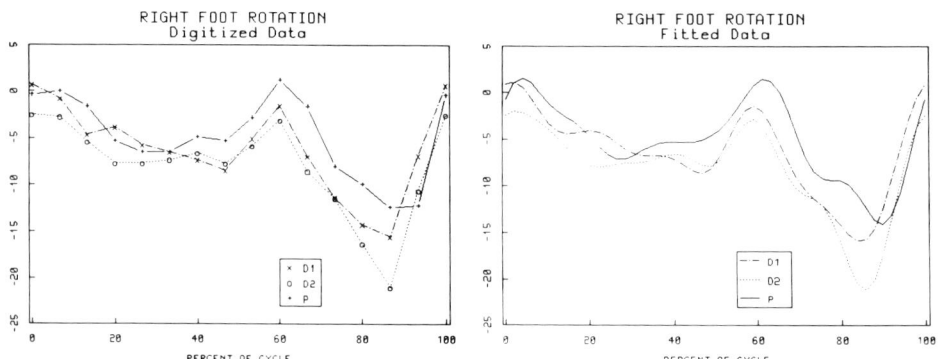

Fig. 2.10. Right foot rotation. Repeated digitization of same cycle by one observer (D1, D2) and digitization of same cycle by a different observer (P).

What, then, are the differences one should expect from cycle to cycle in normal children? Lasko (1986) studied this question in her Ph.D. dissertation, the data for which were derived in part from those reported in this book. Working with 2- and 7-year-old children, she digitized about 10 walks per child and fitted the Fourier series model described above. She found that the harmonic components of the curve were qualitatively similar, but that in the worst case a joint angle at a given percentage of the gait cycle could vary considerably from the joint angle of the same subject at the same point in a different cycle. In many cases the differences appeared to be related to the timing and choice of the frames indicating particular events rather than to digitizing errors. Generally the worst-case difference for repeated walks for a single subject was about half that observed for a group of normal children of the same age.

The ideas described above must be modified somewhat if modern automatic or semi-automatic digitizing techniques are employed. The first consideration is that the resolution of the system is likely to be somewhat different from that of the cine systems used to collect the data from which our work proceeded. Secondly, whereas the human sitting at the digitizing screen is an excellent 'image processor' and is not stymied by missing or badly placed markers, the automatic or semi-automatic system can only record what is read by its sensors. Work done in our lab in conjunction with several other gait facilities (Biden *et al.* 1987) indicates that automated systems can measure the harmonic components of gait in a generally reproducible fashion, but that the averages across the cycle (the α_0 terms: see Chapter 3) vary considerably depending on the system. This variability seems to be due in large part to the effect of marker positioning. We admonish the skeptical reader that even for a physician or physical therapist, exact reproduction of a given marker placement is extremely difficult.

Equipment

The instruments of measurement are relevant to the results of any study and it is appropriate to list them. Table 2.I provides information as to the types of instruments used for this study and where such instruments can be obtained.

The film digitization method of movement measurement used in this study proved to be well suited even to the smallest children. The surface markers and sticks were not sufficiently cumbersome to produce gross alterations in gait. The greatest drawback to this system is the high requirement for human labor. Even with such technical devices as the sonic digitizer, computer and plotter to speed the process, it is still labor-intensive and costly for humans to make the measurements.

Our laboratory has now supplanted the film digitization system with a five-camera, semi-automated VICON system. We are providing a list of the instruments in our current laboratory (Table 2.II) because we believe that most newly organized facilities will want to employ methods of measurement which minimize human labor. This subject is considered further, and our current system is described in more detail, in Chapter 13. We will not discuss alternative methods of gait analysis or compare competing commercial systems, as such topics are beyond the scope of this manuscript.

TABLE 2.I
Laboratory system used in this study

Item of Equipment	Supplier	Comments
Motion		
2 Photo-Sonics IP 16mm cine cameras	Photo-Sonics, Inc., 820 South Mariposa Street, Burbank, CA 91506	Front camera, 75mm lens; side-view camera, 16mm lens
1 Hycam Model 40 high-speed cine camera	Redlake Corp., 15005 Concorde Circle, Morgan Hill, CA 95037	Right-side camera; zoom lens set at 18mm
1 Bolex H16-KX5 cine camera	Bolex S.A., 15 Route de Lausanne, Case Postale, 1401 Yverdon, Switzerland	Used in pit to photograph foot through transparent forceplate; 25mm lens
2 Vanguard Motion Analyzers	Vanguard Instrument Corp., 1860 Walt Whitman Road, Melville, NY 11746	Only one required
2 Graf-Pen sonic digitizers	Science Accessories Corp., 970 Kings Highway West, Southport, CT 06490	Used in conjunction with Vanguard motion analyzer; only one required
Force		
1 Multicomponent measuring platform with plexiglas top plate	Medical Data Systems, Santa Clara, CA 95051. (No longer in business)	Developed at Shriners Hospital for Crippled Children, San Francisco Unit
1 Bell & Howell CPR-401 magnetic tape recorder/reproducer	Data Tape Inc., Instrument Division, 5430 Van Nuys Blvd. Ste. 314, Van Nuys, CA 91401	
EMG		
8 Beckman surface electrodes	Beckman Instruments, Inc., Schiller Park, IL 60176	
4 MCI surface electrodes	IOMED Corp., 1290 West 2320 South Ste. A, Salt Lake City, UH 84119	
1 Tektronic oscilloscope	Tektronics, Inc., P.O. Box 500, Beaverton, OR	
1 Soltec oscillograph	Soltec Corp., 11684 Pendleton Street, Sun Valley, CA 91352	
2 Footswitches		Made in our laboratory
Computer		
1 EPI 118	Electronics Processor Inc. (Formerly of Denver, CO; no longer in computer business)	
1 DEC PDP 11/44	Digital Equipment Corp., Maynard, MA 01754	Acquired after data had been gathered; used for statistical calculations

TABLE 2.II

Present laboratory system. Two systems are used simultaneously. A five-camera VICON system makes the recordings from which the actual movement measurements are made. A separate video system enables the lab personnel and physicians to watch the motion and gives a permanent record of the subject walking.

Item of Equipment	Supplier	Comments
Movement measurement system		
5 VICON cameras	Oxford Metrics Ltd., Unit 8, 7 West Way, Botley, Oxford OX2 0JB, England. Oxford Metrics, 14206 Carlson Circle, Tampa, FL 33626	Five cameras are needed to enable all the body markers to be seen at all times from both sides of the body. For further description of this system, see Chapter 13, pp. 207–208
1 Panasonic AG-6200e VHS video cassette recorder	Panasonic Industrial Co., Audio-Video Systems Division, One Panasonic Way, Secaucus, NJ 07094	
1 Memscan V2516SE input source encoder	Vicon Industries, Inc., 525 Broadhollow Road, Melville, NY 11747	Switches between the five VICON cameras so that every fifth frame from each is videotaped
2 NEC JB-1201 M(A) 12-inch monitors	NEC Home Electronics 1401 Estes Avenue, Elk Grove Village, IL 60007	
Motion viewing system		
3 Sharp XC-800 professional ENG/EFP video cameras	Sharp Electronics Corp., Professional Products Div., 10 Sharp Plaza, Paramus, NJ 07652	For front, left- and right-side views. (Used to provide a permanent record of the subject walking)
3 Fujinon TV zoom lenses (f/1.6, 10–100mm)	Fujinon, Inc., 672 White Plains Road, Scarsdale, NY 10583	
1 RCA TC2000 closed-circuit video camera with 25mm lens	RCA Closed-circuit Video Eqpt., New Holland Avenue, Lancaster, PA 17604	Used under transparent force platform to view feet
3 Sony VO-5600 video cassette recorders	Sony Corporation of America, Video Communications Div., Sony Drive, Park Ridge, NJ 07656	
1 Sony VO-5800 video cassette recorder		
1 Sony RM-555 multi remote-control unit		
1 Sony RM-580 remote-control unit		
2 Panasonic BT-S1300N color video monitors	Panasonic Industrial Co. (see above)	
Force		
2 Kistler multicomponent measuring platforms with glass-top plates	Kistler Instruments, 75 John Glenn Drive, Amherst, NY 14120	
EMG		
(As present study)	See Table 2.I	
Computer		
DEC PDP 11/44	See Table 2.I	

3
MODELING AND PREDICTION REGIONS FOR MOTION DATA

In this chapter we give details regarding the mathematical and statistical analysis of the motion data generated in our study. Necessarily, the prerequisites to an understanding of some of this material are different from those required for the rest of the book. However, the chapter was written with varying mathematical levels in mind, in the hope that each reader might find something informative and interesting.

Statistical analyses of the motion data in this study have hinged upon having adequate means of describing their variation, both across the gait cycle for individual children and among the total sample in each age-group. Free-speed walking on a level surface by normal children is approximately periodic, and our analyses proceeded from the assumption that angular rotations are periodic waveforms. Any periodic waveform can be constructed by superimposing a combination of waveforms that have the proper amplitudes, phases and harmonics. Thus, the angular data can be subjected to Fourier analysis, which mathematically resolves the data into these component waveforms (see Anderson 1971).

The advantages of the Fourier approach are that it permits one to: (a) interpolate values for joint movements at percentages of the walk cycle for which no data are available; (b) extrapolate values for rotations beyond the cycle observed; (c) record slightly smoother joint-motion curves than might be obtained by crudely connecting the digitized points; and (d) theoretically, separate individual waveforms that comprise the whole of each movement.

A more precise description of our model can be given as follows. We denote by θ a percentage point between one foot-strike and the next, so $0 \leq \theta \leq 100$. A generic angular rotation is denoted by the function f; the value of f at θ is written $f(\theta)$. Thus:

$$(1) \quad f(\theta) = \alpha_0 + \sum_{j=1}^{6} \left[\alpha_j \, cos \left(\frac{2\pi j \theta}{100} \right) + \beta_j \, sin \left(\frac{2\pi j \theta}{100} \right) \right],$$

where j is the frequency of the harmonic[1] and α_0 is the mean rotation across all phases of the cycle. Much of the remainder of this chapter is devoted to explaining which aspects of this model (**1**) are fitted to our data, and how.

---

[1]The subscripts of the Fourier coefficients α_1 to α_6 and β_1 to β_6 identify the first to sixth fundamental harmonics of the waveform and thus the events that occur, respectively, one to six times per cycle.

We think of each α and β as being characteristic of a particular child and gait, and therefore random. This simple observation has been an important key to the successes we have enjoyed in fitting prediction regions. Also, since walking involves compensating actions of limbs, joints and muscles in order to maintain balance and direction, it stands to reason—and is amply borne out by data—that the coefficients which apply to any individual subject are highly dependent on one another. [Ignoring this lack of independence is a significant flaw in the analyses of Capozzo et al. (1975).]

If the children in a particular age-group are indexed by i ($i = 1, \ldots, N$), then the ith child's respective f and Fourier coefficients are written $f^{(i)}$ and $\alpha_0^{(i)}, \ldots, \beta_6^{(i)}$. The random vectors $\{v^{(i)}\}_{i=1}^N = \{(\alpha_0^{(i)}, \alpha_1^{(i)}, \ldots, \beta_6^{(i)})^t\}_{i=1}^N$ are assumed to be independent. The variance of $f(\theta)$ is the quadratic form $\sigma_f^2(\theta) = T^t(\theta)\Gamma T(\theta)$, where the superscripted t denotes 'transpose', $\Gamma = [\gamma_{i,j}]$ is the covariance matrix of $v = (\alpha_0, \alpha_1, \ldots, \beta_6)^t$ (see footnote[1] for clarification), and

$$T^t(\theta) = \left(1, \cos\left(\frac{2\pi\theta}{100}\right), \sin\left(\frac{2\pi\theta}{100}\right), \ldots, \sin\left(\frac{12\pi\theta}{100}\right)\right).$$

In fact, each $f^{(i)}$ is observed at a discrete set of $d(i)$ θ values, $\theta_1^{(i)} < \theta_2^{(i)} < \ldots < \theta_{d(i)}^{(i)}$ where we take $\theta_k^{(i)} = 100(k-1)/d(i)$. (In Chapter 2 we have addressed problems that arise from the failure of the digitized points to be equally spaced.) What are 'observed', then, are:

$$\{f^{(i)}(\theta_k) + \varepsilon_k^{(i)}\}, k = 1, \ldots d(i),$$

where the errors of measurement $\{\varepsilon_k^{(i)}\}$ are assumed to be independent, and independent of the $\{v^{(i)}\}$, with mean 0 and variance σ^2. (All random variables here are assumed to have more than eight finite moments[2]; see Olshen et al. 1988.)

Occasionally, isolated digitized values are greatly out of keeping with our model for any believable distribution of errors. For example, this can occur as the foot strikes the ground and the sticks are shaken (a problem which is more acute in obese children). If the θ_k values are as we have described and a digitized value at, say, θ_l is aberrant but those at $\theta_{l-2}, \theta_{l-1}, \theta_{l+1}$ and θ_{l+2} are not, then we replace the value at θ_l as follows. One quadratic is fitted to values at $\theta_{l-2}, \theta_{l-1}$ and θ_{l+1} and another to those at $\theta_{l-1}, \theta_{l+1}$ and θ_{l+2}. The two fitted values at θ_l are averaged, and this average replaces the digitized value at θ_l. It follows from the

---

[1]The expression $\gamma_{i,j}$ refers to the number in the ith row of the jth column of Γ, the 13-by-13 covariance matrix of v. Therefore, it is the covariance of the ith and jth entries of v. For example, if $i = 2$ and $j = 13$, then $\gamma_{i,j}$ is the covariance of α_1 and β_6. Note also that because the covariance of two random variables does not depend on the order in which they appear, $\gamma_{i,j} = \gamma_{j,i}$ for all i and j. Moreover, $\gamma_{i,i}$ is the variance of the ith entry of v.

[2]*Finite moment* refers to the finiteness of a certain integral that quantifies in part how heavy the 'tails' of a probability distribution are. The higher the finite moment, the lighter the tails, and thus the less likely one is (upon sampling from the distribution) to see observations far removed from 'central' values. The normal (Gaussian) distribution has all positive moments finite and even more (a so-called 'moment generating function'). Even though it is possible to draw values from a Gaussian distribution that are arbitrarily large (positive or negative) multiples of the standard deviation away from the center, it is not likely.

Lagrange interpolation formula (Powell 1981, Section 4.1) that this interpolation scheme is exact for cubics if the digitized points are equally spaced.

The expectation of the Fourier coefficients ($E(v)$) is estimated for each child by the method of least squares. [The least-squares fit is that which minimizes the sum of the squares of the vertical distances between the digitized points and the fitted curve in the model (**1**).] This is possible because $d(i) \geq 16$ for all children, and there are only 13 terms to the model. The estimate of $E(v)$ computed from the data of the ith child is used to estimate the expectation of $f(\theta)$; call this estimate $\hat{f}^{(i)}(\theta)$. It follows from Raò (1965) that this approach is best linear unbiased within subjects, that is, for each individual child. Combining the $\hat{f}^{(i)}(\theta)$ across subjects to form an overall estimate $\bar{\hat{f}}(\theta)$ is potentially difficult, since the best method of averaging is dependent on the value of θ. There are two extreme possibilities. One is to average with each child weighted equally, but this ignores the fact that the $d(i)$ are unequal. The other is to weight $\hat{f}^{(i)}$ proportional to $d(i)$. This, which is our chosen method, ignores the intrinsic variability across subjects. Fortunately, this is not a major problem; for around 99 per cent of subjects, $d(i)$ is between 16 and 23. In any case, the two extreme methods of combining the $\hat{f}^{(i)}$ produce estimates $\bar{\hat{f}}$ whose graphs as functions of θ are visually indistinguishable.

The number of times a cycle is digitized is the limiting factor in determining how many harmonics can be fitted. Our model, with an upper limit of six to the summation in (**1**), has 13 terms. Thus, there are 13 'degrees of freedom'[1] remaining for assessing the fit for each child and rotation. Because it is important for statistical reasons to leave some degrees of freedom for assessing errors, and because some rotations are digitized at as few as 16 approximately equally spaced points, our model is about as detailed as the data allow. In fact, multiple correlations calculated by child and rotation for data digitized at many more than 16 points indicate that harmonics beyond the sixth contain almost no information. Both Capozzo *et al.* (1975) and Sutherland *et al.* (1980*a*) used the same number of harmonics as we have chosen. Finally on the question of the numbers of harmonics, analyses using the Shibata (1981) model selection criterion (reported by Olshen *et al.* 1988) suggest that in many instances it would be unwise to use *fewer* than six sine and cosine coefficients.

One might ask whether the distributions of the α and β terms are of the familiar bell-shaped Gaussian type. Generally speaking, for normal children the higher up the body the rotation, the older the children, and the lower the harmonic (*i.e.* the lower the value of j), the more Gaussian are the distributions (Olshen *et al.* 1988).

While mean values are a *sine qua non* in our analyses, the process of comparing test children to normal subjects requires estimates of the variability of rotations. We address this by finding boundaries around the mean curves—that is, prediction regions. Initial attempts to define such regions led to several important observations. For many rotations, the variability of the mean is larger than that of the sum of the (six sine and cosine) principal harmonic components of the curves.

---

[1] For an explanation of the concept of *degrees of freedom*, see Kotz and Johnson (1982), pp. 293–294.

(To explain, during the gait cycle a joint has both a 'pattern' of motion and an average angular value—*e.g.* in 7-year-olds the average knee flexion over the cycle is around 30°.) Therefore, for each rotation we separated the process of prediction into two (not entirely independent) components: one for the overall average across the cycle (α_0) and one for the sum of the harmonics (*i.e.* the pattern of motion). This is reasonable from a physiological point of view, since the former is primarily a function of body alignment and the latter is largely dependent on muscle control. Also we know from recent work (Biden *et al.* 1987) that estimation of α_0 is much more sensitive to marker placement than is determination of the pattern of movement.

We denote the sum of harmonics in (**1**) by $f_h(\theta)$; its corresponding least-squares estimate by $\tilde{f}_h(\theta)$; the 12-dimensional vector that corresponds to $T^t(\theta)$ save a deleted 1 by $T_h^t(\theta)$; and by obvious analogy we introduce the random vector v_h, its 12-by-12 covariance Γ_h, and $\sigma_{f,h}^2(\theta) = T^t(\theta)\,\Gamma_h\,T_h(\theta)$. For convenience we now take $d(i) \equiv d$. (That is, we assume that all subjects are digitized at the same number of points for the rotation f. This is not of course true in practice, but it is not so far from true as to have any real bearing on what we do.) Write the sample covariance of the N separate estimates of $E(v_h)$ as $\widehat{cov}_h$. This estimates $\Gamma_h + (2\sigma^2/d)I$ where I is the 12-by-12 identity. Now, define $\hat{\sigma}_{f,h}^2(\theta)$ to be $T_h^t(\theta)\,\widehat{cov}_h\,T(\theta)$.

For nearly all ages and rotations $\sigma_{f,h}^2(\theta)$, the variance of the sum of harmonics, is far from constant across the gait cycle. Typically, it is greater in swing phase than in stance phase. Our prediction regions are defined to be equal multiples of the estimated standard deviation ($\hat{\sigma}_{f,h}^2(\theta)$) above and below the mean curve at each point in the gait cycle (*i.e.* at each θ).

Actually, much can be inferred in regard to these regions. For any fixed multiple of the standard deviation function, there can be associated a percentile for the normal child; the multiple corresponding to the 95th percentile is generally of most interest. For a given multiple, we estimate what percentage of Fourier fits for normal children fall completely within a band defined by the mean curve plus or minus that number of standard deviations. To adjust for biases inherent in estimating the cited percentile from the raw data, we adapted the 'bootstrap' technique developed by Bradley Efron of Stanford University (see Efron 1982).

The term 'bootstrap'[1] derives from the expression 'to pull oneself up by one's bootstraps', meaning to do something by oneself, without outside assistance. Here, the 'doing' is by the data. To implement the bootstrap, one draws randomly from one's data to create a 'sample' the same size as the original study sample. This random sample is then regarded as though it were the actual data and the real data were 'nature'. The intuitive justification for this is that the bootstrap sample bears

---

[1] Efron had a precedent for the lighthearted name he gave the process, since the bootstrap is closely related to an earlier technique, introduced by M. Quenouille in 1949, and dubbed the 'jackknife'. In his original publication on the bootstrap (Efron 1979), he remarked upon his choice of terminology: 'I also wish to thank the many friends who suggested names more colorful than *Bootstrap*, including *Swiss Army Knife*, *Meat Axe*, *Swan-Dive*, *Jack-Rabbit*, and my personal favorite, the *Shotgun*, which, to paraphrase Tukey, "can blow the head off any problem if the statistician can stand the resulting mess."'

approximately the same relationship to the real data as the real data do to nature. Therefore, since the real data are known, whereas nature is not, it seems that by bootstrapping one might infer something of the relationship between the real data and nature from the relationship between the bootstrap sample and the real data. This proposition can be supported by much mathematics, as well as by computer simulations and practical experience.

We turn now to a more precise description of bootstrapping in our prediction context. To this end we introduce a 'test case' $f_h^{(0)}(\theta)$ and its corresponding fit $\hat{f}_h^{(0)}(\theta)$. The bootstrap process for the sum of harmonics is our attempt to estimate this probability for various positive values of m:

$$(2) \quad P\left\{ \max_\theta \left| \frac{\hat{f}_h^{(0)}(\theta) - \bar{\tilde{f}}_h(\theta)}{\hat{\sigma}_{f,h}(\theta)} \right| \leq m \right\}$$

Bootstrapping begins with the selection, from our study group of children of a given age, of a random sample with replacement the same size as the study group. (Although this process is, of course, carried out on the computer, it is as though one had written each child's data on a separate slip of paper and then put all the slips of paper into a hat. A slip is drawn from the hat, the data are recorded, and the slip is returned to the hat. Then another slip is drawn and so on until a sample as large as the original population is produced.) It is possible to include the same data more than once, and in practice an average of about 63 per cent of the original subjects will be represented in any given 'bootstrap' sample.

We compute from this bootstrap sample estimates $\bar{\tilde{f}}_h^*(\theta)$ and $\hat{\sigma}_{f,h}^{2*}(\theta)$. (In this notation, superscripted asterisks always refer to the bootstrap.) The bootstrap distribution of $f_h^{(0)}(\theta)$ is the empirical distribution of the $f_h^{(i)}(\theta)$ values (see Olshen et al. 1988). Therefore, a bootstrap estimate of the probability given by (2) is

$$(3) \quad \hat{F}^*(m) = N^{-1} \# \left\{ \hat{f}^{(i)} : \max_\theta \left| \frac{\hat{f}_h^{(i)}(\theta) - \bar{\tilde{f}}_h^*(\theta)}{\hat{\sigma}_{f,h}^*(\theta)} \right| \leq m \right\}.$$

Now repeat the bootstrap sampling and computation of (3), and average the values of $\hat{F}^*(m)$. In practice, a series of 25 bootstrap samples seems to be adequate. Call this average $\bar{\tilde{F}}^*(m)$. If $0 < p < 1$, define m_p by $m_p = \min\{m : \bar{\tilde{F}}^*(m) \geq p\}$; m_p is our estimate of the 100th quantile of the distribution of our index of departure from 'normal'

$$(4) \quad \max \left| \frac{\hat{f}_h^{(0)} - \bar{\tilde{f}}_h(\theta)}{\hat{\sigma}_{f,h}(\theta)} \right|.$$

Furthermore, for any positive m, if $\bar{\tilde{F}}^*(m) = p_m$, then the region encompassed by $\bar{\tilde{f}}_h(\theta) - m\hat{\sigma}_{f,h}(\theta)$ to $\bar{\tilde{f}}_h(\theta) + m\hat{\sigma}_{f,h}(\theta)$ as θ runs from 0 to 100 constitutes our estimated $100p_m$ per cent simultaneous prediction region for f_h. If $\hat{f}_h^{(0)}(\theta)$ ever passes outside this region, then we say that the 'test case' departs from 'normal' at beyond the $100p_m$th percentile. Alternatively, one computes (**4**); call it M. Then one finds $\tilde{\hat{F}}^*(M)$ from a graph and imputes a $100\,\tilde{\hat{F}}(M)$ percentile to the 'test case'. The cited paper by Olshen *et al.* (1988) contains some mathematical details regarding asymptotic properties of these prediction regions, and several applications (see also Chapter 12).

The bootstrap procedure that has been described for the harmonic component of (**1**) can also be conducted for the overall mean, that is, for α_0. In this context what was a prediction region becomes a prediction interval.

Recent work by Søren Johansen of the University of Copenhagen and Iain Johnstone of Stanford University indicates that analytical approximations to our bootstrap-based prediction regions for f_h are possible (Johansen and Johnstone 1988). Their work utilizes $\hat{f}$ and $\hat{\sigma}^2_{f,h}$ but avoids most of the computing that the bootstrap approach entails.

4
STUDY PLAN

Introduction
This study includes physical examinations and gait analyses of 309 normal, term children aged 1 to 7 years. The examinations comprised an assessment of ranges of motion, gross manual muscle strength testing, a developmental screening exam, and tests of laterality and of reflex development, all performed by a physical therapist. The gait analysis portion of the study consisted of movement measurements (including time/distance parameters), force-plate measurements, and surface electromyography (EMG) measurements of seven muscle groups in one lower extremity. Some children were studied more than once, at different ages, for a total of 449 visits.

Subject selection and recruitment
Subjects for this project were volunteers. The criteria for inclusion were designed to ensure that we tested 'normal' children, since 'normal' gait patterns were the topic of interest. To be included in the study a child had to have: (1) been the product of a full-term pregnancy; (2) walked independently by 14 months of age; (3) had no orthopaedic problems or treatments; (4) displayed normal growth and development as judged by the parents and family physician; and (5) experienced no major medical problems or hospitalizations.

Several avenues were pursued to obtain appropriate subjects for the study. First, letters were sent and announcements made to the practicing pediatricians at the Children's Hospital, San Diego. They were asked to post notices in their offices and to solicit patients during 'well-child' check-ups. Second, an effort was made to work with the San Diego elementary school system to ensure a wide cross-section of subjects. With the school board's permission a notice was sent home with students in kindergarten, first and second grades in all the public schools within a 10-mile radius of the Children's Hospital. This notice explained the basic purpose of the study and gave a telephone number for the family to call for further information. A similar scheme was initiated to solicit younger subjects from area nursery schools. In addition, the Motion Analysis Laboratory staff attended several parent-teacher association meetings to describe the project and request support. Families who entered the study group themselves became an excellent source of referral by telling their friends and encouraging them to participate. Appeals for assistance were also published in the hospital newsletter and on bulletin boards, and this too proved to be a successful avenue of recruitment.

Parents calling the Motion Analysis Laboratory to volunteer their children were sent a health screening questionnaire (Appendix A). Each questionnaire was reviewed by an orthopaedist or physical therapist to determine whether the child had medical problems which would disqualify him/her from the study.

TABLE 4.I
Number of completed physical therapy (PT) examinations, movement measurement (MM), time/distance parameter (TD), force-plate (FP) and electromyographic (EMG) studies, by age-group

Age	PT	MM	TD	FP	EMG
1	54	49	51	12	24
1½	44	39	40	10	28
2	49	44	45	13	34
2½	37	36	36	23	35
3	51	47	47	37	44
3½	41	38	40	36	36
4	41	36	39	37	38
5	42	39	42	38	42
6	44	44	44	39	44
7	46	43	46	43	44
Total*	449	415	430	288	369

*The variation in totals in part reflects differing abilities at walking, and different degrees of willingness to cooperate in testing among subjects.

If the child was accepted, the family was contacted and a date was arranged so that the study could take place within 30 days of the child's birthday or 'half-birthday' (*i.e.* the date midway between two successive birthdays). This strict scheduling was designed to ensure uniformity of each age-group. A parent or guardian of each selected child signed an informed consent (Appendix B) before that child was studied. Each study session lasted approximately 1½ to 2 hours.

In addition to the health questionnaire, as part of the study each subject was examined by a physical therapist. If any question of orthopaedic abnormality or developmental delay was found, the child's data were eliminated from the data base.

Number of subjects; age and sex distribution
The original study plan was to examine 50 children (25 boys and 25 girls) in each of 10 age-groups, for a total of 500 subjects. The age-groups were 1, 1½, 2, 2½, 3, 3½, 4, 5, 6 and 7 years. Also, the plan was to study some children longitudinally.

A total of 309 different children were studied, some more than once, for a total of 449 studies. The total numbers of physical therapy examinations, movement measurement studies, time/distance parameter calculations, force-plate studies and EMG studies in each of the 10 age-groups are listed in Table 4.I.

More studies were filmed than are included in the final data. A total of four sets of data were deleted due to the following examination findings: (1) excessive drooling and poor coordination; (2) soft neurological signs consisting of: positive Babinski sign, residual asymmetrical tonic neck reflex and incomplete protective extension reflex at age 6 years; (3) significant leg-length inequality (2.5cm); and (4) clinically significant scoliosis. We were unable to obtain any meaningful data on three children who were utterly unable to cooperate with testing. Film data and subsequent movement measurement data were unobtainable for 19 children who cooperated for the physical therapy evaluation but were unable to cooperate for the

TABLE 4.II

Sex distribution by age-group for the 415 completed movement measurement studies*

Age	Male	Female	Total
1	26	23	49
1½	22	17	39
2	20	24	44
2½	17	19	36
3	24	23	47
3½	18	20	38
4	17	19	36
5	22	17	39
6	20	24	44
7	24	19	43
Total	210	205	415

*A χ^2 test, applied to see whether the proportions of boys and girls differed from 50 per cent by more than would be expected by chance, showed definitively that in none of the 10 age-groups was this the case. Therefore we did not need to consider making allowances for differences in the sex distribution across age-groups.

filming. This was a more frequent problem in the younger children who objected to our skin markers, had short attention spans, or who would not walk the length of the walkway without stopping. In addition, 11 sets of movement measurement data were lost during computer analysis.

Table 4.II shows the sex distribution by age-group for the 415 completed movement measurement studies. While the initial goal of obtaining equal numbers of male and female children in each of the 10 age-groups was not realized, all the respective boy/girl ratios were close to unity, so that it was possible to analyze the data for possible sex differences.

Race

An effort was made to ensure that the racial and ethnic composition of the sample matched that of the population of the San Diego area. Despite this effort and the cooperation of the public school system, this was not achieved, the Hispanic, Black and Asian communities being under-represented. The total study-group comprised: Caucasian 91.5 per cent, Hispanic 6.4 per cent, Black 1.4 per cent and Asian 0.7 per cent.

Summary

Subjects for this project were normal children who had walked by 14 months of age. They were studied within 30 days of their birthdate or half-birthdate. 309 children were studied, some more than once, for a total of 449 visits. From these studies both longitudinal and cross-sectional data on the maturation of normal gait were obtained. All subjects were screened and examined carefully to ensure that these data would be representative of 'normal' children.

5
ANTHROPOMETRIC MEASUREMENTS AND DEVELOPMENTAL SCREENING

Introduction
The goal of this research was to establish normal gait values for children aged from 1 to 7 years. Why, then, did we also gather anthropometric data on our subjects?

Physical measurements of the children were needed to allow correlations of form and function and to permit comparisons of our study group with those of other investigators. Some of the gait measurements, such as stride length, are directly related to growth. Growth and weight are affected by many variables including nutrition, genetics, history of frequent illness, and possibly environmental factors such as available sunshine. Some of the available height and weight tables were old and may not have reflected normal standards for the Sunbelt community in which our subjects live. While we were gathering gait data it was natural and relatively easy to carry out anthropometric measurements on the same subjects. We also included measurements of passive joint rotations, tests of joint laxity and tibial torsion, and developmental screening tests. Including this information with the gait data in a single volume will make it easier to compare the child who may be abnormal with a normal study population.

The anthropometric measurements and developmental screening tests were all conducted by a registered physical therapist. The data were appraised by two individuals, recorded on a single form (Appendix C), and later entered into the computer data base on the PDP 11/44.

As they were usually conducted first and required less co-operation from the children than the subsequent gait studies, the number of completed examinations exceeded the number of film studies obtained. In all, 449 anthropometric and developmental screening evaluations were conducted (see Table 4.I, p. 31).

Height and body-proportion measurements
All height measurements were taken with a tape measure and recorded in centimeters. For the *standing-height* measurement, a square was held on the crown of the head, parallel to the floor, with the subject standing barefoot against a wall to which a metal tape measure was fixed. Standing height was defined as the distance from the square to the floor.

The *crown-to-pubis* and *pubis-to-toe* measurements were made with the subject supine. The superior border of the pubis symphysis was marked with a felt-tip pen and the measurements were made from this point: for the crown-to-pubis length, to a square placed on the crown of the subject's head; for the pubis-to-toe length, to the dorsal surface of the great toe with the ankle in neutral dorsiflexion/plantar flexion and neutral eversion/inversion.

Sitting height was measured with the subject sitting erect on a wooden box with the hips in approximately 90° flexion and the bare feet flat on the floor. (Wooden boxes of various sizes had been built for use in taking this measurement.) The square was placed on the crown of the head and the sitting height measured as the distance from the square to the box.

Figure 5.1 gives the standing height for each age group. If we compare the respective medians (50th percentiles) with those reported by Hamill *et al.* (1977), there is close agreement in spite of some difference in the mode of display of data. Hamill *et al.* separated boys and girls, whereas we grouped them together because there were no sex-related differences in the 1 to 7 year age-span. Due to the similarity of the two sets of data, we feel that our population is representative of normal children. There does not appear to be any competitive height advantage for children growing up in San Diego.

Figure 5.2 gives the sitting height for each age-group. The ratio of standing to sitting height varies between approximately 1.6 and 1.8, with the lower ratios occurring in the younger age-groups. The trunk occupies a greater percentage of the total height in the youngest children.

Figure 5.3 gives the crown-to-pubis heights. Comparing these to the pubis-to-toe measurements (Fig. 5.4), it is apparent that the ratio between upper body and lower body gradually diminishes. Based on the median values for each measurement, this ratio is 1.4 at age 1 year and drops progressively to 1.0 at 5 years. The median upper-body and lower-body heights within groups are equal in the 5, 6 and 7 year age-groups.

Weight
With the subject dressed in only underclothes or bathing suit, body weight was measured (in kilograms) by means of a calibrated balance scale.

The median body weight (Fig. 5.5) increases by approximately 2kg per year. Our data are in very close agreement with those of Hamill *et al.* (1977). Again, although we have combined the data from boys and girls, such comparisons can be made because there were no significant inter-sex differences up to the age of 7 years.

Arm span
Arm span was measured with the subject seated and the arms abducted to 90°. It was defined as the distance (in centimeters) from the tip of the longest finger of one hand to the tip of the longest finger on the other hand, measured across the back. The results are shown in Figure 5.6. Median arm span approximates median standing height in all age-groups.

Passive range of motion
Eight ranges of motion were measured. The examiner, a physical therapist, moved the joint through its available range. Each motion was measured once on each side (left and right), using a goniometer. An assistant stabilized proximal joints when necessary and entered data on the recording sheet. No measurement data were

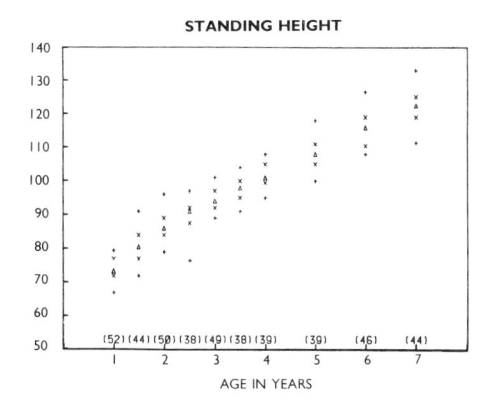

Fig. 5.1. Standing height (cm) vs. age (yrs.) (N = 439).

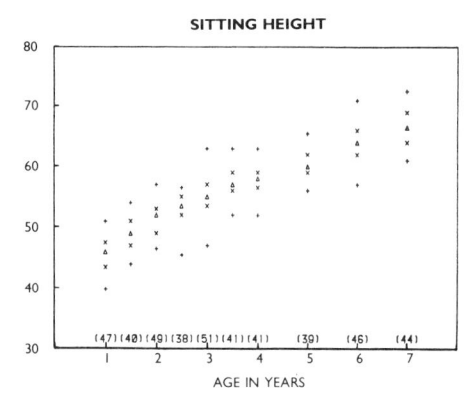

Fig. 5.2. Sitting height (cm) vs. age (N = 435).

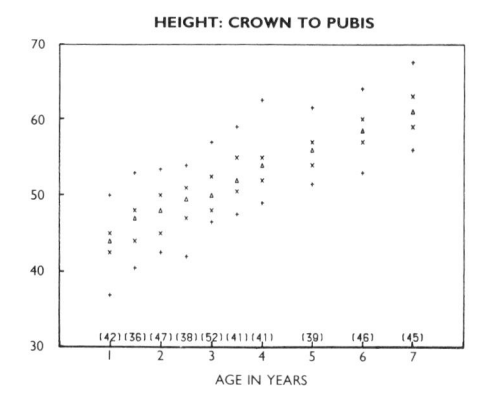

Fig. 5.3. Crown-to-pubis height (cm) vs. age (N = 427).

In Figures 5.1 to 5.6, at each age the two '×' markers encompass the middle 50 per cent of subjects, the triangle indicates the median, and the upper and lower marks respectively show the greatest and least values recorded. Numbers of subjects in each age-group are given in parentheses along the horizontal axis.

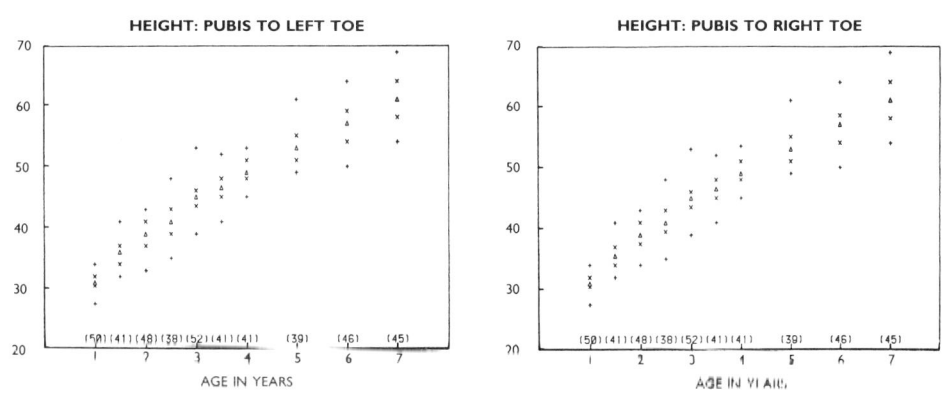

Fig. 5.4. Height (cm) from pubis to left toe (A) and right toe (B) vs. age (N = 441).

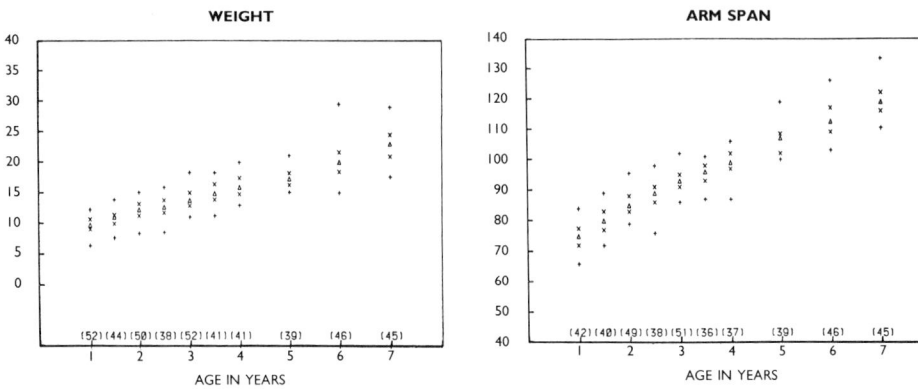

Fig. 5.5. Body weight (kg) *vs.* age (N = 448).

Fig. 5.6. Arm span (cm) *vs.* age (N = 423).

recorded if the child was not able to relax during the test maneuver. The following ranges of motion were measured: (1) straight-leg raising; (2) hip extension; (3) hip internal rotation; (4) hip external rotation; (5) hip abduction; (6) hip adduction; (7) knee extension; (8) ankle dorsiflexion.

Comparisons between right and left sides showed no significant differences at the $p<0.01$ level for range of motion for any age-group for either sex.

Hip flexion with knee extended (passive straight-leg raising)
For this test, the subject was first placed supine, with both legs extended and resting flat on the table. For right straight-leg raising, the right leg was passively elevated until the knee began to flex. The goniometer was positioned with the pivot over the greater trochanter of the femur, and with one arm parallel to the table-top and the other arm pointing toward the lateral femoral condyle. The angle between the two goniometer arms was designated as the right straight-leg raising angle. The process was repeated for the left leg.

At age 1 year, the median straight-leg elevation was 100° (Fig. 5.7). There was a gradual decrease in the range of elevation until age 5, when the median was 80°. This change represents a gradual tightening of the hamstrings. At 7 years, passive straight-leg raising still exceeded that of most adults.

Hip extension
With the subject supine with the knees over the edge of the examining table, the contralateral hip and knee were flexed until the lumbar lordosis was flattened. The goniometer was placed with the pivot over the right greater trochanter, one arm parallel with the table-top and the other pointing toward the lateral femoral condyle. If the hip lacked full extension, the angle formed was designated a negative value.

The median range of hip extension was 10° at 1 year, with very little change observed in the older subjects (Fig. 5.8).

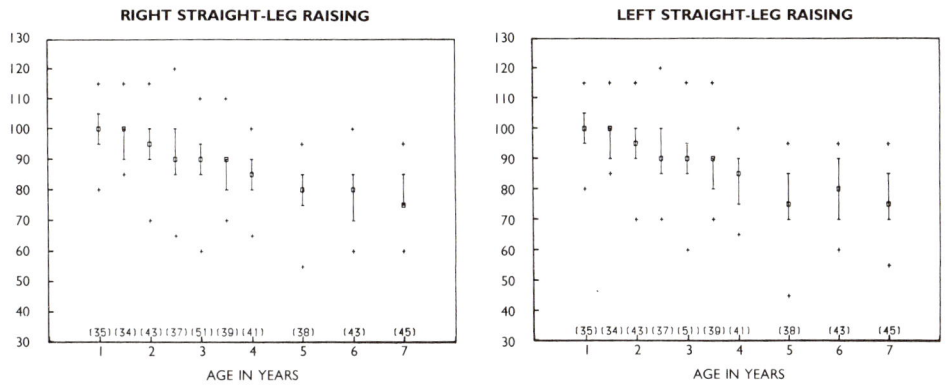

Fig. 5.7. Range of passive right (A) and left (B) straight-leg raising (degrees) *vs.* age (N = 406).
In this and in subsequent figures in this chapter, at each age the vertical bar encompasses the middle 50 per cent of subjects and the box indicates the median. The upper and lower markers respectively show the greatest and least values recorded. Numbers of subjects in each age-group are given in parentheses along the horizontal axis.

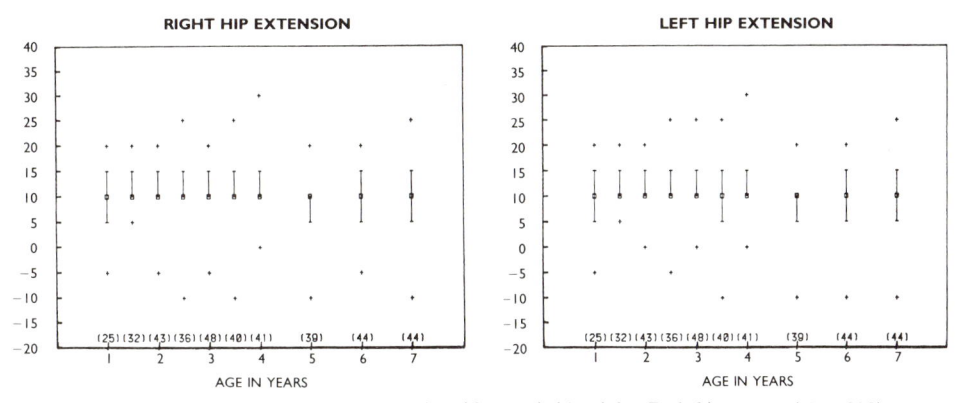

Fig. 5.8. Range of passive hip extension (degrees) (A: right; B: left) *vs.* age (N = 392).

Hip internal rotation
For this test the subject was prone with the knee flexed and the calf perpendicular to the table-top. An assistant stabilized the pelvis while the examiner rotated the hip. The goniometer was placed with the pivot over the tibial tuberosity, one arm on the shaft of the tibia and the other perpendicular to the table-top.

The median range of internal rotation across the 10 age-groups varied between 53° and 60° (Fig. 5.9). There was substantial variability throughout.

Hip external rotation
With the subject prone, the knee was flexed to a right-angle; an assistant stabilized the pelvis, and the examiner externally rotated the hip. The goniometer was placed

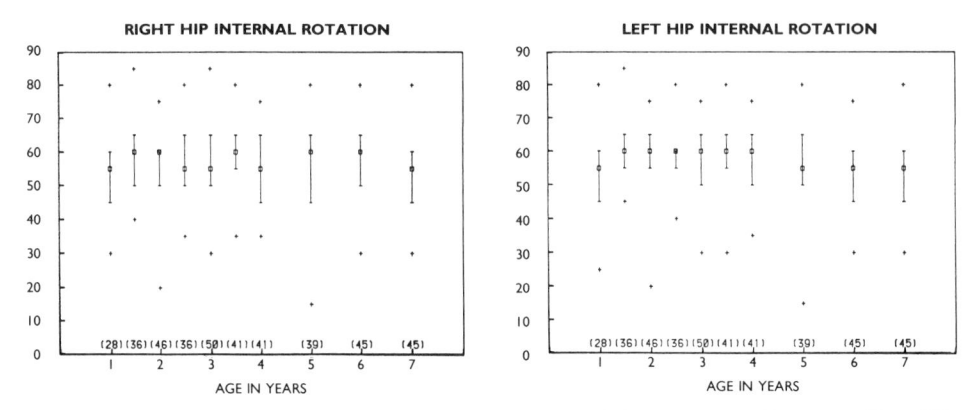

Fig. 5.9. Range of passive internal rotation of the hip (degrees) (A: right; B: left) *vs.* age (N = 407).

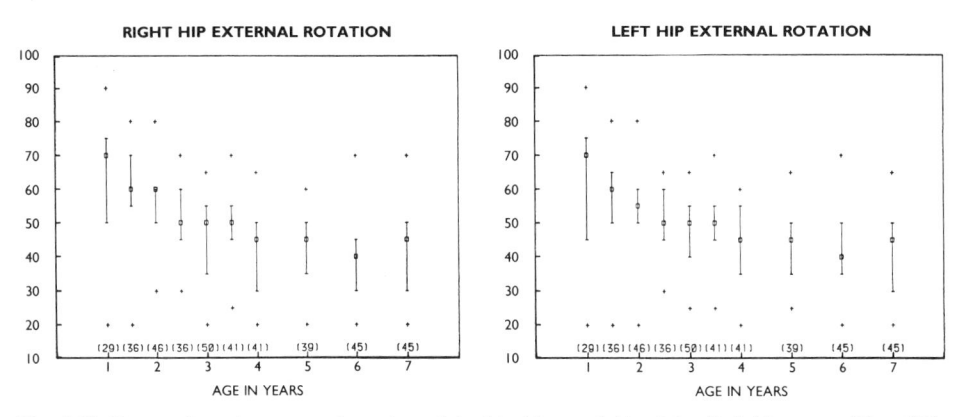

Fig. 5.10. Range of passive external rotation of the hip (degrees) (A: right; B: left) *vs.* age (N = 408).

with the pivot over the tibial tuberosity, one arm on the shaft of the tibia and the other perpendicular to the table-top.

There was a clear change in the range of external rotation across the age-groups, with a median of 65° at 1 year, diminishing gradually to 45° at 7 years (Fig. 5.10). Stated simply, the range of external rotation was exaggerated at 1 year but declined steadily thereafter, with the greatest change occurring between 1 year and 2½ years.

Hip abduction
Hip abduction was tested with the subject supine, and with the hips and knees extended parallel with the midline axis of the body. The goniometer was placed with the pivot over the anterior superior spine of the ipsilateral side, one arm pointing toward the contralateral anterior superior iliac spine and the other along

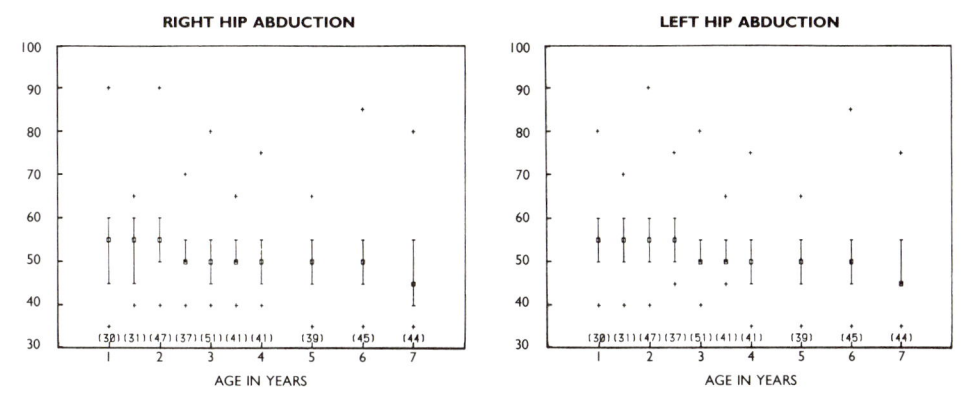

Fig. 5.11. Range of passive abduction of the hip (degrees) (A: right; B: left) *vs.* age (N = 406).

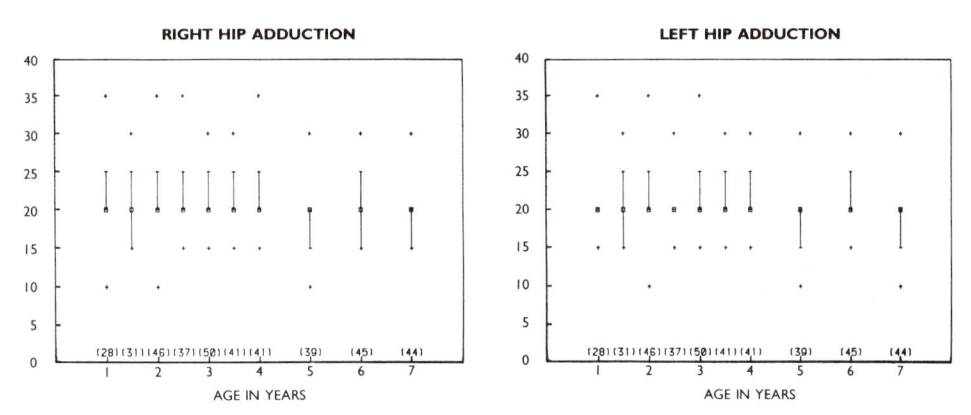

Fig. 5.12. Range of passive adduction of the hip (degrees) (A: right; B: left) *vs.* age (N = 402).

the longitudinal axis of the femur.

The median abduction range was 55° at 1 year, gradually diminishing to 45° at 7 years (Fig. 5.11). This reduction was fairly evenly distributed across the age-groups. We suppose this to be due to a gradual tightening of the hamstring and adductor muscles. It is well known that both muscle sets influence hip abduction in extension.

Hip adduction
Hip adduction was tested with the subject supine, hips and knees extended, hips in neutral rotation and the contralateral hip abducted. The goniometer was placed as in the test of hip abduction.

There was very little change with age, the median value in all age-groups being 20° (Fig. 5.12).

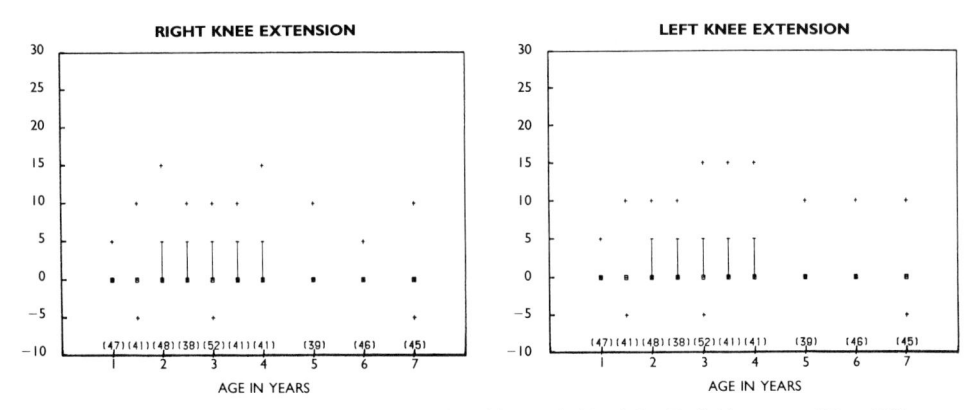

Fig. 5.13. Range of passive knee extension (degrees) (A: right; B: left) vs. age (N = 438).

Knee extension
Knee extension was tested with the subject supine, hips extended in neutral rotation. The goniometer was placed with the pivot over the midpoint of the lateral knee-joint line, one arm pointing toward the greater trochanter of the femur and the other toward the lateral malleolus of the fibula. Negative extension values were used to denote lack of full extension and positive values to indicate hyperextension.

Throughout the 10 age-groups, the range between the 25th and 75th percentiles was only 5°, with a median of 0° (Fig. 5.13). Maximum and minimum recorded values were +15° and −5° respectively. Virtually all the children demonstrated full extension and many showed hyperextension to 10°. In the 2 and 4 year age-groups, maximum extension to 15° was recorded.

Flexion contractures of 5° were observed in the 1½, 3 and 7 year age-groups; these were the minimum values for knee extension. The only trend was a reduction in the number of subjects showing hyperextension after the age of 4. This correlates well with straight-leg raising. Both tests relate to flexibility of the hamstring muscles.

Ankle dorsiflexion
This test was conducted with the subject supine, knee extended and hip in neutral rotation. The goniometer was placed with the pivot over the lateral ankle joint, one arm along the shaft of the fibula and the other parallel with the fifth metatarsal. Care was taken to restrict inversion or eversion. Right-angle alignment was designated as neutral dorsiflexion (0°). Dorsiflexion falling short of neutral was given a negative notation, that above neutral a positive one.

A significant decline in median dorsiflexion occurred with increasing age, from 25° at 1 year to 15° at 7 years (Fig. 5.14). The greatest change was between 1 and 4 years, indicating diminishing flexibility of the triceps surae between these ages.

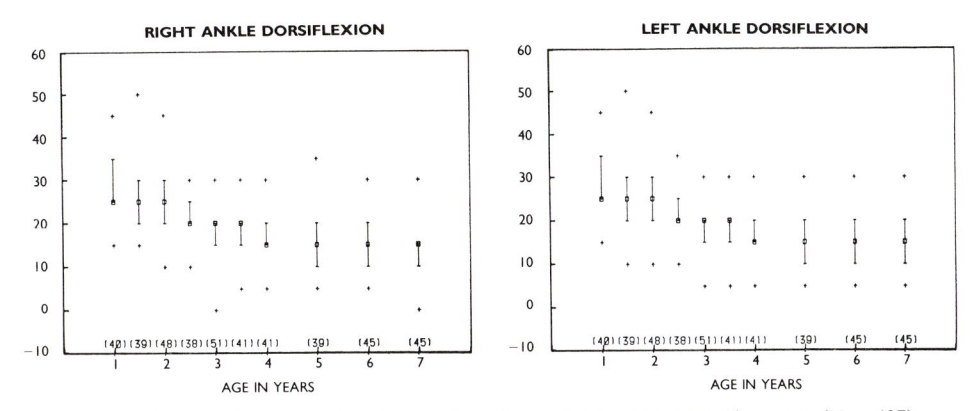

Fig. 5.14. Range of passive ankle dorsiflexion (degrees) (A: right; B: left) *vs.* age (N = 427).

Discussion
The ranges of motion presented above are helpful if used as guidelines. However, it would be unwise to label as abnormal a child who shows minor deviations from these values. If the variability in subjects is recognized and the tests are performed as described, useful comparisons can be made. These tests can be a part of the complete assessment necessary to establish deviation from normality.

The data for straight-leg raising, hip abduction, hip external rotation and ankle dorsiflexion show a gradual decrease with age. We cannot say with certainty that these motions actually decrease with age because this was primarily a cross-sectional study. We believe that they do.

Our study shows that external rotation of the hip is greater than internal rotation at 1 year and internal rotation exceeds external rotation after 2½ years. Engel and Staheli (1974) and Pitkow (1975) published similar conclusions; Crane (1959), however, reported that external rotation is greater than internal rotation at all ages.

Our finding of full extension of the hip to 10° across all the age-groups in our study is in disagreement with Hoffer (1980), who reported hip extension to only −10° to −12° at 15 months, and Boone and Azen (1978) who stated that hip extension under 5 years was less than 0°.

Tibial torsion
Tibial torsion was measured by the method of Staheli and Engel (1972). The subject was seated on a wooden box with the hips and knees flexed 90° and the ankles neutral with the heels in contact with the box. The width of each ankle (the distance between medial and lateral malleoli) was measured with a caliper, and the distance from the center of each malleolus to the box was measured with a ruler. Tibial torsion was then calculated using the graph provided in the article by Staheli and Engel. External tibial torsion was designated a positive value and internal tibial torsion a negative one.

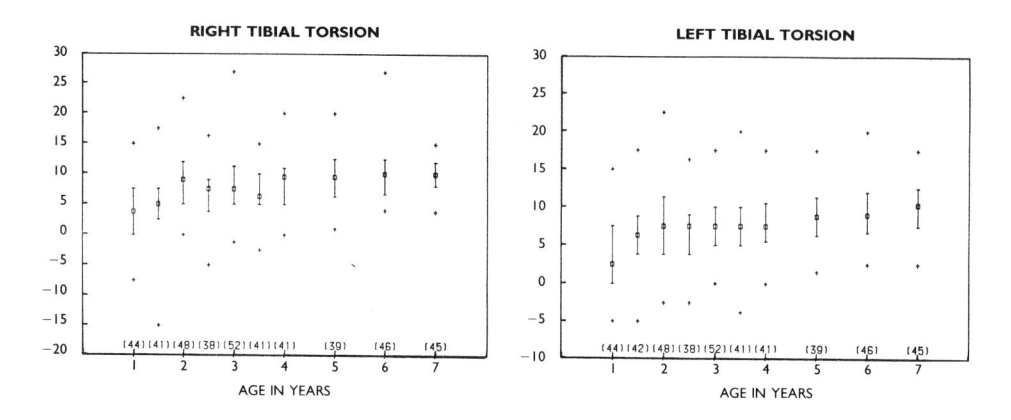

Fig. 5.15. Tibial torsion (degrees) (A: right, N = 435; B: left, N = 436) *vs.* age.

The median values displayed a pattern of gradually increasing external rotation with age (Fig. 5.15). This pattern is best seen in the diagram for left tibial torsion (Fig. 5.15B). At 1 year, the transmalleolar axis is externally rotated by approximately 4°. This increases by 2° at 1½ years, then very gradually to 10° at 7 years. There are minor differences in the median values for right (Fig. 5.15A) and left sides, but the difference is never greater than 2°.

It is appropriate to compare our measurements with those of Staheli and Engel (Fig. 5.16). Our results are quite similar, differing primarily between the ages of 2 and 4 years. The external torsion in our subjects is lower by approximately 4°. It should be noted that our data are presented differently from those of Staheli and Engel. Those authors quoted mean values as opposed to medians; we give right and left sides separately whereas they combined the two. Their study included adult measurements (the mean adult transmalleolar axis was 10°). Finally, the total number of tibial torsion measurements in our series of 1- to 7-year-old subjects was 871, compared with only 140 in the comparable age-range in their study. Our results provide a substantial normal data base.

Femoral/tibial alignment
This measure was obtained by aligning the lower extremities with the subject supine, and measuring the gap between the femoral condyles (genu varum) or between the medial malleoli (genu valgum). Two examiners, or one examiner and the parent, were usually required to minimize movement during the test. The measurement data are plotted in Figure 5.17. Intercondylar distance is shown as varus and intermalleolar distance as valgus.

The median alignment at age 1 was approximately neutral (*i.e.* with little distance between either the femoral condyles or the medial malleoli). The distribution of the middle 50 per cent of 1-year-olds shows both varus and valgus alignment. Valgus increases with age until 2½ years, then diminishes slightly. Note that there are very few children over the age of 1 year with varus alignment.

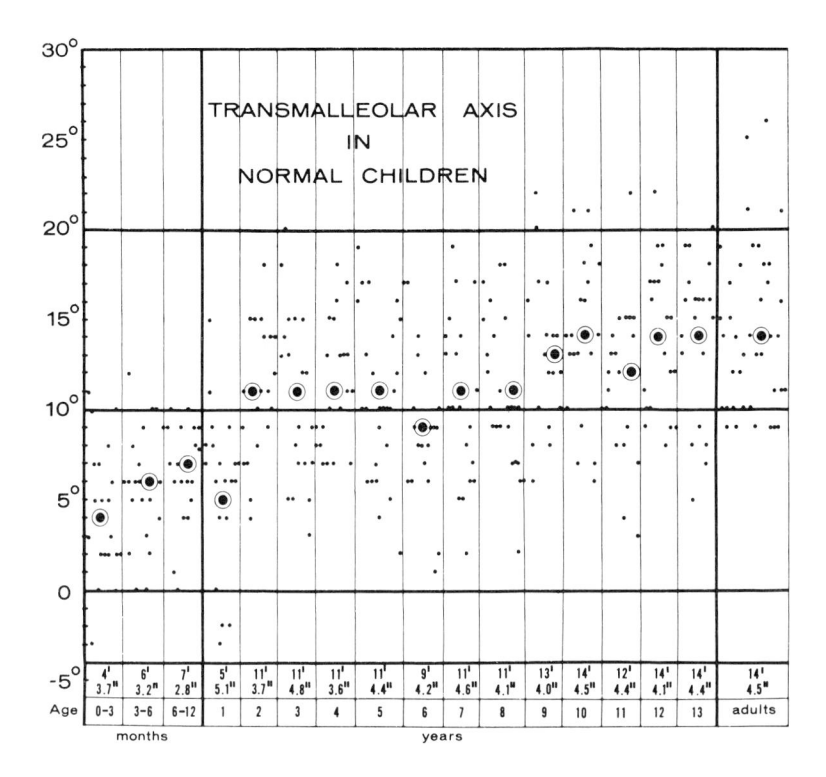

Fig. 5.16. The transmalleolar axis (tibial torsion) in normal children and adults. The mean in each age-group is indicated by the larger dot and circle (^{I}) is the mean by age-group and (^{II}) is the standard deviation. (Staheli and Engel 1972; reproduced by permission.)

Salenius and Vankka (1975) reported measurements of 1480 tibial/femoral angles of subjects between birth and 13 years of age (Fig. 5.18). All the children had varus alignment until late in the second year of life. The mean time of transition from varus to valgus was 22 months. The mean age of maximus valgus was 3 years; after this valgus decreased, leveling off at approximately 6 years. Our study shows similar trends but greater variability. The two studies are not comparable, however, because Salenius and Vankka X-rayed their subjects whereas we did not. With current awareness of the dangers of irradiation, non-urgent X-ray of the limbs should be reserved for those children suspected to have a pathology such as Blount's disease (and as this seldom occurs before the age of 2 years, it is appropriate to delay X-ray examination until that age or older). The measurement of intercondylar or intermalleolar distance is a practical alternative, or a supplement, to radiography in monitoring changes in lower-limb alignment. It should be emphasized that our subjects, all of them normal by our standards, showed considerable variability. The greatest spread of data was in the direction of valgus.

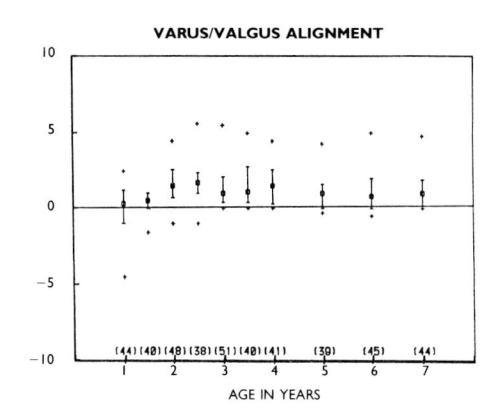

Fig. 5.17. Varus/valgus alignment of the knees, measured (in cm) with the subject supine, *vs.* age (N = 430).

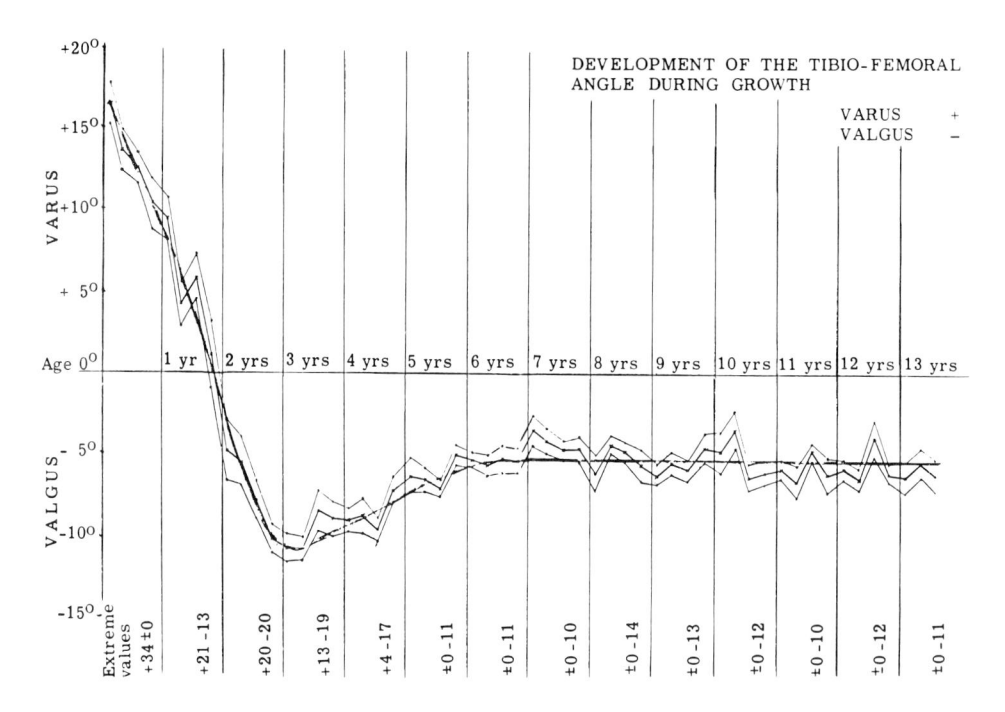

Fig. 5.18. Development of the tibiofemoral angle in children during growth. (Results based on 1480 measurements in children at different ages. The middle line shows the mean, and on both sides of this is the error of the mean (average 4.4°). Standard deviation was 8°.) (Salerius and Vankka 1975; reproduced by permission.)

Muscle strength
Upper- and lower-extremity muscle strength and tone were evaluated by an experienced physical therapist as part of the study screening procedure. Baseline data for muscle strength at each age are scarce if not non-existent, and we depended entirely on the skills and experience of the physical therapist to make the judgments.

By criterion, all children included in the study were rated as normal. If the goal had been to establish standards for muscle strength at each age it would have been necessary to use other methods and devote much more time to the individual tests, but this was not done as it was not part of the study design.

Joint laxity
Subjects were screened for ligamentous mobility at the fingers, wrists, elbows, knees and ankles. The tests for joint laxity are subjective and likely to be greatly affected by interobserver differences. The results of this testing therefore must be viewed as the opinions of experienced observers rather than as well-defined measurements. Hyperextension of elbows and knees were the only two easily measured evidences of hypermobility.

Children with pathological hypermobility such as is found in Ehlers-Danlos syndrome (McKusick 1972) were not admitted to the study. Children with benign hypotonia and delayed walking (Dubowitz 1968) also were excluded by the requirement that independent walking must have occurred by 14 months of age.

Three categories of mobility were anticipated: (1) within normal limits of laxity; (2) greater than normal; (3) less than normal. As few subjects were rated in the 'less than normal' category, we are presenting graphs only of those showing hypermobility (in terms of percentages of numbers tested in each age-group).

Fingers
Ninety per cent or more of the subjects in each age-group were designated normal. Results for left and right fingers were identical (Fig. 5.19).

Wrists
Ninety per cent or more of subjects 4 years and under, and virtually all the 5-, 6- and 7-year-olds had normal wrist-joint mobility (Fig. 5.20).

Elbows
A greater proportion of children, particularly in age-groups 4 years and up, had increased elbow-joint laxity. Three subjects, one aged 1 year and two aged 4 years, had restricted elbow extension. Findings for left and right elbows were nearly identical (Fig. 5.21).

Knees
Approximately 12 per cent of the 2-year-olds had increased laxity of the knee. In all other age-groups this figure was 10 per cent or less. Findings for right and left knees were nearly identical (Fig. 5.22).

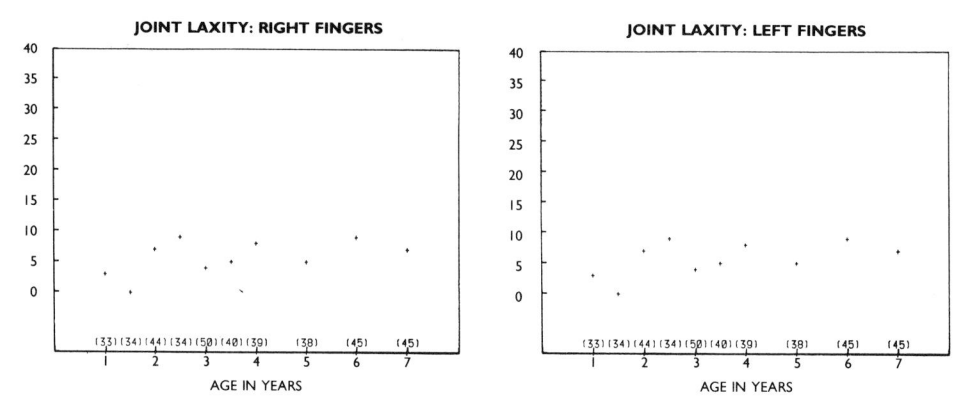

Fig. 5.19. Percentage of subjects (N = 402) with laxity of the joints of the fingers (A: right; B: left) *vs.* age.

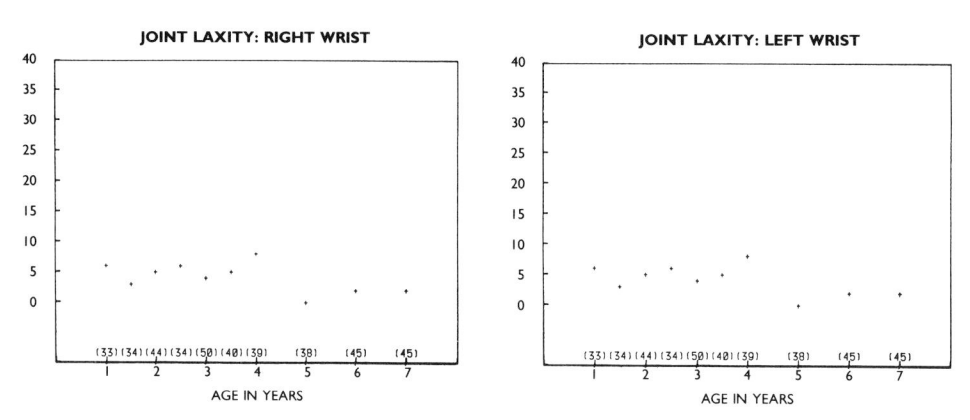

Fig. 5.20. Percentage of subjects (N = 402) showing hypermobility of the wrist (A: right; B: left) *vs.* age.

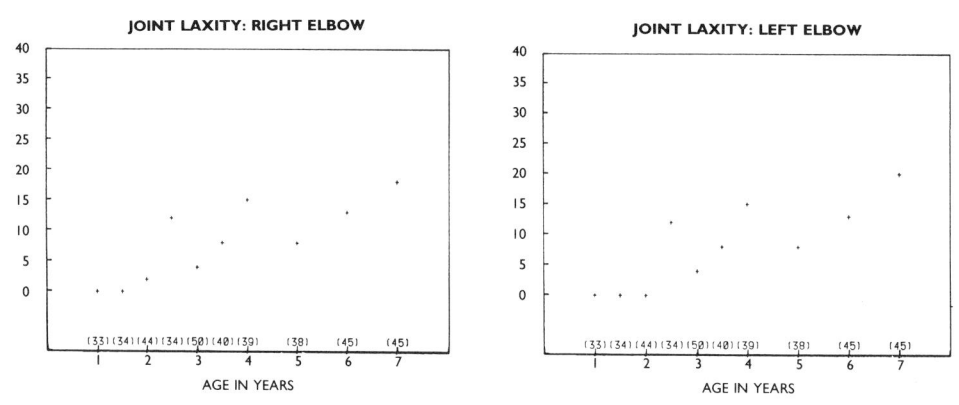

Fig. 5.21. Percentage of subjects (N = 402) showing hyperextension of the elbow (A: right; B: left) *vs.* age.

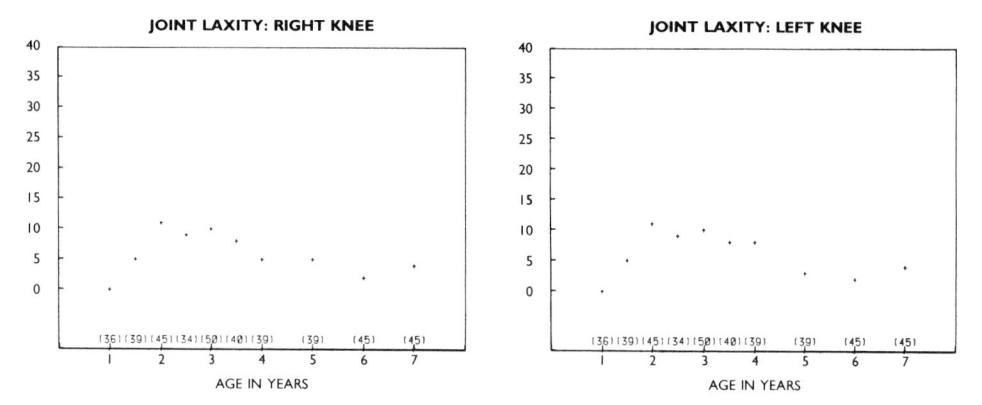

Fig. 5.22. Percentage of subjects (N = 412) showing passive hyperextension of the knee (A: right; B: left) vs. age.

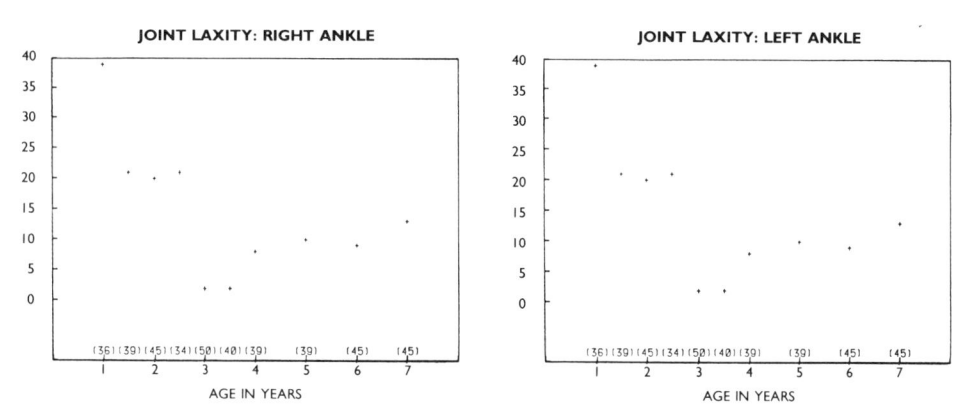

Fig. 5.23. Percentage of subjects (N = 412) with greater than normal ankle dorsiflexion (A: right; B: left) vs. age.

Ankles
Forty per cent of 1-year-olds had increased ankle-joint laxity. This proportion fell to 20 per cent among the 1½-, 2- and 2½-year-olds, and thereafter to around 10 per cent (Fig. 5.23). Restricted dorsiflexion was recorded in six subjects, aged 2½ (one), 3 (one), 4 (two) and 7 (two).

Discussion
Hypermobility of joints unrelated to injury in normal children is generally thought to be an inherited trait. 7 per cent of normal subjects in a study by Carter and Wilkinson (1964) were found to be hypermobile in more than three joints. Hupprich and Sigerseth (1950) examined correlations among 12 measures of general body flexibility and concluded that flexibility was a joint-specific function and not a generalized trait. By contrast, Marshall *et al* (1980) assessed 13 measures of flexibility in boys and girls aged 6 to 18 years and determined that children who

were flexible on one measure tended to be flexible on many measures; they concluded that joint looseness is an individual characteristic or trait. Any other conclusion would be very difficult to explain.

In general, our results confirm the conclusions of Carter and Wilkinson and of Marshall and colleagues. 10 per cent or less of the children in all age-groups demonstrated hypermobility of the right and left fingers, right and left wrists, and right and left knees. 20 per cent of children up to the age of 2½ had hypermobility of the ankle. A careful study of ankle dorsiflexion (see p. 40) reveals an age-related decline due to decreased flexibility in the triceps surae.

Hypermobility does not appear to be age-related. We looked at the peak incidence of hypermobility in the right knee and ankle. Comparisons of the outcomes of these tests indicated some examiner bias. One therapist rated a higher proportion of children as hypermobile than the other. Increases in hypermobility were noted in the 2, 2½, 3 and 3½ year age-groups. The 'bump' in the curves for these age-groups appeared to be related to the numbers of examinations performed by the first therapist. Of the total number of children exhibiting hypermobility, 48 showed it in two joints, usually paired (left and right). 35 showed it in three or more joints, and in most cases this was also in joint pairs. Only three children showed hypermobility in a single joint.

There were no instances of restricted mobility in the 1½, 2, 3½, 5 or 6 year age-groups. One 1-year-old had restricted elbow extension. One 2½-year-old had restricted ankle dorsiflexion. Of the 4-year-olds, two had restricted ankle dorsiflexion and two had restricted elbow extension. In the 7 year age-group one subject had restricted ankle dorsiflexion and one other had restricted elbow extension.

Developmental screening and mobility
Age of walking
Subjects' parents were asked to recall as accurately as possible the age at which their child began independent walking (Table 5.I).

The mean age of walking for our study population was 11.2 months. This compares with: 11.3 months, Denver Developmental Screening Test (Frankenberg and Dodds 1967); 11.7 months, Bayley Scales of Infant Development (Bayley 1969); 12 months, Revised Denver Developmental Screening Test (Frankenberg *et al.* 1981); and 15 months, Nelson Textbook of Pediatrics (Vaughan and Litt 1987).

In our study, parents of the 5-, 6- and 7-year-olds gave a date of independent walking for their children that was approximately one month earlier than that quoted by parents of the 1½- to 4-year olds. Possibly parents' memories are less accurate several years after the event, or it may be that there is a natural tendency to exaggerate as the time between event and recall lengthens. Hart *et al.* (1978) noted that the proportion of mothers able to recall the timing of developmental milestones decreased with increasing time after the event; however, walking was the best recalled milestone. With the exception of smiling, all milestones were reported as occurring earlier than they actually did.

TABLE 5.I
Estimated age of independent walking (in months) in each age-group

Age-group	N	Age started walking	
		Mean	S.D.
1	51	10.6	2.0
1½	40	11.8	1.5
2	45	12.1	1.5
2½	36	11.4	1.1
3	47	11.4	1.7
3½	40	11.1	2.0
4	39	11.3	1.6
5	42	10.6	1.8
6	44	10.7	1.6
7	46	10.9	2.4

Dominance

Upper-extremity dominance was tested by placing a crayon or pencil on a flat surface in front of and at midline to the subject, who was then asked (depending on his/her age) either to draw a shape or to write his/her name. This was repeated three times, and the hand chosen to hold the crayon or pencil was noted as the dominant upper extremity. For the youngest children dominance was determined by asking the parent or guardian whether the child had a hand preference for eating. If a child made equal use of both hands, the description was 'no preference'.

Lower-extremity dominance was evaluated by getting the subject to kick a ball. The younger children were asked to place-kick a soccer ball, and the older children were asked to drop-kick the ball. This was repeated at least three times and the foot most often used to kick the ball was defined as the dominant lower extremity. If a child used both feet equally, again the description was 'no preference'.

Upper-extremity dominance was established in the majority of children by the age of 1 year; however, at 2½ years, 14 per cent of subjects still showed no preference. By 3 years, only 1 per cent showed no preference. Lower-extremity dominance was established in the majority of subjects by the age of 2, although 17 per cent of 2½-year-olds, 13 per cent of 3-year-olds and 12 per cent of 3½-year-olds still had no preference. It was not until the age of 4 that this proportion dropped to 8 per cent.

The dominance patterns in each age-group are shown in Table 5.II. The relationship of right *vs.* left dominance was approximately constant across those age-groups in which subjects were old enough for this to be tested.

Combining the upper-extremity data for all subjects aged 3 and over, 87 per cent were right-hand and 11 per cent left-hand dominant. 2 per cent showed no preference. To establish the pattern for lower-extremity dominance we combined only the data of subjects aged 4 and over. This was because lower-extremity dominance developed later than upper-extremity dominance. 89 per cent were

TABLE 5.II

Upper- and lower-extremity dominance in subjects who participated in movement measurement studies (N = 415)

Age-group	Upper extremity			Mixed Dominance††	Lower extremity		
	Right	Left	None†		Right	Left	None†
1	29	7	13	0	9	4	9*
1½	29	4	6	2	16	17	14**
2	32	7	5	4	25	5	14
2½	28	3	5	1	26	4	6
3	39	5	3	1	36	5	6
3½	36	2	0	0	32	3	3
4	33	3	0	0	33	3	0
5	33	6	0	2	35	3	1
6	39	5	0	1	38	6	0
7	36	6	1	0	38	4	1

†Unknown or no preference.
††*Mixed dominance* refers to a preference for one upper extremity and the contralateral lower extremity.
*27 unable to kick.
**2 unable to kick.

right-foot dominant, 10 per cent left-foot dominant, and 1 per cent showed no preference. Thus, right-hand and right-foot dominance occurred in roughly equal numbers of subjects. Left-foot dominance occurred in slightly fewer subjects than left-hand dominance. No foot preference was shown by a slightly higher proportion of subjects than showed no hand preference.

'Mixed' dominance (upper and contralateral lower) was very rare, occurring in only 11 subjects: two at age 1½, four at 2, one at 2½, one at 3, two at 5 and one at 6 years.

Statistical analysis of the movement measurements showed no effect due to dominance.

Squatting
The subject was asked to squat on the floor without support. 95 per cent of the 1-year-olds and all the older children were successful. It is clear that this is an easy function for even a very small child to perform, and that the ability is present from the time of the onset of walking.

Standing up without support
The subject was asked to sit on the floor, and then to stand up again without receiving support from either the parent or therapist. Over 90 per cent of the 1-year-olds and all of the other children could perform this task. This is not surprising, since the ability to pull up to stand and cruise* precedes the onset of independent walking.

Cruising. A US expression referring to the act of standing upright and moving around independently by clutching on to furniture, crib railings, etc.

Running

The subject was asked to run from one end of the laboratory to the other, a distance of around 17 meters. Just over 30 per cent of the 1-year-olds were able to do this, rising to 78 per cent among the 1½-year-olds and 97 per cent among the 2-year-olds. All children in the remaining age-groups were able to run (Fig. 5.24).

Toe-walking

The subject was asked to 'walk on your tiptoes'. The therapist demonstrated this by walking on the metatarsal heads with heels raised. The success rate was less than 15 per cent among the 1-year-olds, rising to 65 per cent at 1½, and 90 per cent at 2. By 2½ years, all children could toe-walk (Fig. 5.25).

Touwen (1979) stated: 'Children over three years of age should be able to walk on tiptoe; some younger children are also able to do so'. Our results indicate an earlier ability for this task.

Heel-walking

The subject was asked to 'walk on your heels'. The therapist demonstrated by walking on the heels with the toes raised. None of the children in either the 1 or 1½ year age-groups could perform this task. Among the 2-year-olds, less than 10 per cent were successful. At 2½ years, this figure rose to 60 per cent, at 3 to 80 per cent, at 3½ to 90 per cent, and from 4 years upwards to 100 per cent (Fig. 5.26).

Touwen (1979) stated: 'Children over the age of three years should be able to walk on their heels, and some younger children may also be able to do so.' We are in agreement that by 3 years most children can heel-walk, but our study indicates that over one-half of 2½-year-olds also are able to carry out this task.

Standing on one leg

Subjects were asked to stand on one leg for as long as they could. Few of the children aged 2½ years or under could perform this task at all; by 3 years the success rate was 95 per cent (Fig. 5.27). Single-limb stance is, of course, an integral part of independent walking, which in most children occurs before 1 year; however, single stance in walking is only of short duration, and it is less demanding than standing still balancing on one leg.

The median times achieved for single-limb stance were, by age-group: 2½ years (3 secs.), 3 years (4 secs.), 3½ years (6 secs.), 4 years (8 secs.), 5 years (15 secs.), 6 years (20 secs.), and 7 years (30 secs.). There is an obvious correlation between duration of single-limb stance and the ability to stand on one leg. This ability does not develop until 2½ years, and at that age the performance time is only very brief. From 4 years on, performance times increase rapidly. There was very little difference in the average times achieved on right and left legs (Fig. 5.28).

Hopping

The subject was asked to hop for a distance of 3 meters, first on one leg then the other. None of the children under 2½ years could do this, and less than 5 per cent

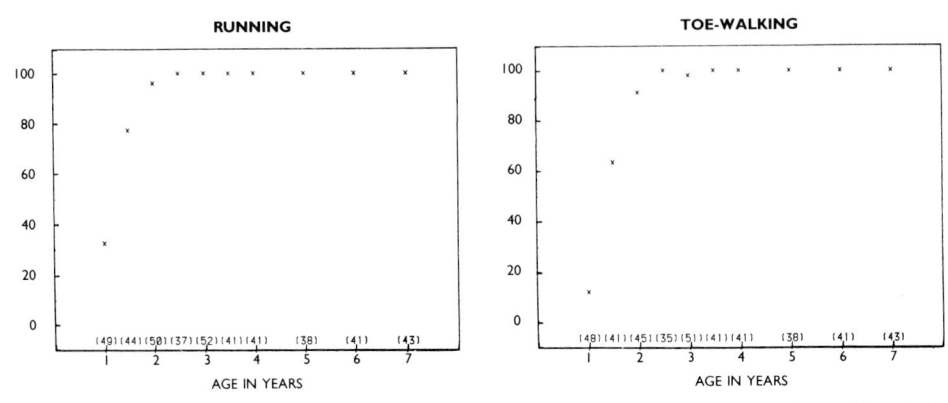

Fig. 5.24. Percentage of subjects (N = 436) able to run the length of the walkway *vs.* age.

Fig. 5.25. Percentage of subjects (N = 424) able to walk on tiptoes *vs.* age.

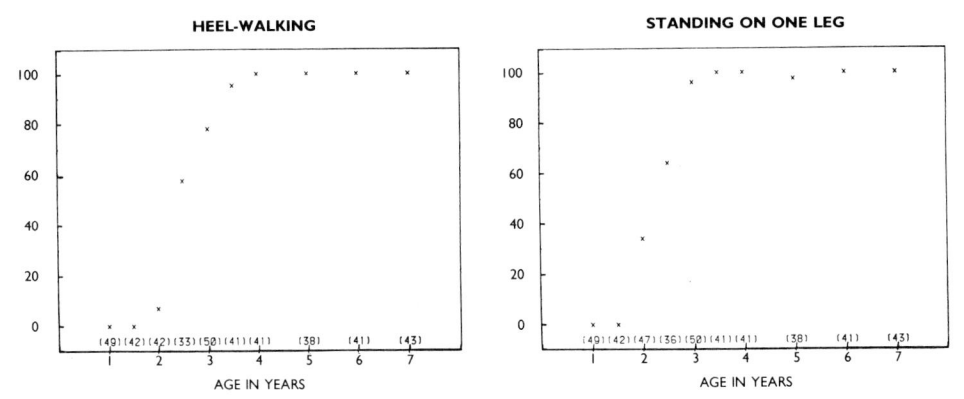

Fig. 5.26. Percentage of subjects (N = 420) able to 'heel-walk' *vs.* age.

Fig. 5.27. Percentage of subjects (N = 428) able to stand on one leg *vs.* age.

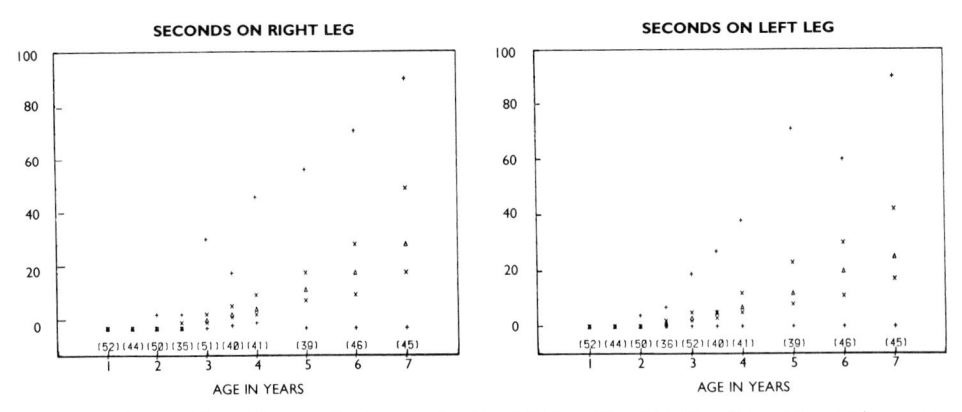

Fig. 5.28. Times achieved for standing on one leg (A: right leg, N = 443; B: left leg, N = 445) *vs.* age. The two '×' markers encompass the middle 50 per cent of subjects; the triangle indicates the median; and the upper and lower marks respectively show the greatest and least values recorded.

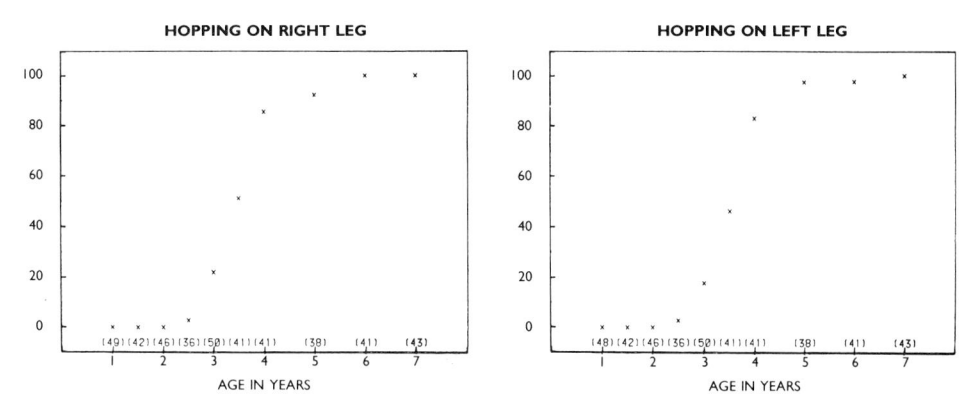

Fig. 5.29. Percentage of subjects able to hop (A: right leg, N = 427; B: left leg, N = 426) *vs.* age.

of the 2½-year-olds were successful. The numbers rose to 23 per cent at age 3, 52 per cent at 3½, 85 per cent at 4, and 92 per cent at 5. All the 6- and 7-year-olds could hop. Comparing these figures with those for standing on one leg, it is clear that in normal children the ability to hop is slower to develop. Landing on one leg and retaining one's balance requires much greater coordination and development than simply standing still on one leg.

Results for right and left legs were very similar (Fig. 5.29). A child who can hop on one leg can also hop on the other. Touwen (1979) points out that the development of this motor function is abrupt and rapid. Our study agrees with this, emphasizing that most children can hop for a distance of 3 meters by the age of 4 years.

Walking and tandem-walking on balance beam
The subject was asked to walk the length of a 3-meter balance beam (comprising a 10cm × 10cm wooden beam, supported 5cm off the floor). If successful, the subject was asked to repeat the walk, this time placing one heel directly in front of the opposite toe (tandem-walking). It is not possible to say how the complexity of tandem-walking on a 10cm balance beam would compare to that of walking along a line painted on a flat surface, since this was not tested. However, it does seem likely that a child might be able to perform this latter task more easily.

Walking on the beam proved a relatively difficult task, with only 7 per cent of 2-year-olds, 30 per cent of 2½-year-olds and 34 per cent of 3-year-olds able to accomplish it. 75 per cent of the 3½-year-olds and 90 per cent or more of the older subjects were successful (Fig. 5.30).

Very few children younger than 3½ years could perform the tandem-walking task. The success rate at 4 years was 20 per cent, rising to 80 per cent at 5 years and 100 per cent at 6 and 7 years (Fig. 5.31). This task was the most difficult of our developmental screening tests as attested by general lack of performance until 5 years of age.

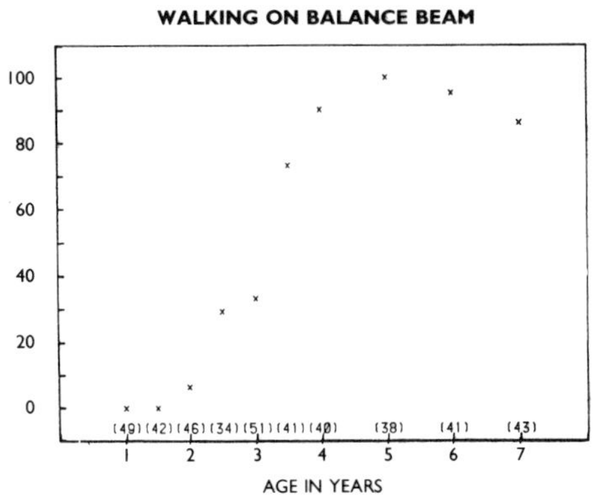

Fig. 5.30. Percentage of subjects (N= 425) able to walk the length of the balance beam *vs.* age.

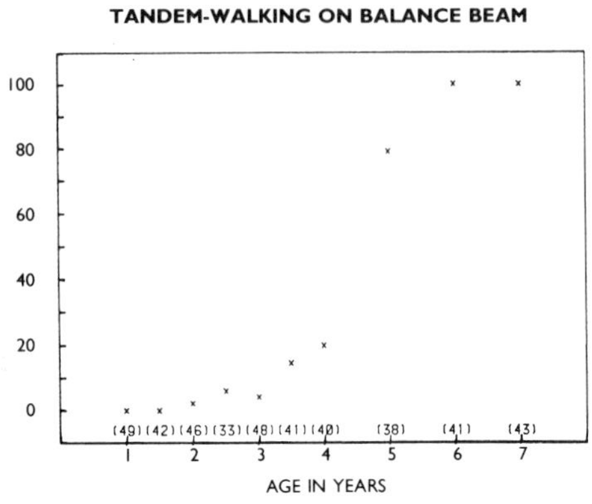

Fig. 5.31. Percentage of subjects (N = 421) able to 'tandem-walk' the length of the balance beam *vs.* age.

Reflexes

Neonatal

Subjects were screened by the physical therapist for retained neonatal reflexes. Specific tests were applied to determine the presence or absence of the following neonatal reflexes: (1) symmetrical tonic neck reflex; (2) asymmetrical tonic neck reflex; (3) Moro reflex; (4) positive supporting reaction in extension. The presence of any of these reflexes was cause for exclusion from the study. One child was excluded because of retained asymmetrical tonic neck reflex.

Protective extension

Subjects were also tested for the presence of the upper-extremity protective extension reflex. The child was suspended by the waist and tilted forward. The reflex was deemed to be present if the arms and hands were extended toward the floor. All children selected for study demonstrated this reflex.

6
TIME/DISTANCE PARAMETERS BY AGE

Introduction
Each gait cycle contains events that subdivide it into manageable components for detailed inspection of the constituent movements, timing of muscle activity, and ground-reaction forces. These events, periods and phases are described in Chapter 2 (and illustrated in Figure 2.7, p. 17). However, for those readers who never turn back, or for those who may be beginning at this point, we shall provide a brief summary.

A gait cycle begins and ends with foot-strike of the same foot. Foot-strike and toe-off for each limb comprise the events that subdivide the cycle into: initial double-limb support, single-limb stance, second double-limb support, and swing phase. The right gait cycle is started by right foot-strike, followed by left toe-off to begin the period of single-limb stance. Single stance is ended by left foot-strike, which begins the period of second double support. Right toe-off begins the swing phase, which is divided into initial swing, mid-swing and terminal swing. Initial swing ends when the right tibia reaches the vertical, and terminal swing ends with right foot-strike.

This chapter is concerned with the measurements of the times of occurrence of these events, their inter-relationships, and the time/distance parameters for each of the 10 age-groups. Throughout the study all measurements were based on free-speed walking. The measurements are: step length, stride length, opposite toe-off, opposite foot-strike, toe-off, duration of single-limb stance, cycle time, cadence, and walking velocity. Cycle time was measured in real time. The other time measurements were normalized by conversion to percentage of gait cycle to facilitate subject-to-subject comparisons.

These measurements are important because they are sensitive indicators of gait maturation and also of gait deficits in pathological gait. Our data provide a 'normative' set for comparison with pathological gait measurements. There are many changes in the time/distance parameters of children from age 1 to 7 years; while some of these changes are related primarily to changes in the size of body segments, others probably are caused by maturation of the motor control system.

Height, leg length and step length
Table 6.I lists the means and standard deviations of the heights, right and left leg lengths, and stride lengths among the 10 age-groups. Height measurements are included in order to emphasize the relationship between leg length and step length. Since right and left step lengths are approximately equal in the children in this study, either step length or stride length could be compared to leg length; we have arbitrarily chosen to use the former. Stride length (the sum of right and left step lengths) divided by cycle time equals walking velocity. This table will be useful for

TABLE 6.I

Means and standard deviations for height, right and left leg lengths, right and left step lengths, and stride length in each age-group. All measurements are in centimeters.

Age	N	Height		Right leg		Left leg		Right step		Left step		Stride	
		Mean	SD	Mean	SD	Mean	SD	Mean	SD	Mean	SD	Mean	SD
1	51	74.5	3.0	31.6	1.4	31.6	1.4	21.6	3.9	21.4	3.5	43.0	6.7
1½	40	80.2	4.1	35.5	2.2	35.5	2.2	25.1	3.6	24.4	3.4	49.5	6.6
2	45	86.2	3.6	38.9	2.0	38.9	2.0	27.5	3.2	27.4	3.6	54.9	6.3
2½	36	89.9	3.9	41.4	2.5	41.5	2.6	30.7	3.9	31.1	3.6	61.8	7.4
3	47	94.8	3.3	44.3	2.1	44.4	2.1	32.9	3.6	33.9	3.7	66.8	7.0
3½	40	98.3	3.9	46.5	2.6	46.5	2.6	36.5	3.9	37.5	4.4	74.0	8.1
4	39	102.6	3.5	49.3	2.1	49.2	2.1	38.5	4.2	39.1	4.0	77.9	8.5
5	42	108.8	4.1	53.4	2.9	53.4	2.9	42.3	4.2	42.9	4.1	84.3	10.2
6	44	115.6	4.6	57.0	3.3	57.0	3.4	44.1	4.4	45.2	4.3	89.3	8.5
7	46	122.2	4.9	61.5	3.8	61.5	3.8	47.9	4.3	48.7	4.1	96.5	8.2

rapid reference. A clearer picture of the changes with age and growth can be got from the graphic representation of the data which follow. Discussion of these changes will accompany the graphs.

Age *vs.* leg length
Between 1 and 7 years, leg length and age are closely related (Fig. 6.1). The correlation coefficient is 0.95. There is a slight decline in the slope beginning at approximately 4 years, which we attribute to altered speed of growth (see Anderson *et al.* 1963, Moseley 1977).

Step length *vs.* height and leg length
Data relating step length and height are depicted in Figure 6.2A. The correlation coefficient is very high (0.91). Step length *vs.* leg length is plotted in Figure 6.2B. There is an obvious linear relationship between the means of step length and leg length between 1 and 7 years of age. The correlation coefficient is 0.91, which yields an exceedingly high t-value of more than 40. An approximate 95 per cent confidence interval extends only from 0.89 to 0.93.

Step length *vs.* age
Between the ages of 1 and 4 years the relationship between step length and age is linear; this applies also between 4 and 7 years but with a reduced slope (Fig. 6.3). The correlation coefficient is 0.90; however, this is an example of data for which a 'significant' correlation is misleading, due to this clear change in the slope at about age 4. Since leg length and step length are related, the explanation for this change is that there is a change in the speed of growth, a fact well described by Anderson *et al.* (1963) and Moseley (1977). We have used chronological age rather than bone age. Changes in the speed of growth are much less evident when bone age is plotted against leg length, but radiographic examination of the hand, necessary for the determination of bone age, was not included in the study plan.

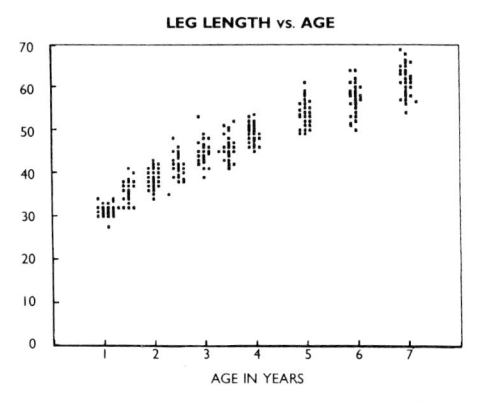

Fig. 6.1. Leg length (cm) *vs.* age (N = 441).

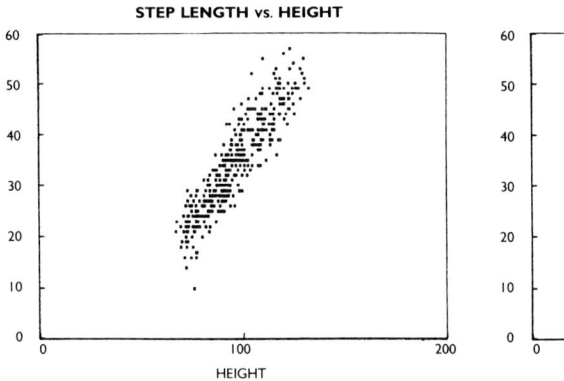

Fig. 6.2A. Step length (cm) *vs.* height (cm) (N = 418).

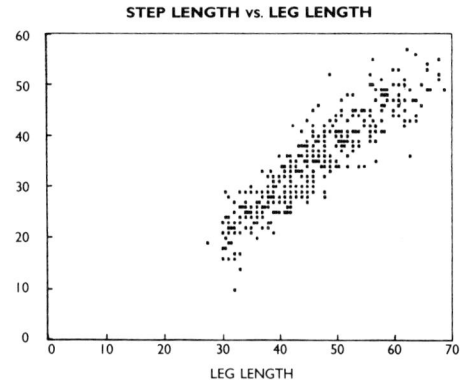

Fig. 6.2B. Step length (cm) *vs.* leg length (cm) (N = 414).

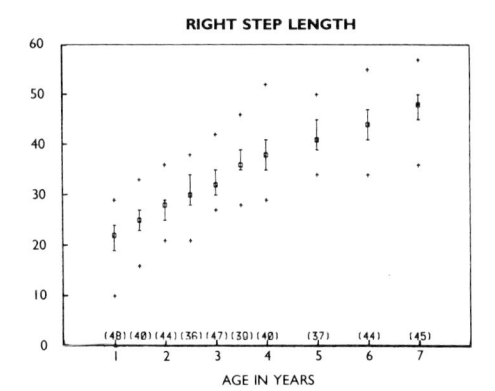

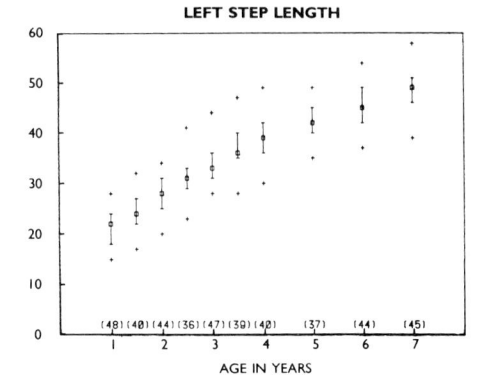

Fig. 6.3. Step length (cm) (A = right; B = left) *vs.* age (N = 420).
    In this and in subsequent figures in this chapter, at each age the vertical bar encompasses the middle 50 per cent of subjects and the box indicates the median. The upper and lower markers respectively show the greatest and least values recorded. Numbers of subjects in each age-group are given in parentheses along the horizontal axis.

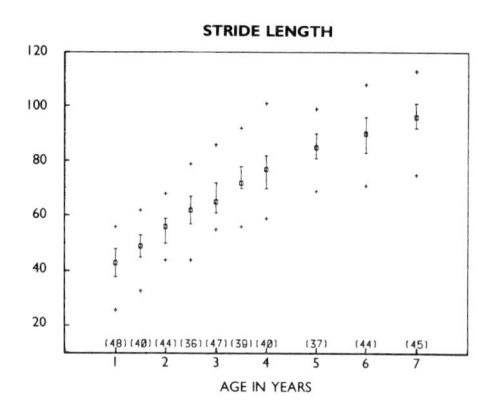

Fig. 6.4. Stride length (cm) *vs.* age (N = 420).

Stride length *vs.* age
Stride length, like leg length, is directly related to age in the 1 to 7 year age-groups. As with step length, there is a linear rise with age from 1 to 4 years, then a linear rise with diminished slope between 4 and 7 years (Fig. 6.4). The explanation is identical. Since right and left step lengths are equal in normal gait, one stride length is equal to two step lengths of the same leg. Thus, stride length and step length are related to age in an identical manner—they differ only in the scale of the ordinate.

Timing of gait events and phases
Table 6.II lists the means and standard deviations for the timing of gait events, and for the duration of right and left single-limb stance, expressed as percentages of the gait cycle. (From these figures, double-stance and swing phase timings also can be inferred.) There were no significant differences in the mean values for right and left sides.

This table will be useful for quick reference. The same data are presented in percentiles, as opposed to means and standard deviations, in the graphs that follow. Since this method of presentation makes it easier to see the changes that occur with maturation, descriptions of these changes will accompany the graphs.

Opposite toe-off *vs.* age
Figures 6.5A and 6.5B show the timings of opposite toe-off for the right and left leg. These times are highest in the two youngest age-groups. Thereafter there is a general downward trend, with the most rapid change occurring between 1½ and 3½ years. A high opposite toe-off time is significant since it indicates prolonged initial double support, which thereby restricts single-limb stance.

Opposite foot-strike
Time of opposite foot-strike appears to have the least variability of all the gait events, occurring regularly at around 50 per cent of the cycle. The median time of left opposite foot-strike closely approximates 50 per cent of the gait cycle in each of

TABLE 6.II

Means and standard deviations for times of gait events, expressed as percentage of gait cycle. (OTO = opposite toe-off; OFS = opposite foot-strike; TO = toe-off; SS = single stance.) There are no significant differences in the mean values for left and right sides.

Age	N	Right OTO Mean	SD	Left OTO Mean	SD	Right OFS Mean	SD	Left OFS Mean	SD
1	51	17.1	4.2	17.9	3.6	49.2	2.1	50.4	2.1
1½	40	17.5	3.6	17.6	3.5	49.5	2.3	50.1	2.2
2	45	16.9	2.7	16.5	2.6	50.4	2.0	49.7	1.9
2½	36	15.5	2.5	15.6	2.3	50.3	1.2	50.2	1.3
3	47	15.6	2.2	15.4	2.3	50.4	1.4	50.2	0.9
3½	40	14.3	1.8	14.5	1.7	50.2	1.1	50.3	1.1
4	39	14.3	1.8	14.0	1.9	50.3	1.0	50.0	1.2
5	42	13.3	2.0	13.6	1.9	49.7	1.7	50.4	1.0
6	44	13.3	1.7	13.5	1.7	49.8	1.0	50.4	0.9
7	46	12.4	1.7	12.3	1.9	50.0	1.1	50.0	1.0

Age	N	Right TO Mean	SD	Left TO Mean	SD	Right SS Mean	SD	Left SS Mean	SD
1	51	67.1	4.0	67.6	4.0	32.1	3.9	32.5	2.7
1½	40	67.6	3.9	67.6	3.4	32.1	3.6	32.4	3.5
2	45	67.1	2.7	66.6	2.6	33.5	3.0	33.3	2.7
2½	36	65.5	2.4	65.9	2.4	34.7	2.5	34.6	2.5
3	47	65.5	2.2	65.4	2.0	34.8	2.1	34.8	2.3
3½	40	64.6	1.7	64.3	2.0	35.9	2.0	35.8	2.2
4	39	64.2	1.8	63.2	4.8	35.9	1.9	36.0	2.0
5	42	63.4	2.1	63.5	2.1	36.6	2.1	36.8	1.8
6	44	63.5	2.0	63.7	1.7	36.5	1.7	36.6	2.1
7	46	62.4	1.7	62.4	1.9	37.6	1.7	37.8	1.6

the age-groups (Fig. 6.6A). The same holds true for right opposite foot-strike with the exception of the 1 and 1½ year age-groups, whose median times are only slightly lower (Fig. 6.6B). For reasons that we do not understand, the distributions appear to be skewed in many age-groups.

Toe-off

Times of right and left toe-off are shown in Figures 6.7A and 6.7B respectively. Values are quite high (>65 per cent) before 2½ years, declining gradually to a normal adult level (around 62 per cent) by 5 years.

Single-limb stance

The durations of right and left single-limb stance are shown in Figures 6.8A and 6.8B respectively. The median for both right and left legs at age 1 year is 32 per cent. No change is evident between 1 and 1½ years; however, the next four age-groups show progressive increases and near-adult levels are attained by 3½ years. Note also that the variability in duration of single stance diminishes with age.

Single-stance time is a powerful indicator of the ability to control the body mass on one limb. The adult mean value is 38 per cent. Lower values reflect

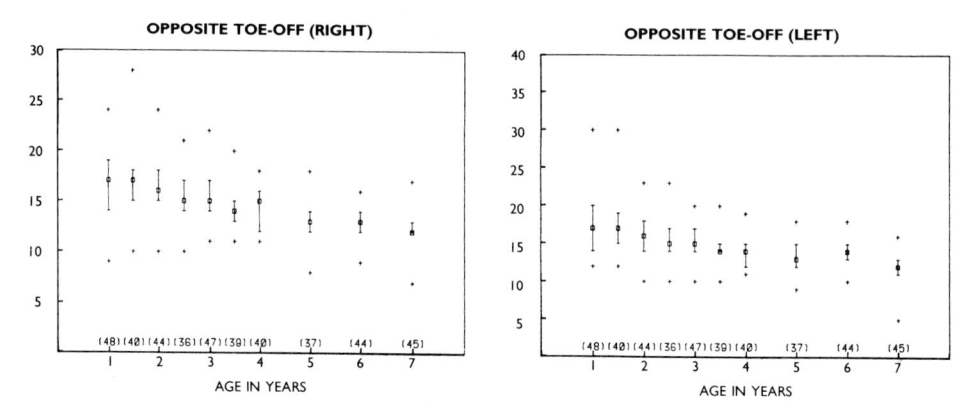

Fig. 6.5. Times of opposite toe-off as percentage of gait cycle (A = right; B = left) *vs.* age (N = 420).

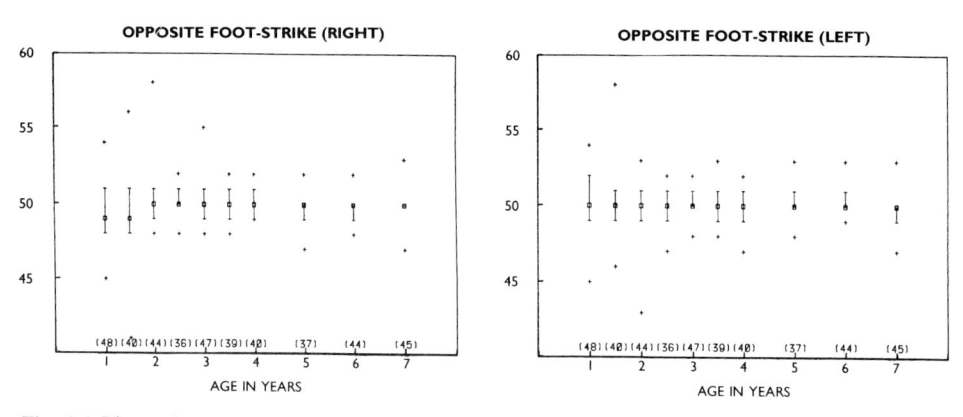

Fig. 6.6. Times of opposite foot-strike as percentage of gait cycle (A = right; B = left) *vs.* age (N = 420).

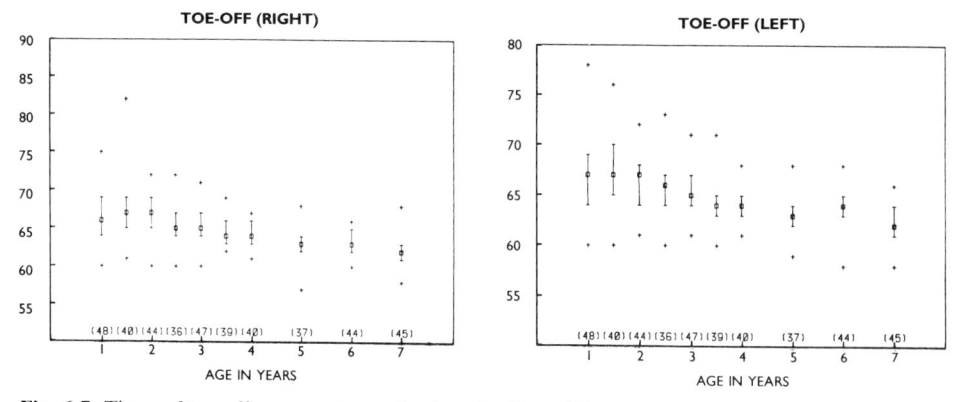

Fig. 6.7. Times of toe-off as percentage of gait cycle (A = right; B = left) *vs.* age (N = 420).

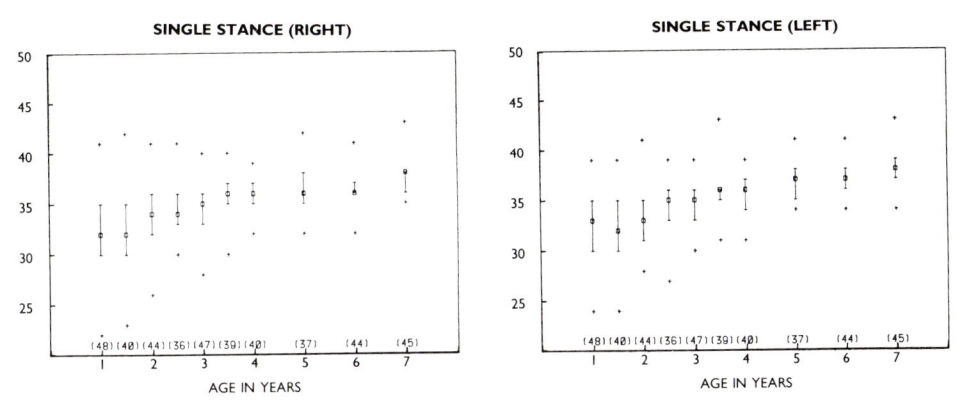

Fig. 6.8. Duration of single-limb stance as percentage of gait cycle (A = right; B = left) vs. age (N = 420).

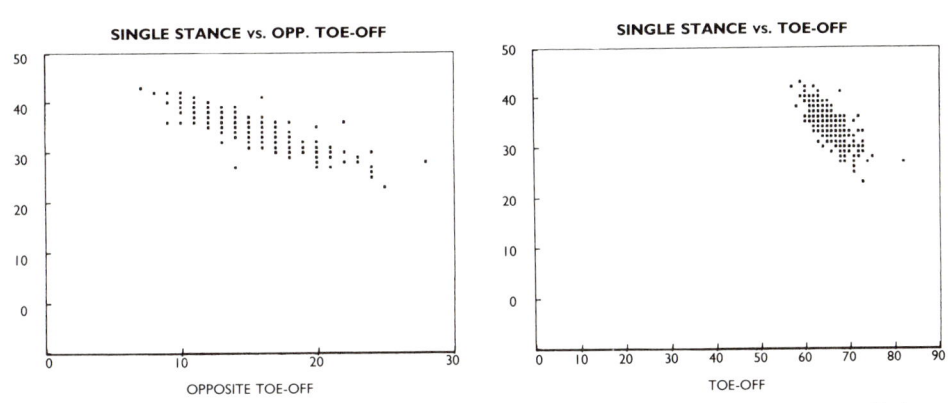

Fig. 6.9A. Single-limb stance vs. opposite toe-off times (percentage of gait cycle) (N = 420).

Fig. 6.9B. Single-limb stance vs. toe-off times (percentage of gait cycle) (N = 420).

instability, which may relate to motor weakness, joint instability, ataxia, or pain with weight-bearing. The lower values found in immature walkers may be due to underdevelopment of the motor control system (Sutherland *et al.* 1980*a*).

Single stance *vs.* opposite toe-off
Obviously, the later opposite toe-off occurs, the shorter single-limb stance will be. In fact, the correlation coefficient is -0.87, with an approximate 95 per cent confidence interval extending from -0.89 to -0.84 (Fig. 6.9A).

Single stance *vs.* toe-off
Single limb stance and toe-off are also inversely related (Fig. 6.9B), with a correlation coefficient of -0.76 and an approximate 95 per cent confidence interval extending from -0.80 to -0.71.

TABLE 6.III
Means and standard deviations for cycle time, cadence and walking velocity in each age-group.

Age	N	Cycle time (secs.)		Cadence (steps/min.)		Velocity (cm/sec.)	
		Mean	SD	Mean	SD	Mean	SD
1	51	0.68	0.09	176	24	64	16
1½	40	0.70	0.08	171	21	71	14
2	45	0.78	0.11	156	25	72	16
2½	36	0.77	0.08	156	17	81	15
3	47	0.77	0.07	154	16	86	14
3½	40	0.74	0.05	160	13	99	15
4	39	0.78	0.07	152	15	100	17
5	42	0.77	0.06	154	14	108	18
6	44	0.82	0.09	146	18	109	19
7	46	0.83	0.07	143	14	114	17

Cycle time, cadence and walking velocity
Means and standard deviations for cycle time, cadence and walking velocity in each age-group are listed in Table 6.III.

Cycle time *vs.* age
A great degree of scatter is evident in the cycle-time data. The median for the 1 and 1½ year age-groups is 0.70 secs. This rises rapidly to 0.80 secs. at age 2, and remains at approximately this level throughout the older age-groups (Fig. 6.10).

Cadence *vs.* age
Cadence in the 1-year-old subjects was approximately 22.5 per cent higher than in the 7-year-olds. The principle reduction occurs between the ages of 1 and 2; thereafter the decrease is gradual (Fig. 6.11). It is important to be aware that at 7 years cadence is still approximately 26 per cent higher than the normal adult mean (Sutherland *et al.* 1980*a*).

Walking velocity *vs.* age
Walking velocity increases with age in a linear manner from 1 to 3 years, at a rate of about 11cm/sec. per year. From 4 to 7 years the rate of change diminishes to 4.5cm/sec. per year; however, the relationship remains linear. The difference in slopes is highly significant (t-test, $p<0.001$). Variability is nearly constant across all age-groups. Two curves are presented (Figs. 6.12A,B). The first gives the walking velocity in cm/sec. The second, for the convenience of readers preferring a measure of meters per minute, is included to eliminate the need for mathematical conversion.

Discussion and summary
Time/distance parameters have been the most frequently reported gait measurements. One reason is obvious: they can be obtained more easily than motion, force

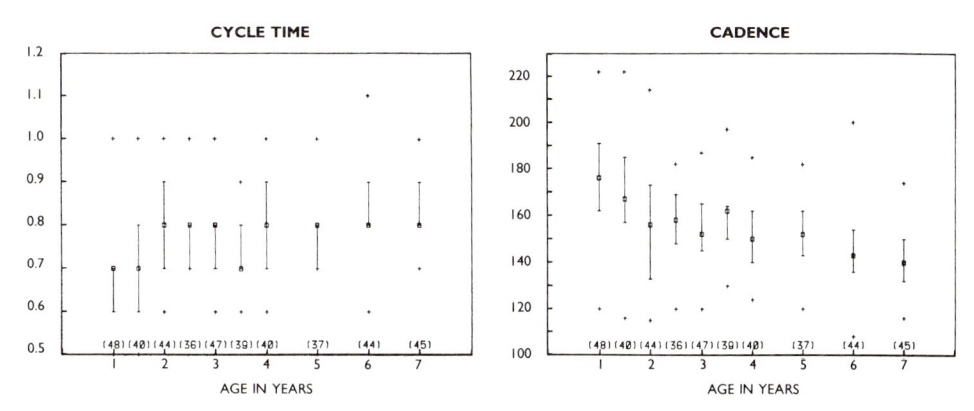

Fig. 6.10. Cycle time (secs.) *vs.* age (N = 420).

Fig. 6.11. Cadence (steps/min.) *vs.* age (N = 420).

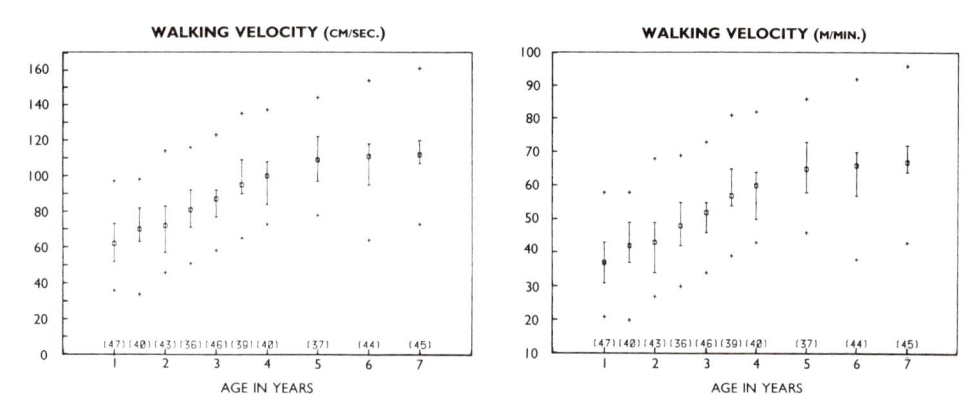

Fig. 6.12. Walking velocity (A: cm/sec.; B: m/min.) *vs.* age (N = 420).

or EMG measurements, and without the need for costly laboratory equipment. Ogg (1963) made measurements of stride length and step length from a roll of paper on which the subject walked with inked corn plasters on the soles of the feet. A similar method, but using talcum powder rather than ink to provide the footprints, was employed by Scrutton (1969). Other investigators have used more sophisticated methods including: footswitches; instrumented walkways; film digitization [the method used in the present study, and also in that of Hennessy and Dixon (1984)]; and optoelectric systems (using advanced technology to collect large amounts of data and needing minimal human intervention to reduce those data).

Grieve and Gear (1966) measured stride length, stature, relative stride length, time of complete cycle of one leg, step frequency, walking speed, relative walking speed, time of swing and relative time of swing. Their subjects were also required to demonstrate progressively faster walking speeds. Their study was comprehensive in scope, but as only nine of the 50 subjects were in the age-groups included in our study, their conclusions regarding immature walkers are based on only a very small sample. Also, their comparisons were directed to the changes observed in the time/distance parameters with progressively faster gaits. They noted that children have a limited ability to increase their speed. In our study the goal was to evaluate free-speed gait, so directions to the child were kept to a minimum. This is not to imply that subjects did not sometimes need some coercion. Many of the youngest children required encouragement and occasionally bribery to complete the walk without making diversions along the way. While we did not attempt to evaluate progressively faster walking, we did test the ability of the children to run. As noted in Chapter 5, this ability developed early and by 1½ years 78 per cent of subjects were able to run. This indicates considerable ability to vary speed; however, we do not doubt that children have less control over walking speed than adults.

Height and leg length are directly related to step length. Age is directly related to leg length and step length; however, because of a change in the velocity of growth, the slope declines, beginning at 2½ years for leg length and at 4 years for step length. This tells us that these two functions are tightly linked to growth, at least under the condition of free-speed walking in the age-groups under study.

The next important observation is that normal children walk symmetrically: right and left step lengths are equal, or nearly so, and gait events also are equal, or nearly so. Walking velocity increases with age and in spite of decreasing cadence; this increase is due to increasing stride length. Cycle time bears an inverse relationship to cadence. Cadence decreases and cycle time increases rapidly between 1 and 2 years. Duration of single-limb stance and time of opposite swing are, by definition, equal. A normal single-stance time is at once an indication of stable weight-bearing and an insurance of adequate time for opposite swing.

Grieve and Gear (1966) observed that, in their subjects, the times of swing were usually less than the calculated half-period for either the lower leg and foot or the whole leg regarded as passive pendulums. Their study adds support to the concept that the movement of the leg in swing cannot be explained by pendular action alone; active muscle contractions must exert a modifying effect. In our study swing time increased rather rapidly up to the age of 2, then more slowly to age 7. An obvious cause for longer swing time is greater limb length, which changes the pendular period, but other explanations based on changes in muscle action may also apply.

With increasing maturity single-limb stance, step length and walking velocity increase as cadence, initial double support and second double support diminish. Hennessy and Dixon (1984) made similar observations regarding single stance, step length, walking velocity and cadence but, in contrast to our findings, they concluded that the proportionality of the phasic events did not change across the 1 to 5 year age-range of their study. This inconsistency may be explained by the much larger sample in our study, and by the advantages offered in using a permanent laboratory as opposed to that study's setting within a primitive African village.

By 4 years the inter-relationships between the time/distance parameters are fixed, though stride length and walking velocity continue to increase with increasing leg length.

7
JOINT ANGLES AND FILM TRACINGS

Introduction
To enable the reader to relate visual observations and measured joint angles, this chapter includes film tracings of a representative child in each of the 10 age-groups studied. The tracings show synchronous front and side views, and the film frames have been selected to show foot-strike (FS), opposite toe-off (OTO), opposite foot-strike (OFS) and toe-off (TO) of one complete gait cycle.

Visual gait observation has not been replaced by laboratory analysis: the two processes are complementary. Scientific analysis of movement serves to verify or correct visual observation.

For each age-group we are also presenting two sets of graphs: one showing the mean joint angles (determined by Fourier analysis) and one giving the 95 per cent prediction regions. Using the familiar format of the first set, joint-angle measurements can readily be related to joint alignment in the film tracings. The second set of curves is entirely unique. What have been estimated by a computer-intensive process (Fourier analysis and the 'bootstrap') are regions within which 95 per cent of normal children should lie throughout the gait cycle. To see the motion with the correct scale of joint rotation, examine the first set of curves; to gain an appreciation of the regions defining the range of movement for 95 per cent of normal children, inspect the processed curves.

It is important to note that unprocessed joint-angle rotations cannot be used for comparisons with these prediction regions. The mathematical techniques of Fourier analysis and the removal of the population average (α_0) must be carried out for each curve before the dynamic joint angle of an individual can be compared with the normal prediction region. This may sound like a complicated process but in reality it is easily performed with the aid of a computer and the appropriate software. Data analysis techniques have been discussed in Chapter 3.

Planes of movement
We have chosen to consider the familiar, laboratory-oriented planes of movement used by physicians and physical therapists rather than more complex concepts such as Eulerian movement* which would be familiar only to engineers, mathematicians or physicists. A brief review will be given for readers who may not be accustomed to the terms. In the context of the laboratory, *sagittal* movement is in the direction of walk progression and is best viewed from the side; *coronal* movement is from side to side and is best viewed from the front or back; *transverse* movement is about a vertical axis and the ideal viewpoint, although impractical, is from above or below

---
*Eulerian movement relates the motion of each segment (rigid body) to another or multiple other rigid bodies in space.

the subject. These planes of movement are illustrated in Figure 7.1. The comments concerning viewing angles relate only to visual inspection of gait. The manner in which movement measurements were made has been detailed in Chapter 2.

Joint-angle graphs and film tracings
On the following pages we present the graphs for each of the 12 joint angles measured. All these graphs are based on right-side measurement data. In each case the curves showing the mean joint angles (with the α_0 terms retained—see Chapter 3) are placed on the left, while the processed curves indicating the 95 per cent prediction regions are on the right. The broken vertical lines indicate approximate timings of (from left to right): opposite (left) toe-off, opposite (left) foot-strike, and (right) toe-off.

To give an overall picture of the expected gait pattern in normal subjects, based on our study-group data, the (unprocessed) joint-angle graphs have also been collected together by age-group and are presented, along with the respective film tracings and time/distance parameters, in Figures 7.2 to 7.11 (pp. 128–147).

Coronal plane
PELVIC OBLIQUITY
Gait events play a dominant role in the production of the pelvic obliquity curve. The anterior superior iliac spine rises during weight-bearing to peak elevation at opposite toe-off. It then drops, reaching a low point halfway through single-limb stance, followed by a smaller peak elevation with opposite foot-strike. After foot-strike, the ipsilateral pelvis drops to its lowest level at toe-off. The peaks correlate with opposite toe-off and opposite foot-strike in all age-groups except the 1-year-olds, in whom the first peak precedes opposite toe-off. The dynamic range of motion varies across the age-groups between 4.2° and 9.4°, with a mean of 7.7° (SD 1.8°).

HIP ABDUCTION/ADDUCTION
While hip abduction/adduction is closely linked to pelvic obliquity, it differs because it includes the thigh segment. By correlating hip abduction/adduction movement, force and EMG data (Winter 1983), we can summarize the action of the principal frontal-plane muscles as follows. The abductor muscles act eccentrically to decelerate hip adduction during initial double support and early single support. The force line (formed by superincumbent body weight and inertia) then moves from the medial to the lateral side of the hip joint, necessitating eccentric action of the hip adductors to stabilize the hip, thus decelerating hip abduction.

The mature hip abduction/adduction curve is characterized by neutral alignment at foot-strike, with rapid adduction during single stance, peaking at opposite toe-off and declining rapidly to a plateau at 30 per cent of the cycle until opposite foot-strike at 50 per cent. The hip then rapidly abducts to a peak of 10° at toe-off. Beginning with swing phase, the hip again adducts, returning to neutral at foot-strike. Maturity in this motion is first evident at 2½ years, and there is no change after that age.

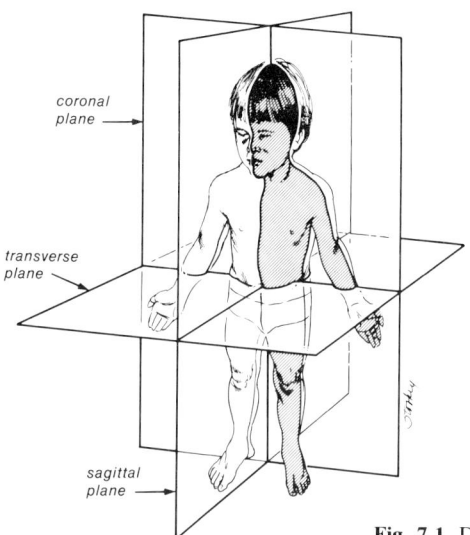

Fig. 7.1. Diagram illustrating the three planes of movement.

The primary differences in the immature age-groups are less adduction in stance phase and a lower overall dynamic range of motion (13° between 1 and 2 years compared to 17° at 2½ years and older). The younger children walk with a wide base, evidenced by a low ratio of pelvic span to ankle spread (Sutherland *et al.* 1980*a*). The relatively wider base of support in children under 2½ years accounts for their lower adduction movements.

Sagittal plane
PELVIC TILT
Sagittal movements of the pelvis are controlled by gravity, inertia, and the action of the hip flexor and extensor muscles. The primary muscles are the gluteus maximus and the hamstrings (extensors), and the iliopsoas, rectus femoris, sartorius and tensor fascia femoris (flexors). The pelvis is inclined downwards anteriorly, and the movements of the pelvis in the sagittal plane consist of very small variations in the degree of anterior pelvic tilt. Two peaks and two valleys are seen. The curve is sinusoidal and the valleys correlate with toe-off and opposite toe-off. The peaks occur in late single stance and in mid-to-late swing phase.

Anterior pelvic tilt diminishes as the limb is loaded during initial double support. It then increases as the body's center of mass moves forward over the supporting foot, decreases again during push-off (between 40 and 50 per cent of the cycle) to a low point at toe-off, and finally increases until following foot-strike.

The greatest tilt is observed in the 1 and 1½ year age-groups; however, the dynamic range of motion is very low (3° to 6°). It is unwise to lay very much importance on very small changes in very limited movement.

(Continued on page 148)

PELVIC OBLIQUITY

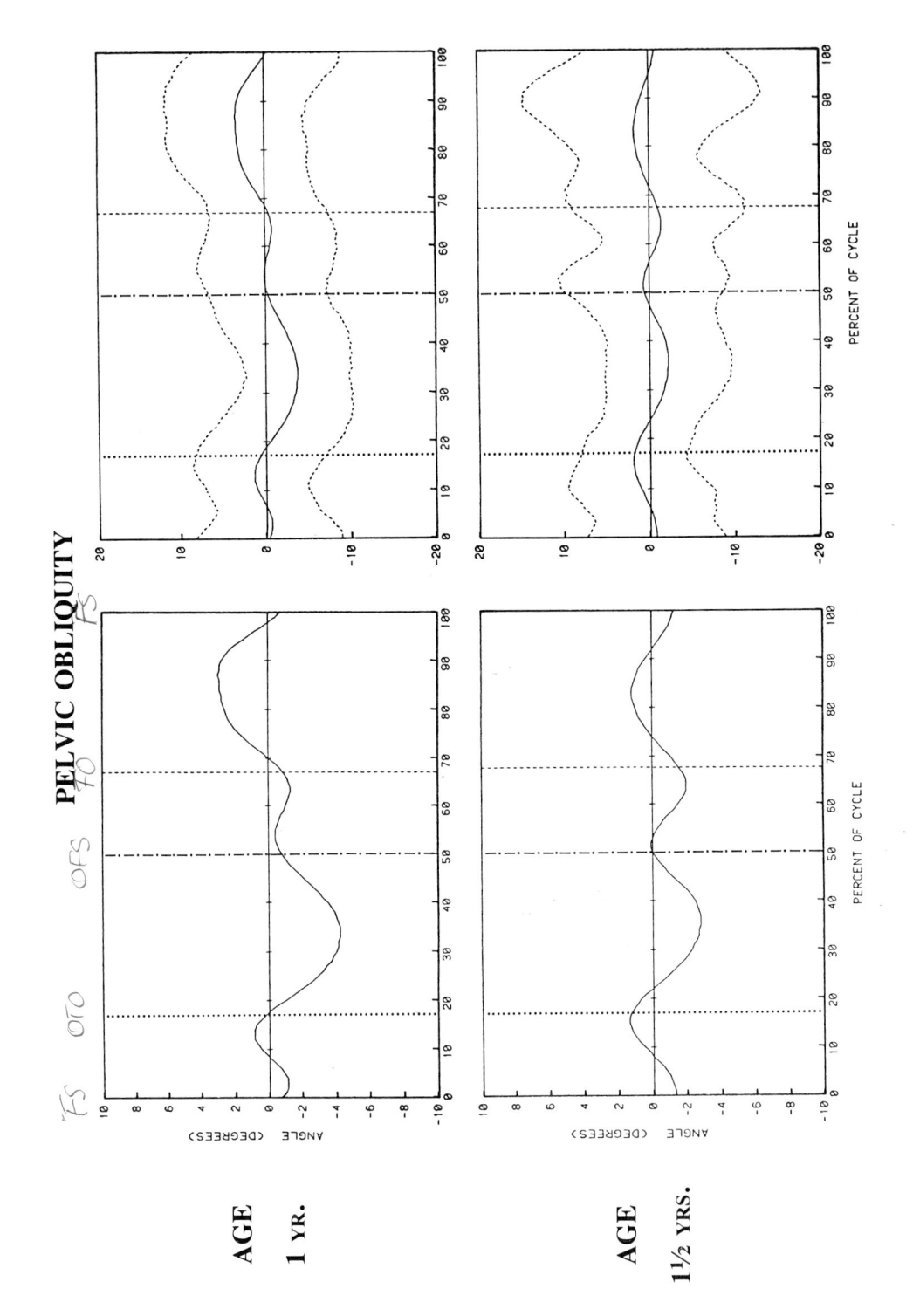

AGE
1 YR.

AGE
1½ YRS.

PELVIC OBLIQUITY

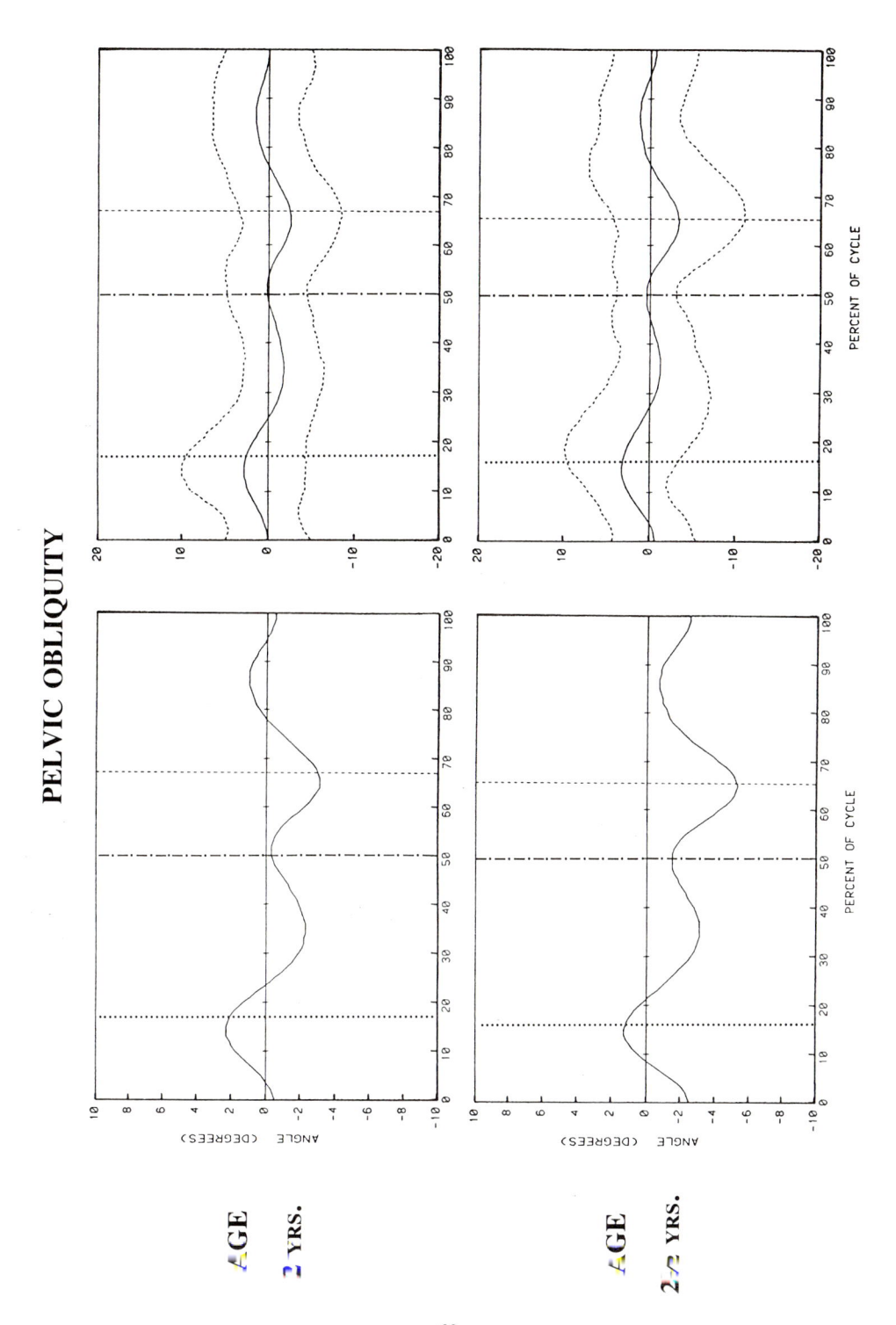

AGE
2 YRS.

AGE
2½ YRS.

PELVIC OBLIQUITY

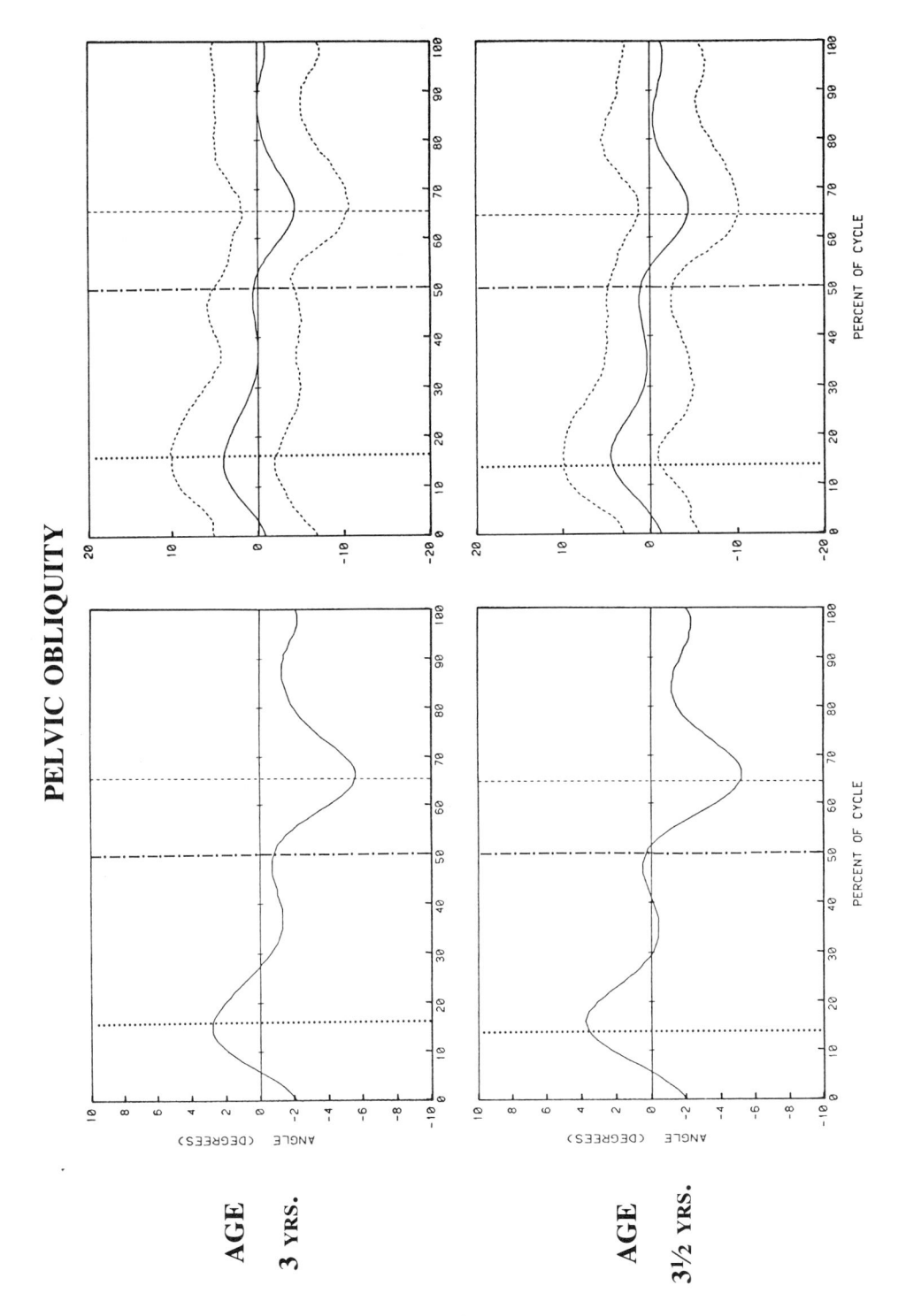

AGE 3 YRS.

AGE 3½ YRS.

PELVIC OBLIQUITY

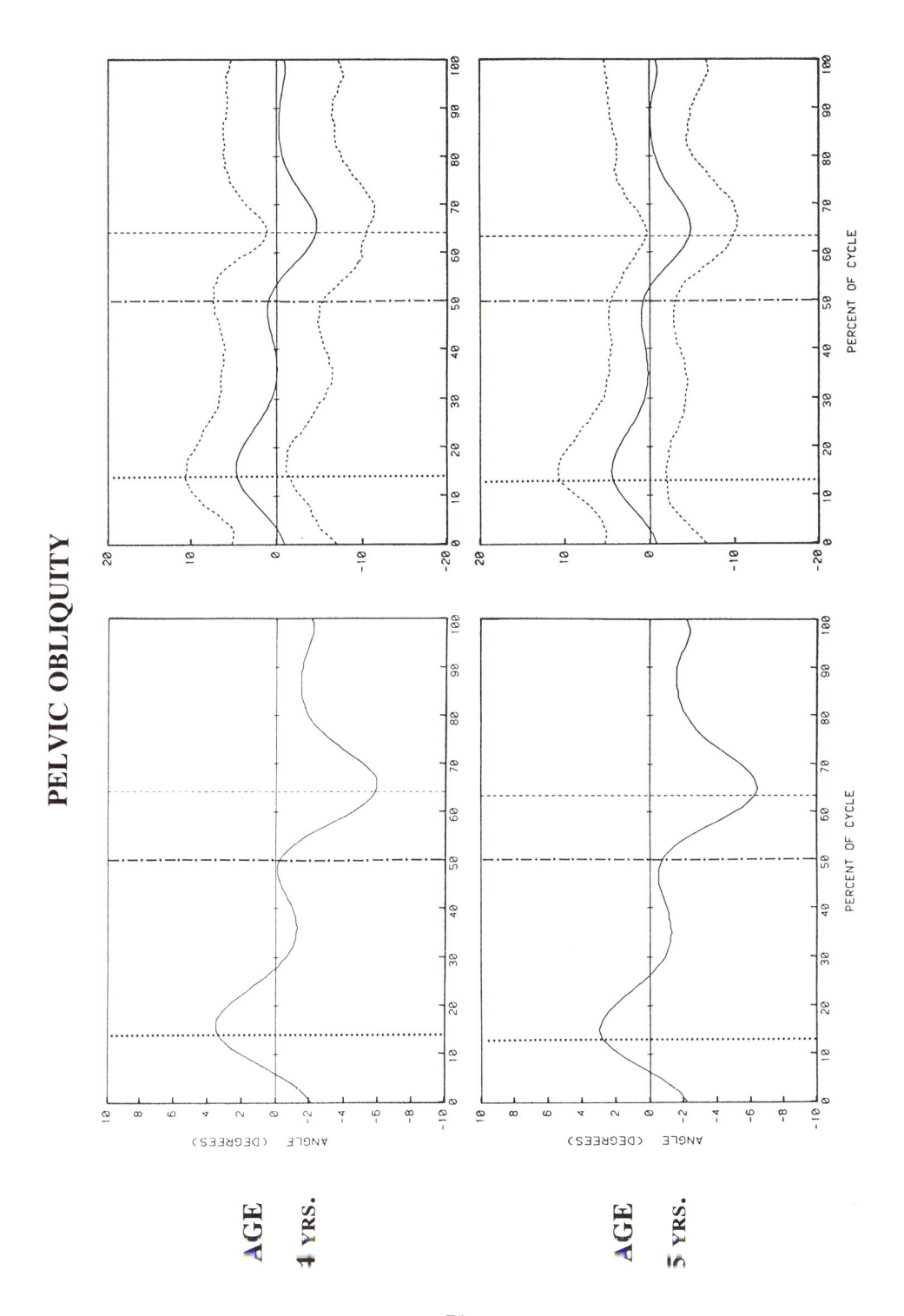

AGE 4 YRS.

AGE 5 YRS.

PELVIC OBLIQUITY

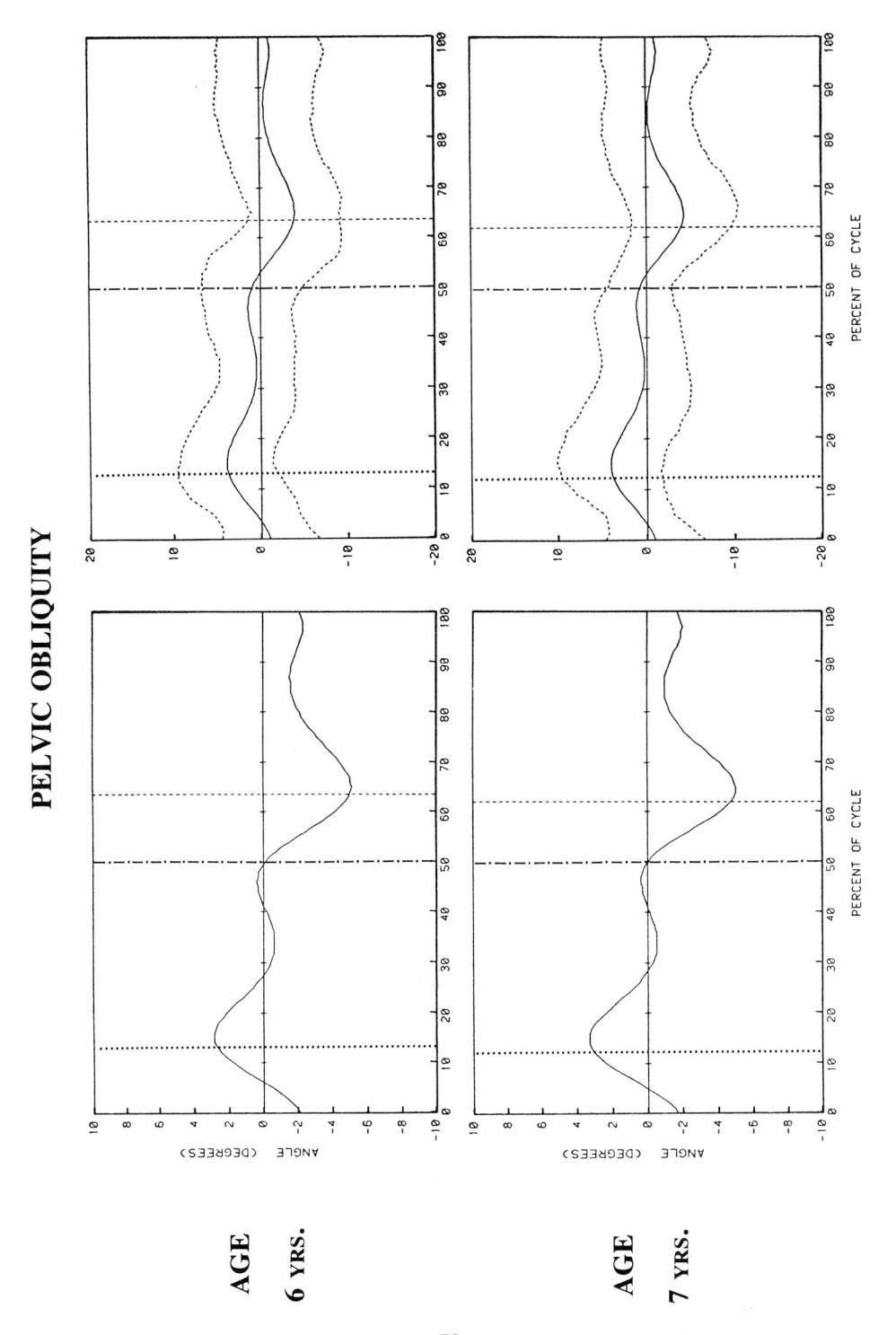

AGE 6 YRS.

AGE 7 YRS.

HIP ABDUCTION/ADUCTION

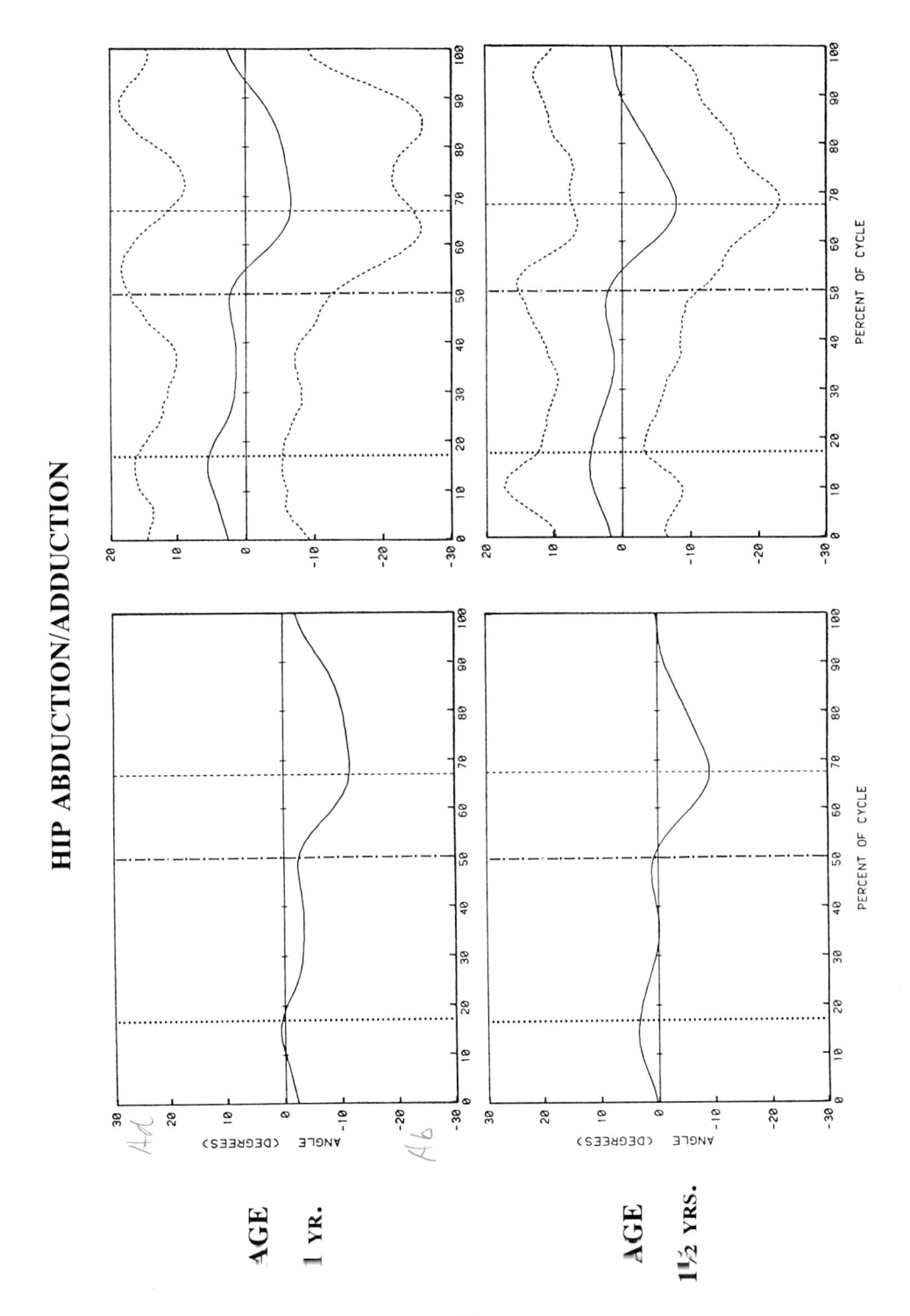

AGE 1 YR.

AGE 1½ YRS.

73

HIP ABDUCTION/ADDUCTION

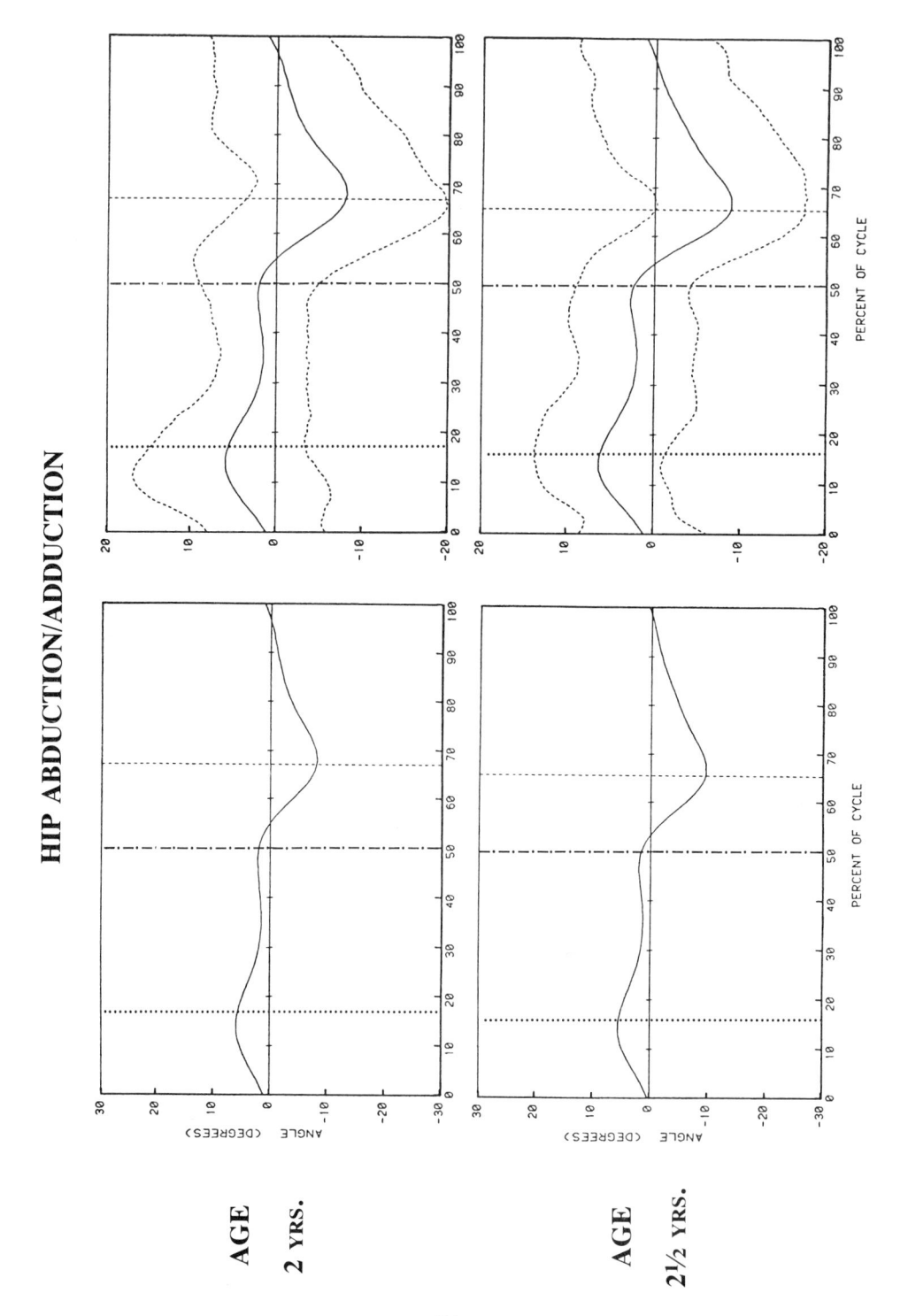

AGE 2 YRS.

AGE 2½ YRS.

HIP ABDUCTION/ADDUCTION

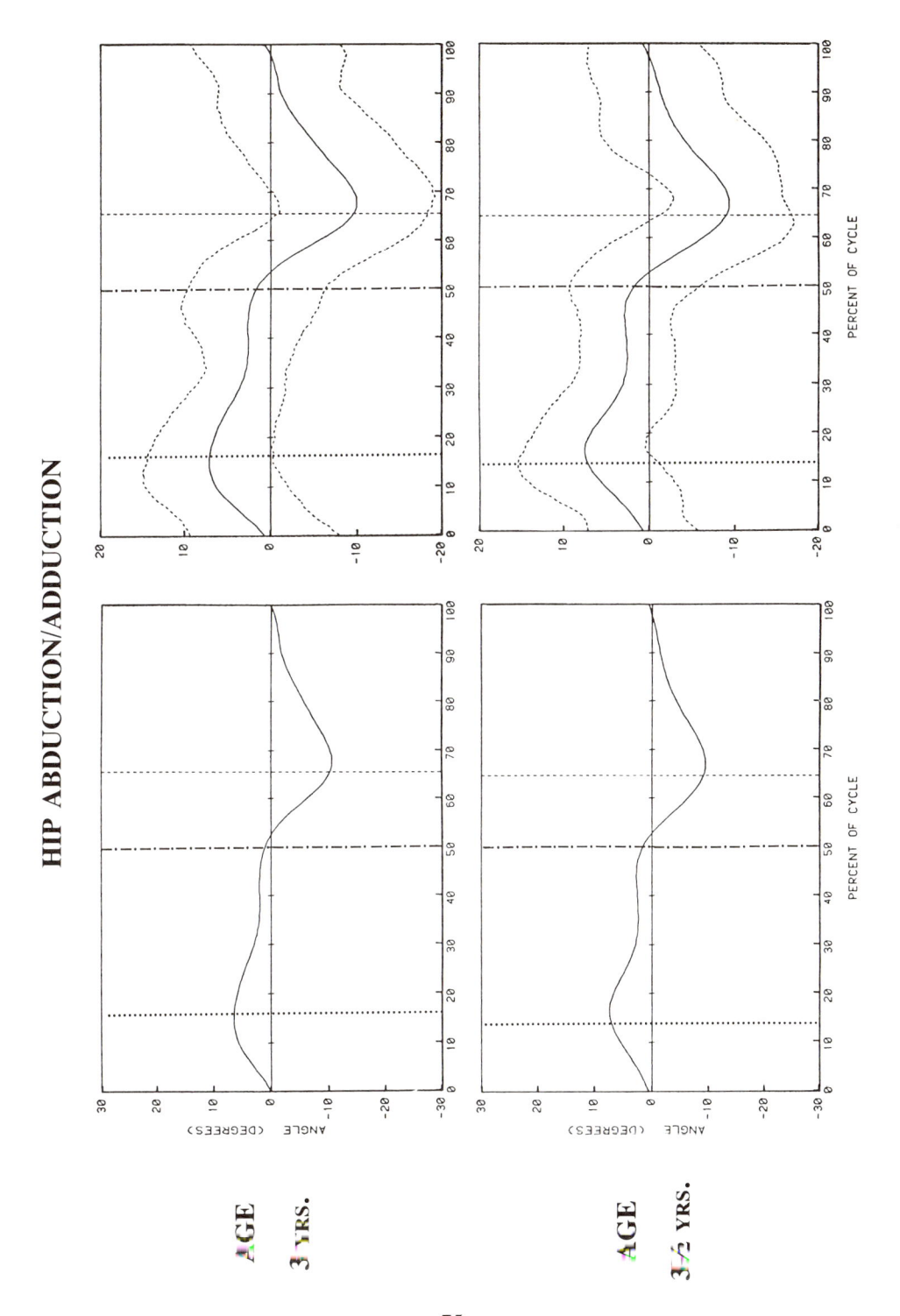

AGE
3 YRS.

AGE
3-1/2 YRS.

HIP ABDUCTION/ADDUCTION

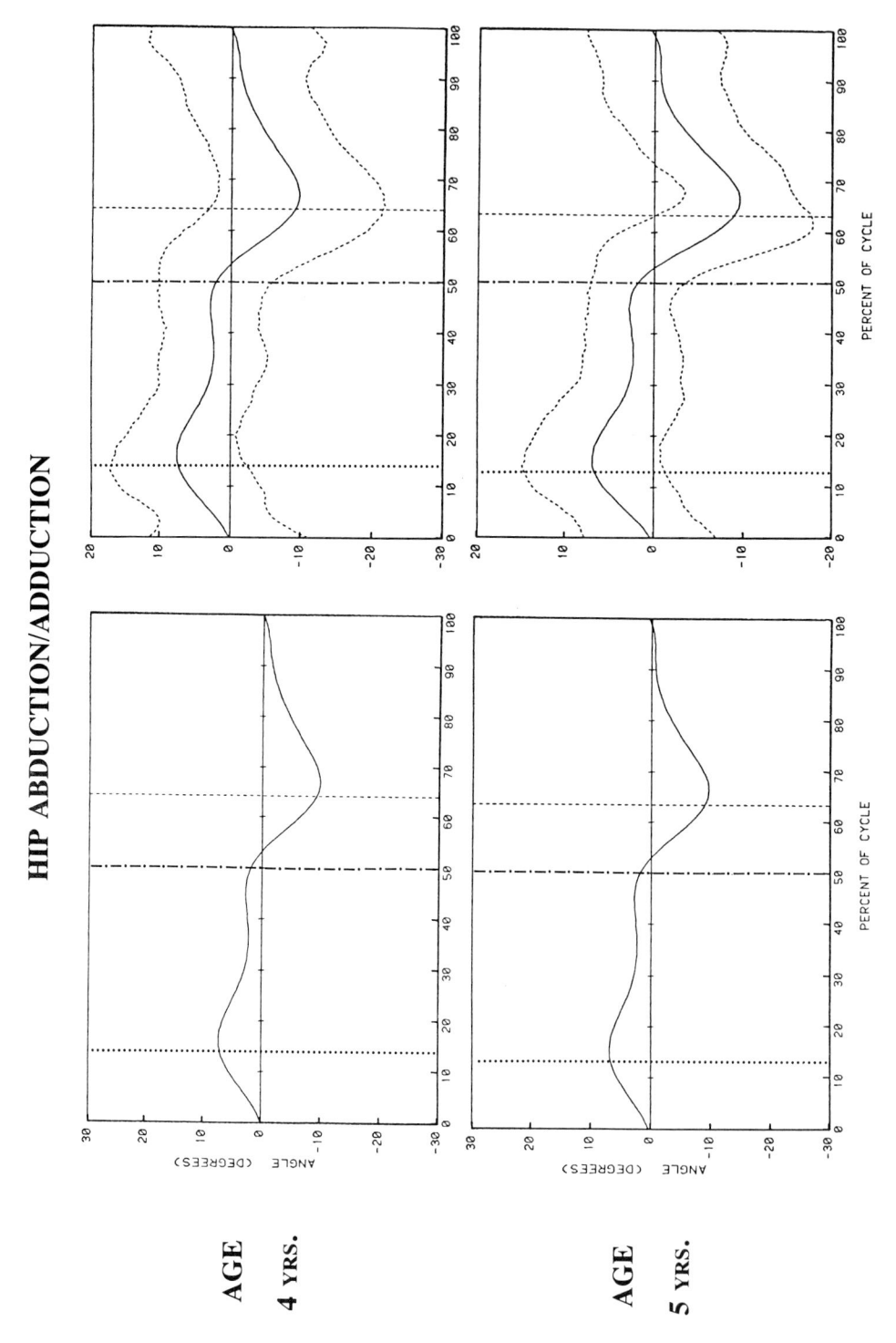

AGE 4 YRS.

AGE 5 YRS.

HIP ABDUCTION/ADDUCTION

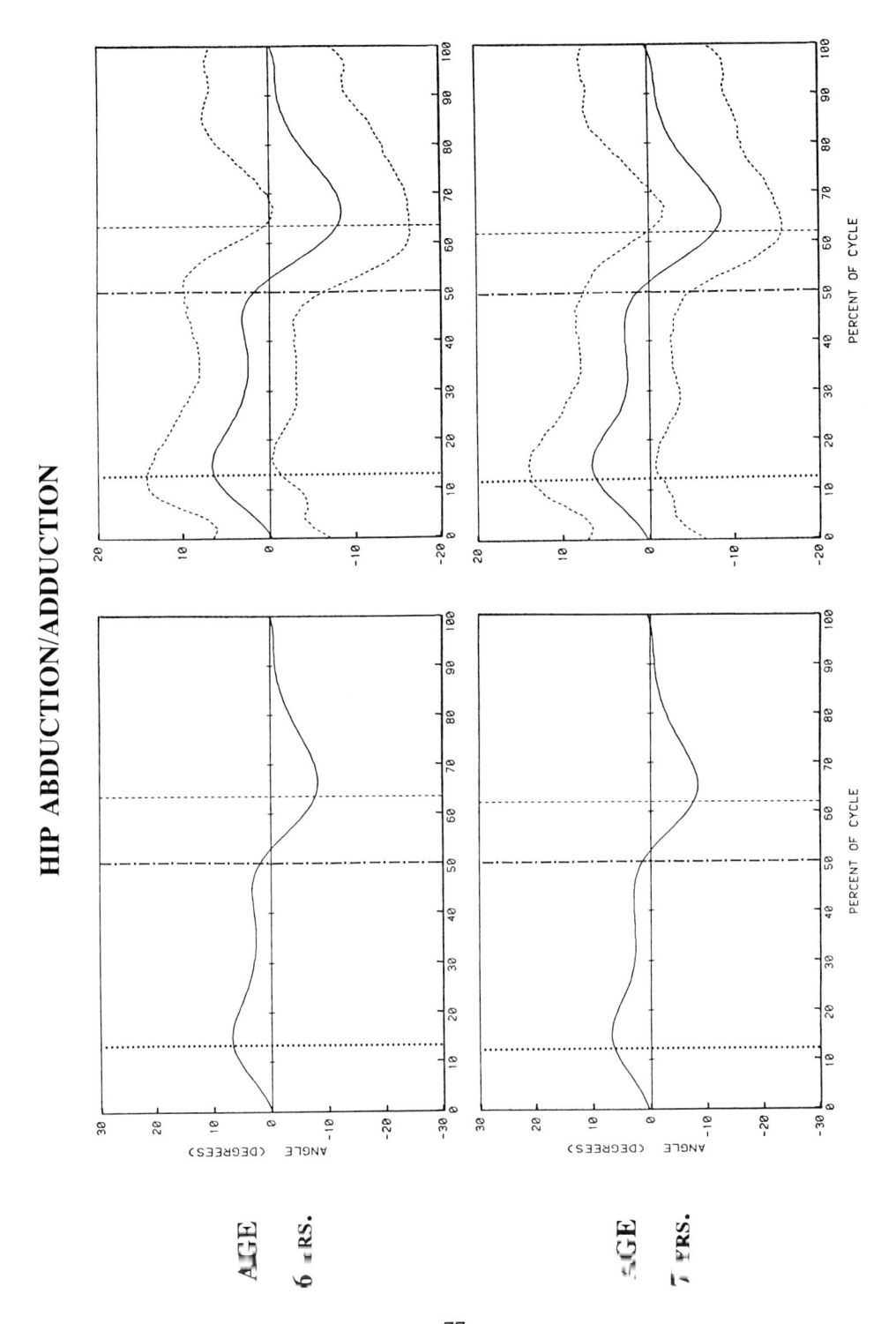

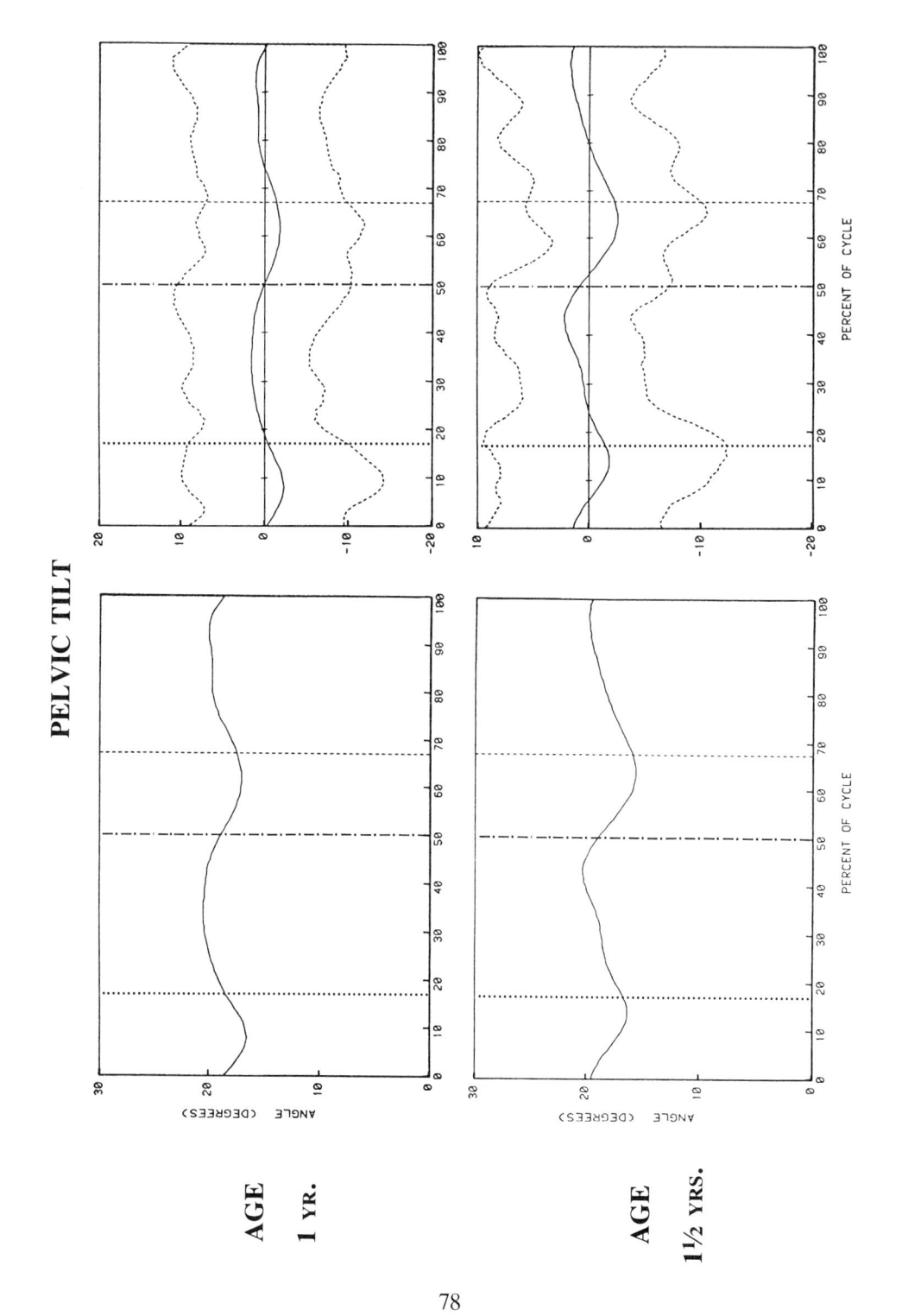

PELVIC TILT

AGE 1 YR.

AGE 1½ YRS.

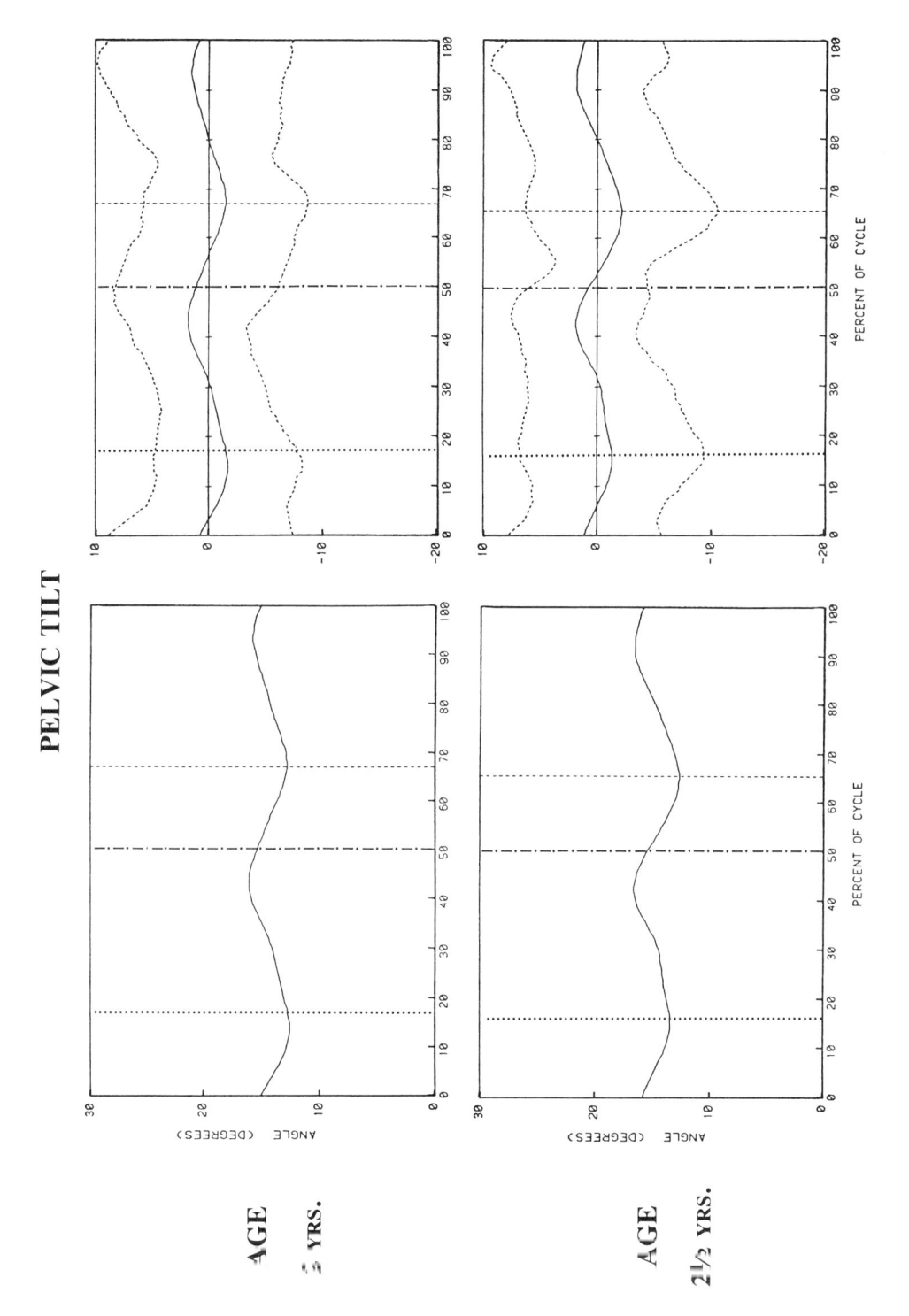

PELVIC TILT

AGE
5 YRS.

AGE
2½ YRS.

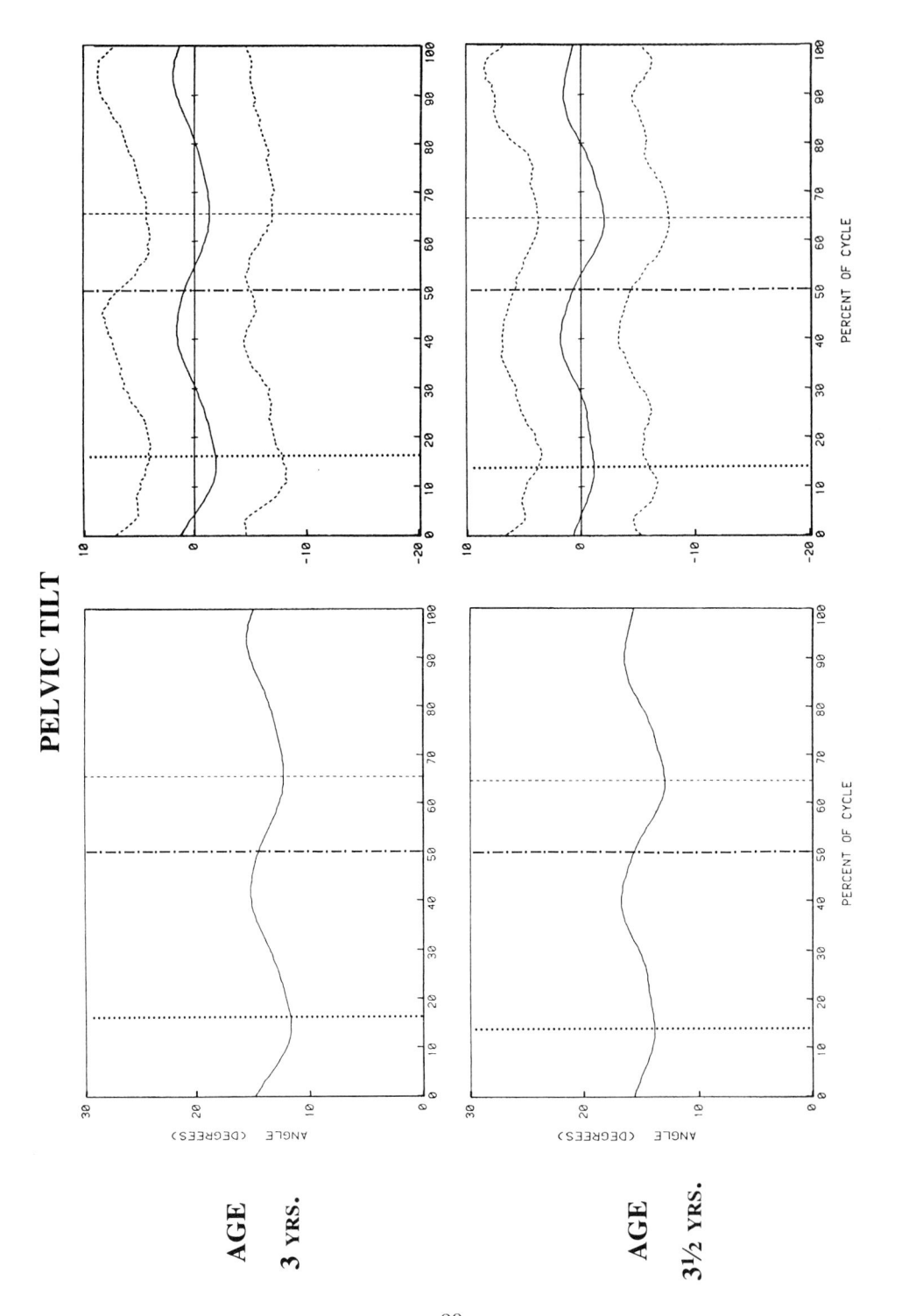

PELVIC TILT

AGE 3 YRS.

AGE 3½ YRS.

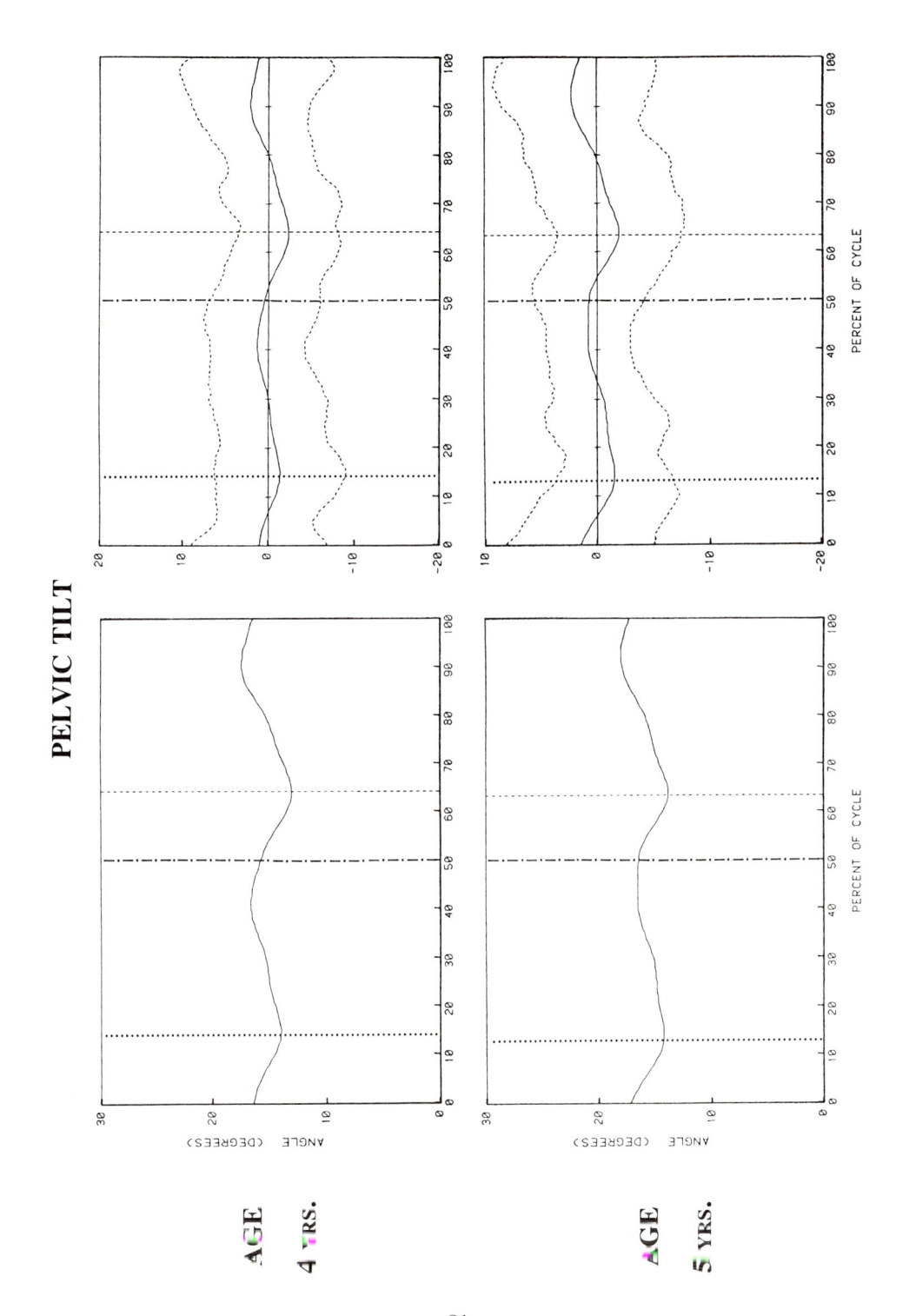

PELVIC TILT

AGE 4 YRS.

AGE 5 YRS.

81

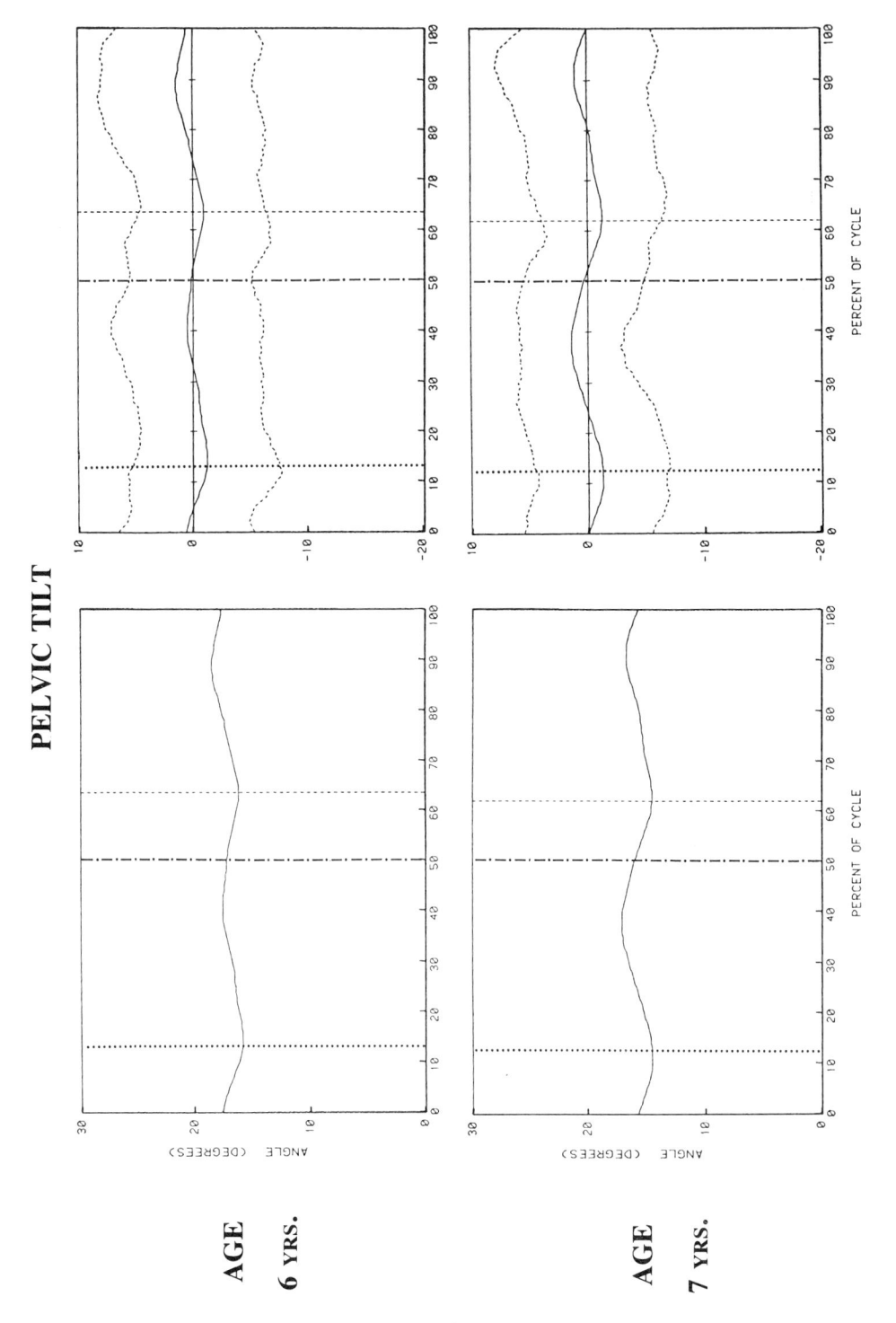

PELVIC TILT

AGE 6 YRS.

AGE 7 YRS.

HIP FLEXION/EXTENSION

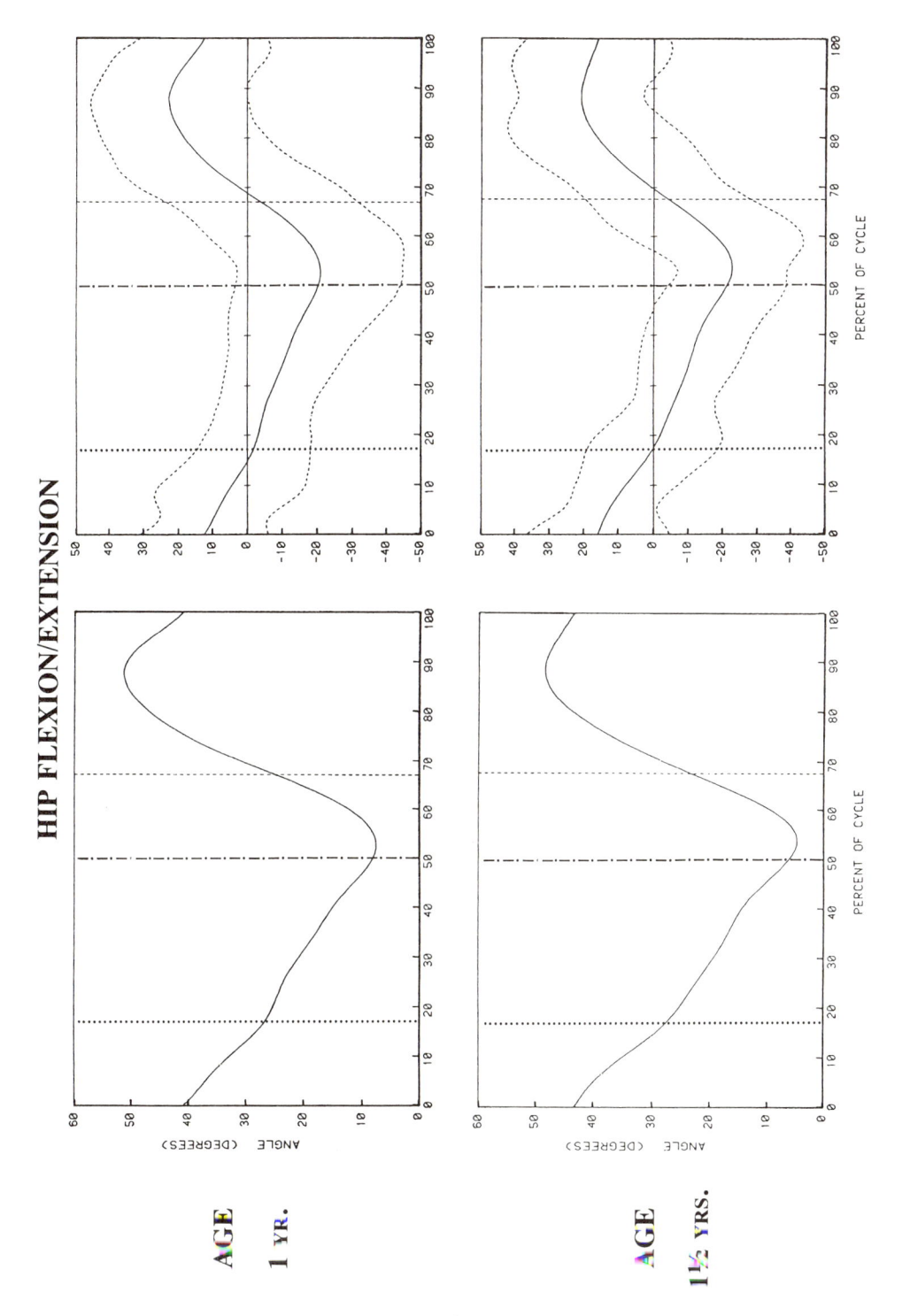

AGE 1 YR.

AGE 1½ YRS.

83

HIP FLEXION/EXTENSION

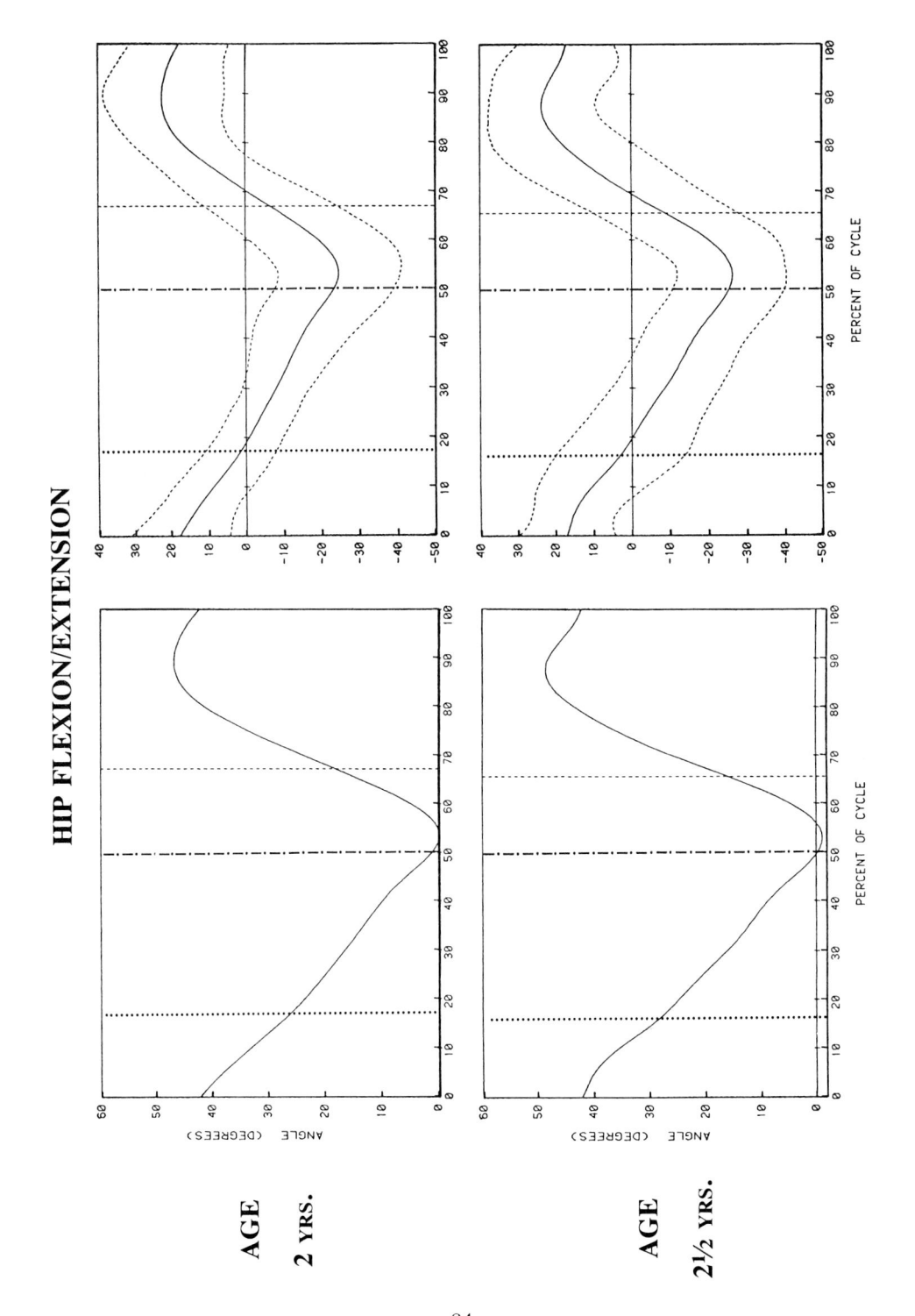

AGE 2 YRS.

AGE 2½ YRS.

HIP FLEXION/EXTENSION

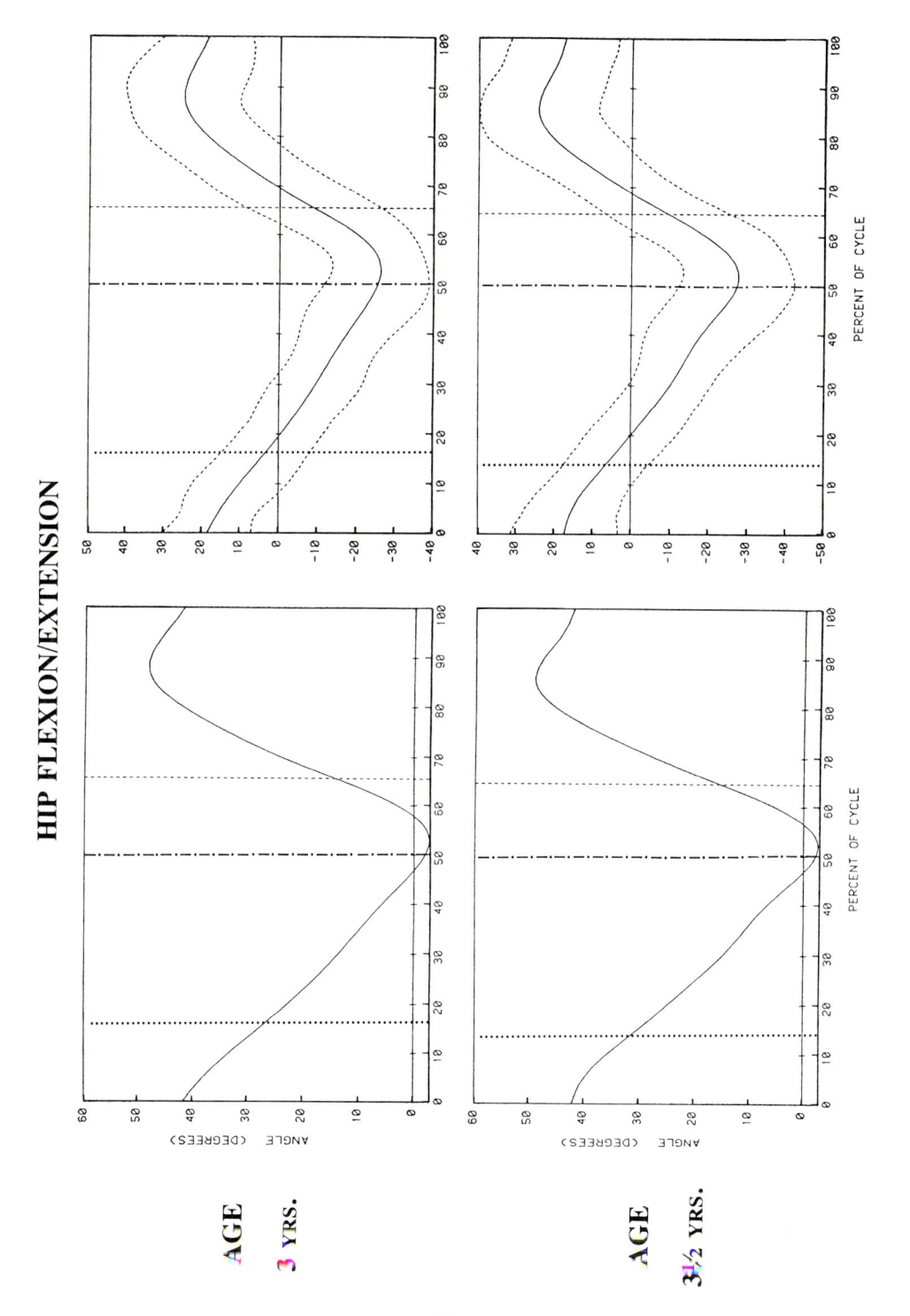

AGE
3 YRS.

AGE
3½ YRS.

HIP FLEXION/EXTENSION

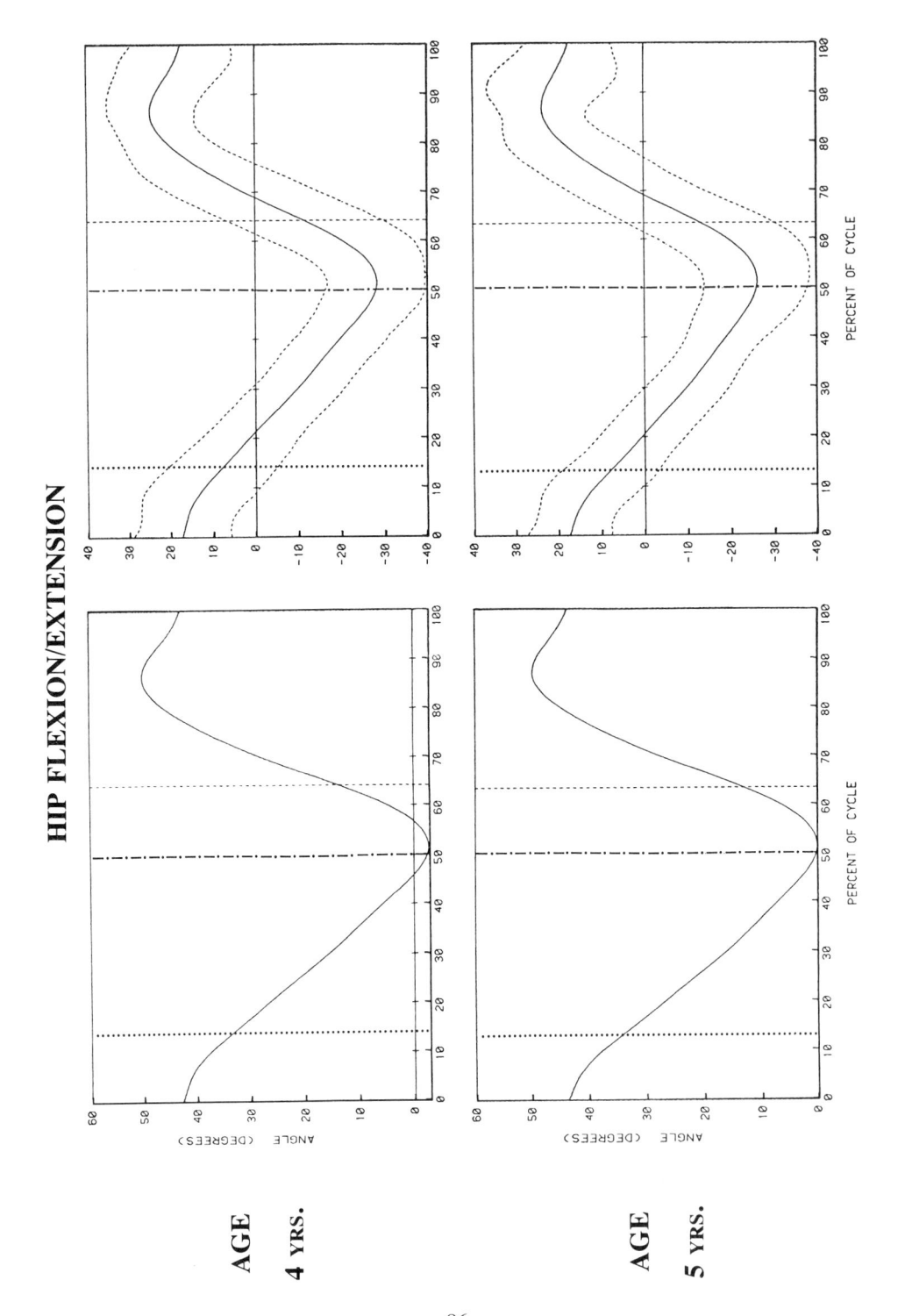

AGE 4 YRS.

AGE 5 YRS.

HIP FLEXION/EXTENSION

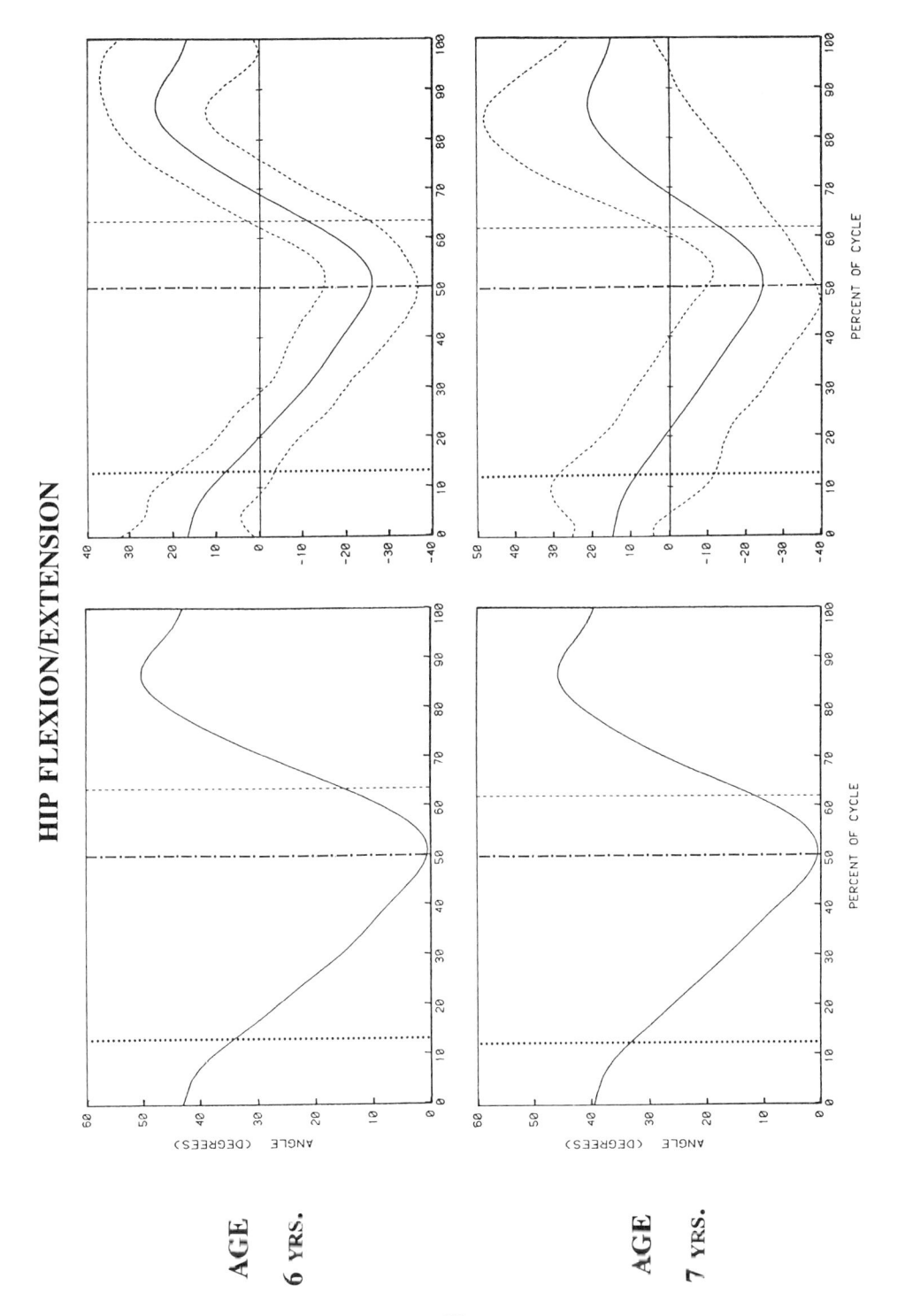

AGE 6 YRS.

AGE 7 YRS.

87

KNEE FLEXION/EXTENSION

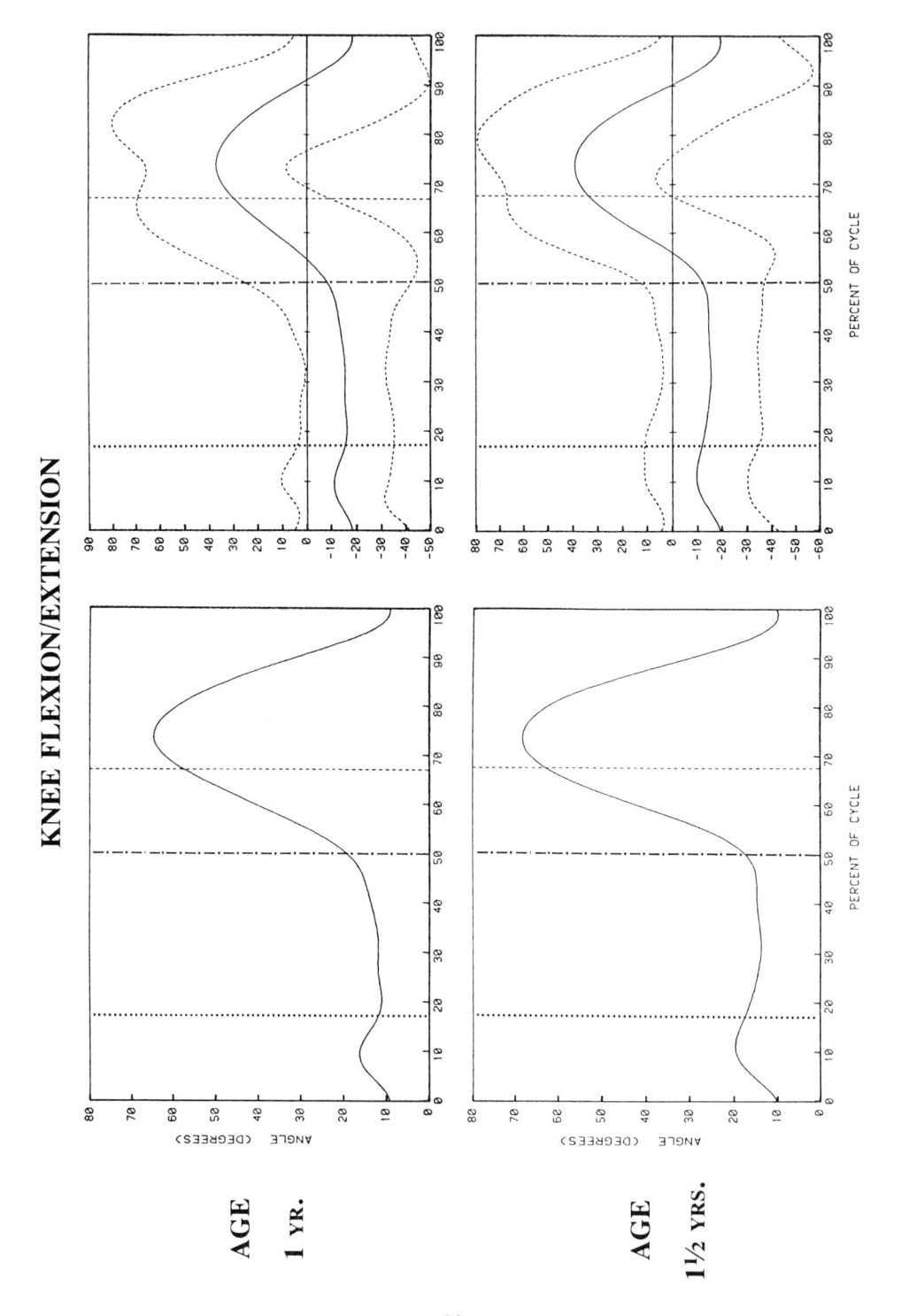

AGE 1 YR.

AGE 1½ YRS.

KNEE FLEXION/EXTENSION

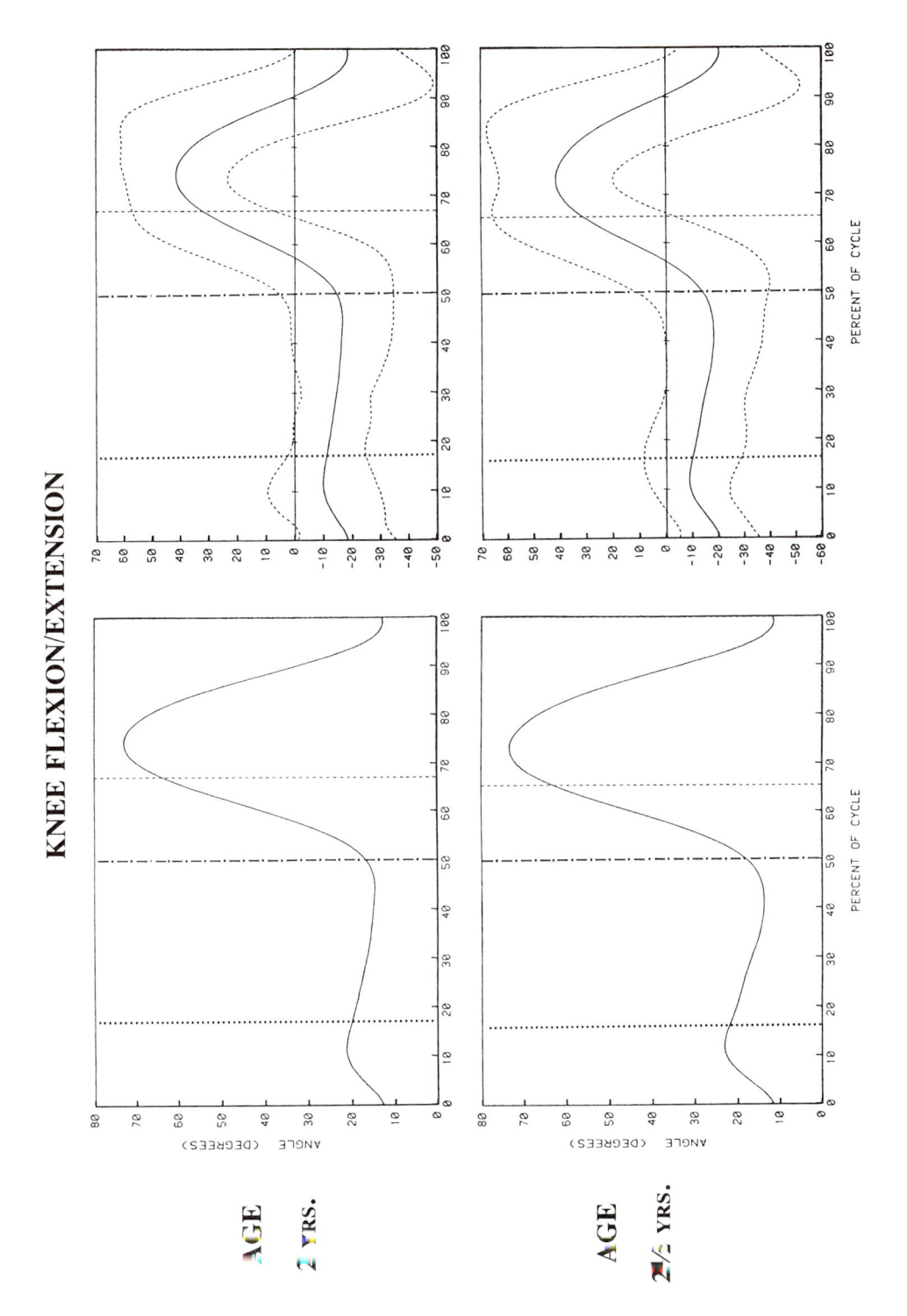

KNEE FLEXION/EXTENSION

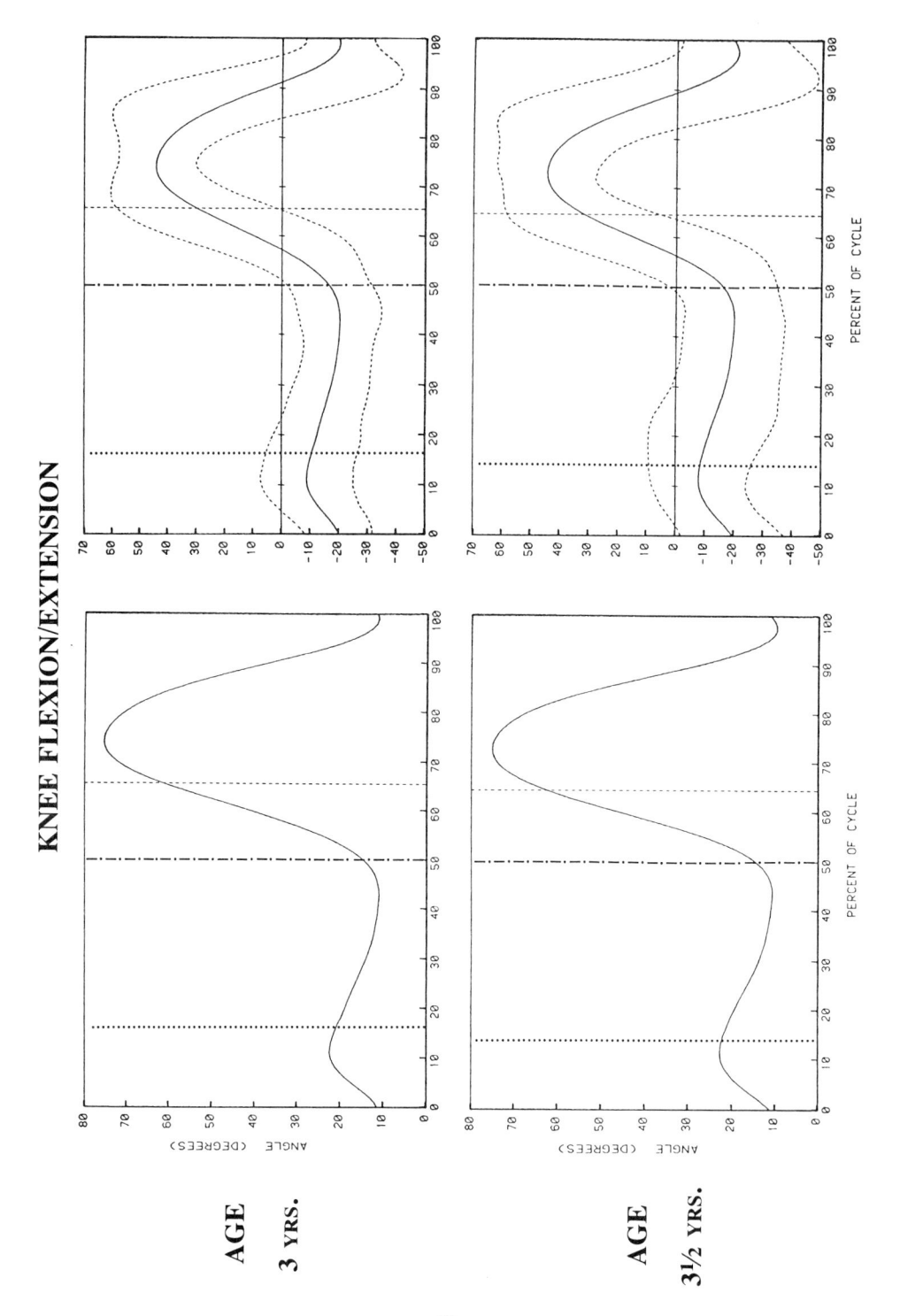

AGE 3 YRS.

AGE 3½ YRS.

KNEE FLEXION/EXTENSION

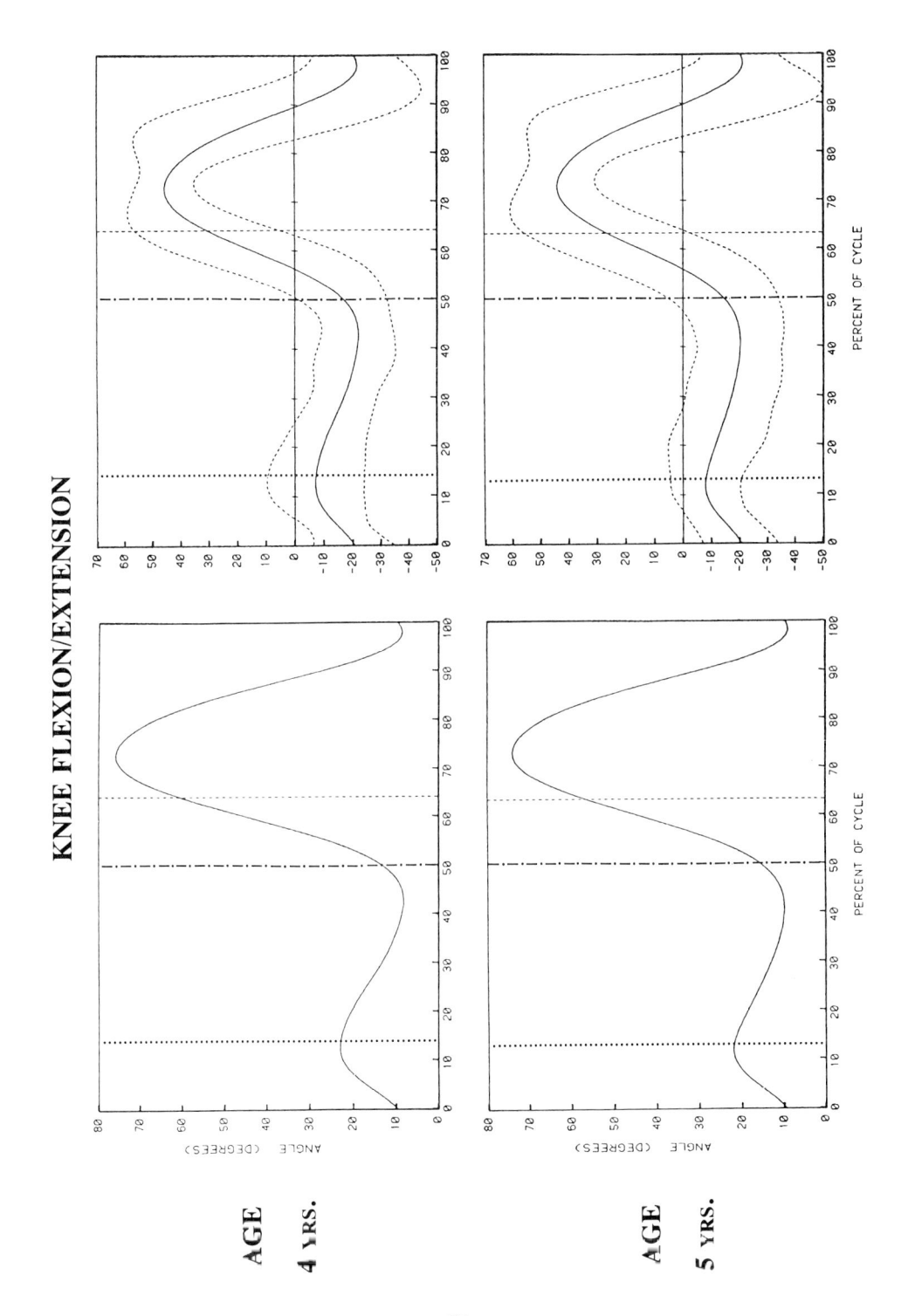

AGE 4 YRS.

AGE 5 YRS.

KNEE FLEXION/EXTENSION

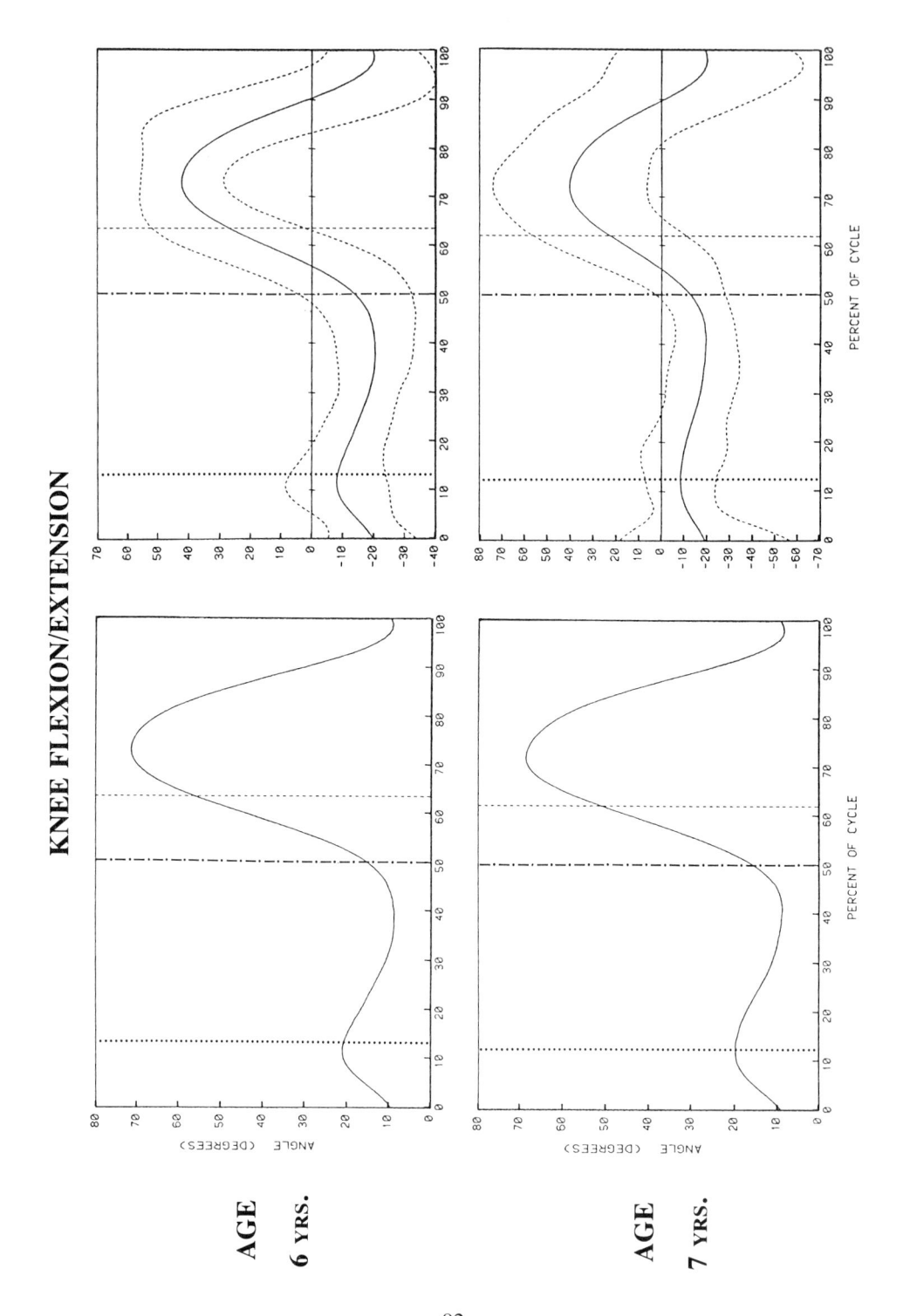

AGE 6 YRS.

AGE 7 YRS.

ANKLE DORSIFLEXION/PLANTAR FLEXION

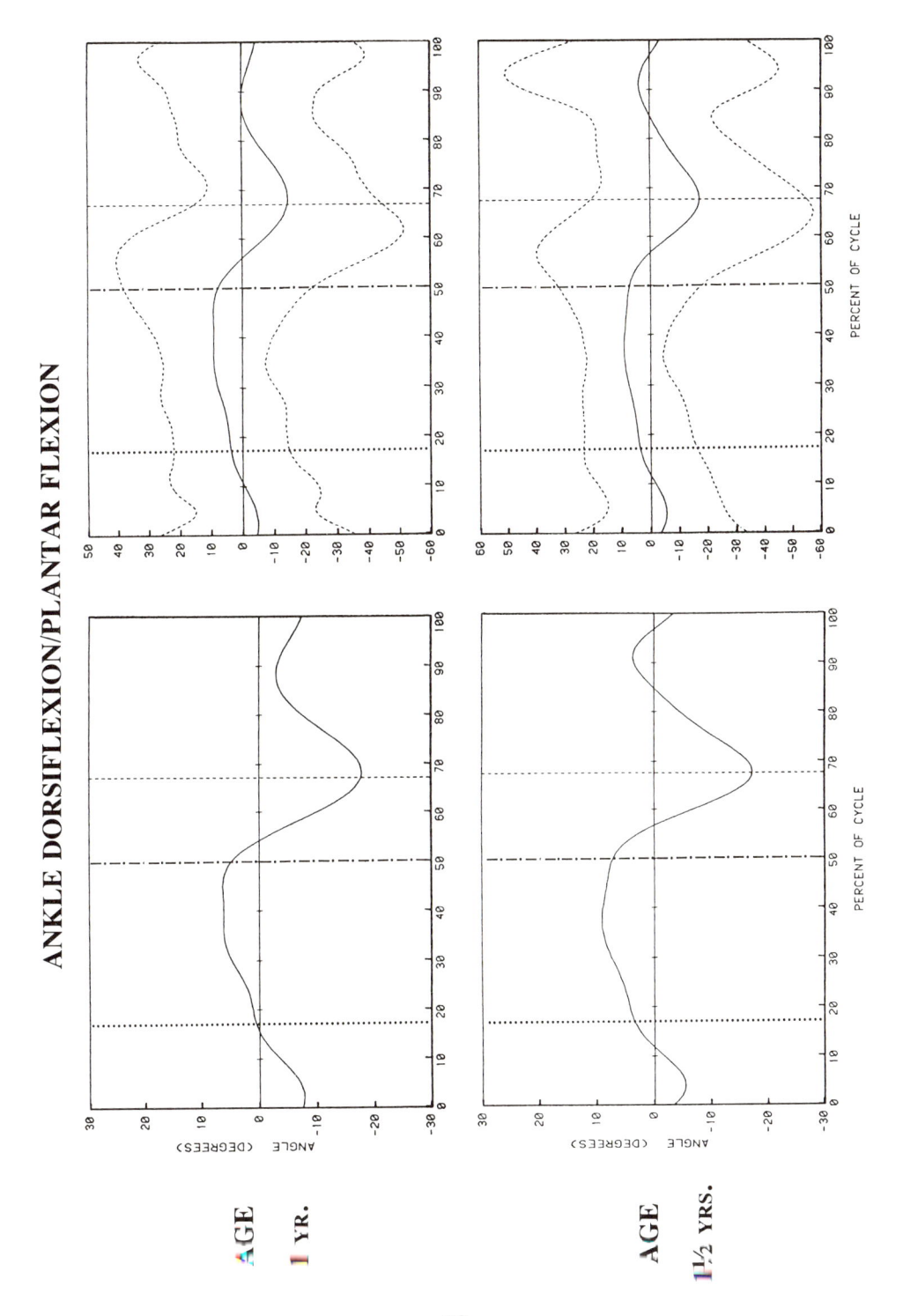

AGE 1 YR.

AGE 1½ YRS.

ANKLE DORSIFLEXION/PLANTAR FLEXION

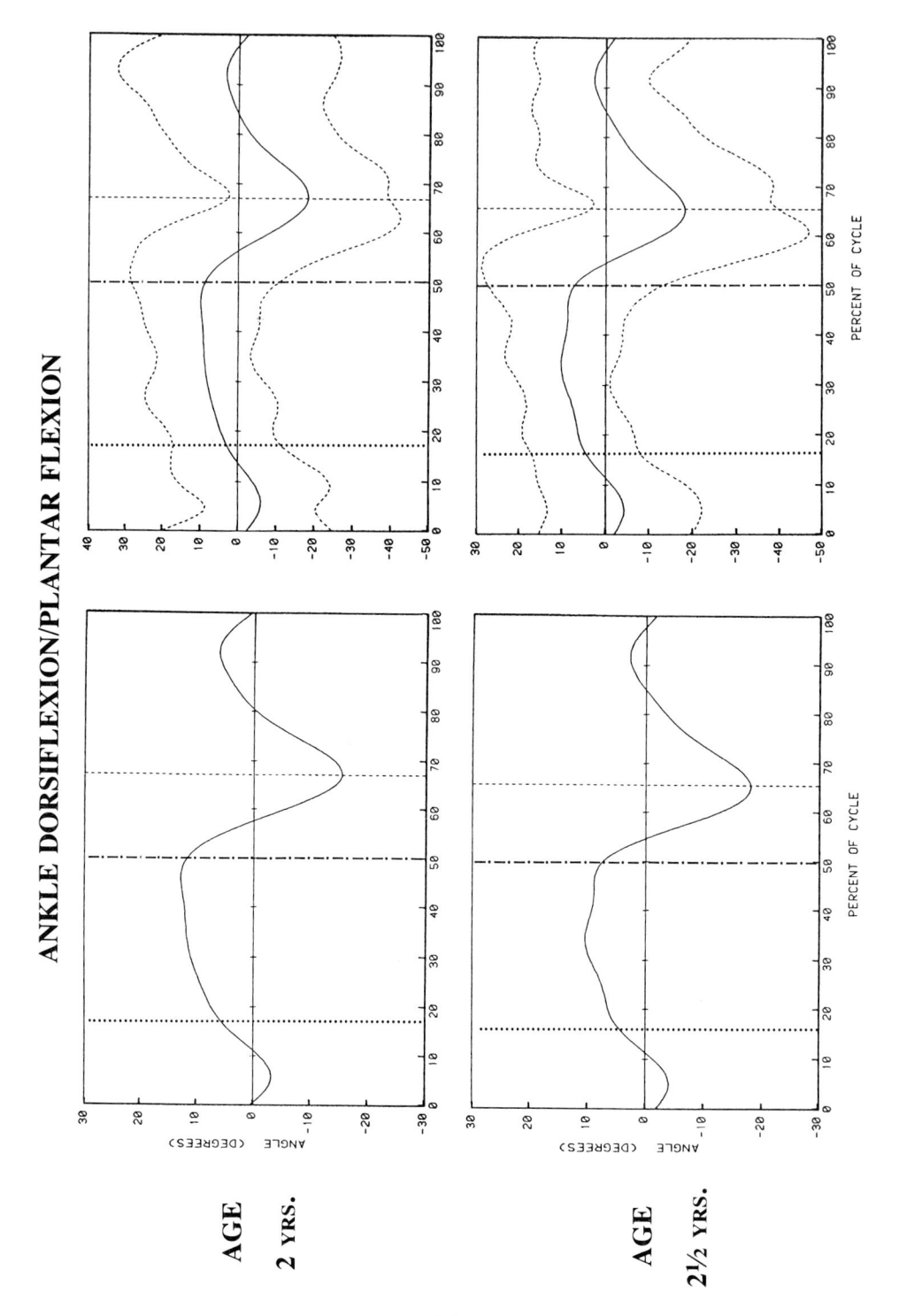

AGE 2 YRS.

AGE 2½ YRS.

ANKLE DORSIFLEXION/PLANTAR FLEXION

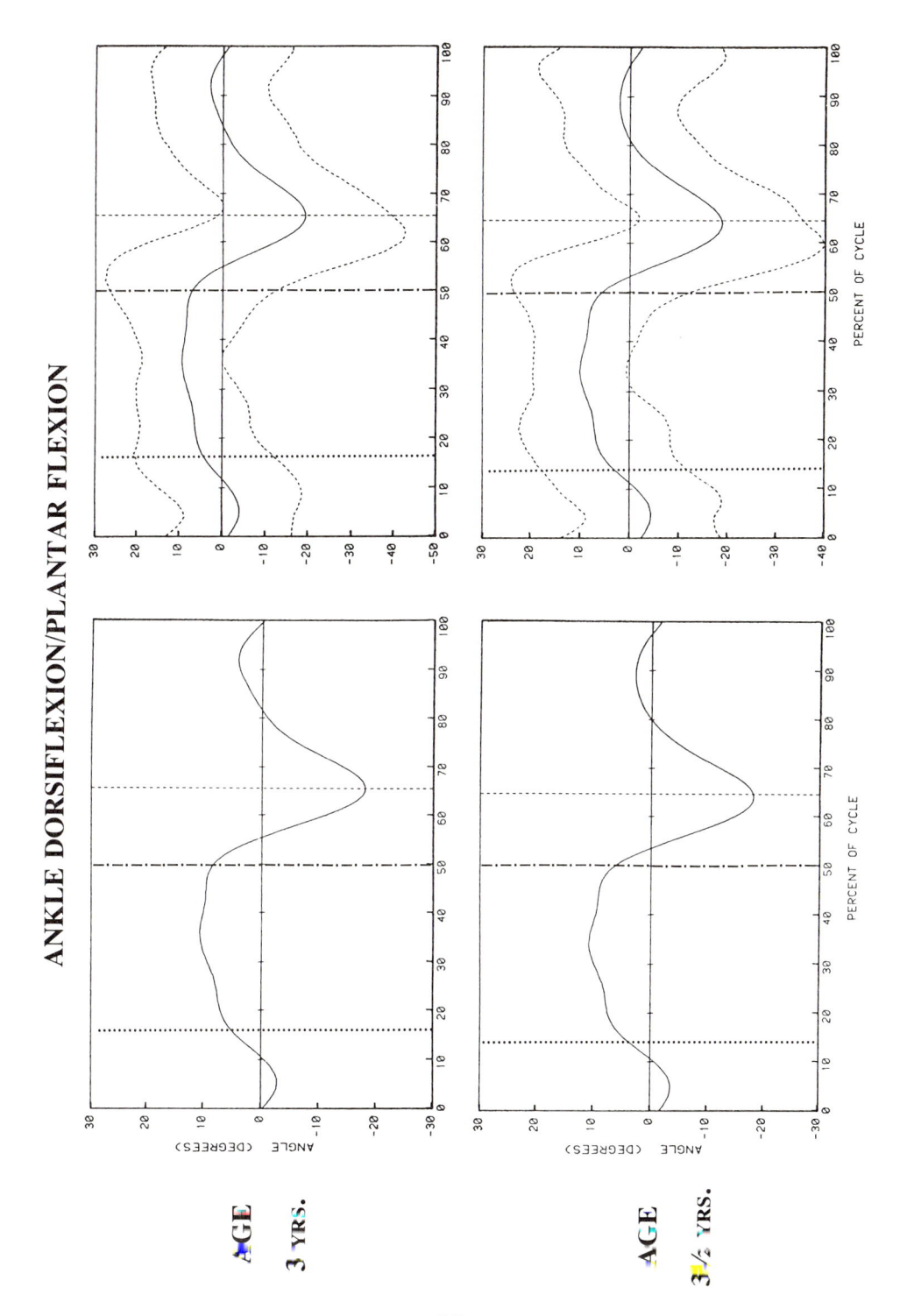

AGE
3 YRS.

AGE
3½ YRS.

ANKLE DORSIFLEXION/PLANTAR FLEXION

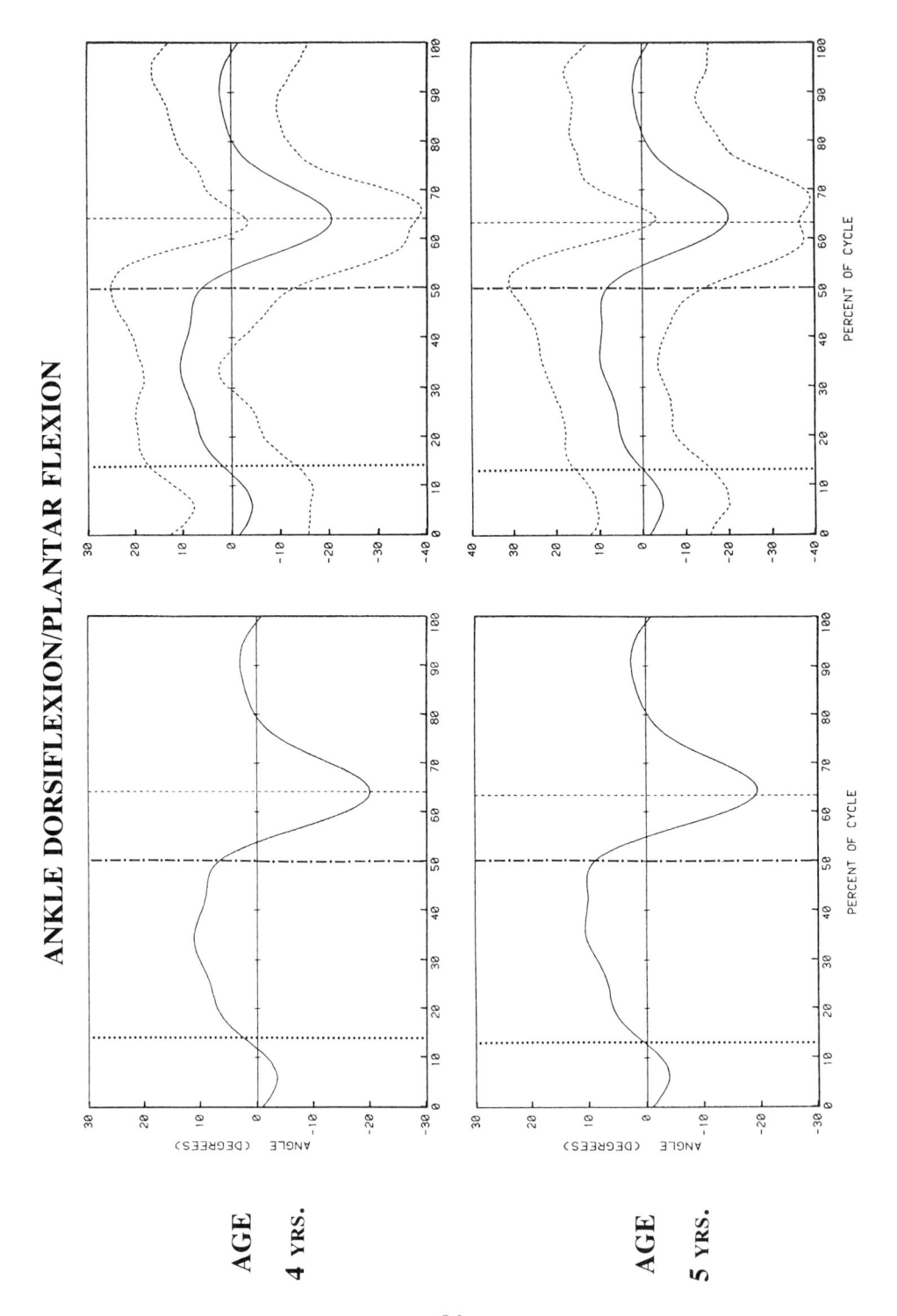

AGE 4 YRS.

AGE 5 YRS.

ANKLE DORSIFLEXION/PLANTAR FLEXION

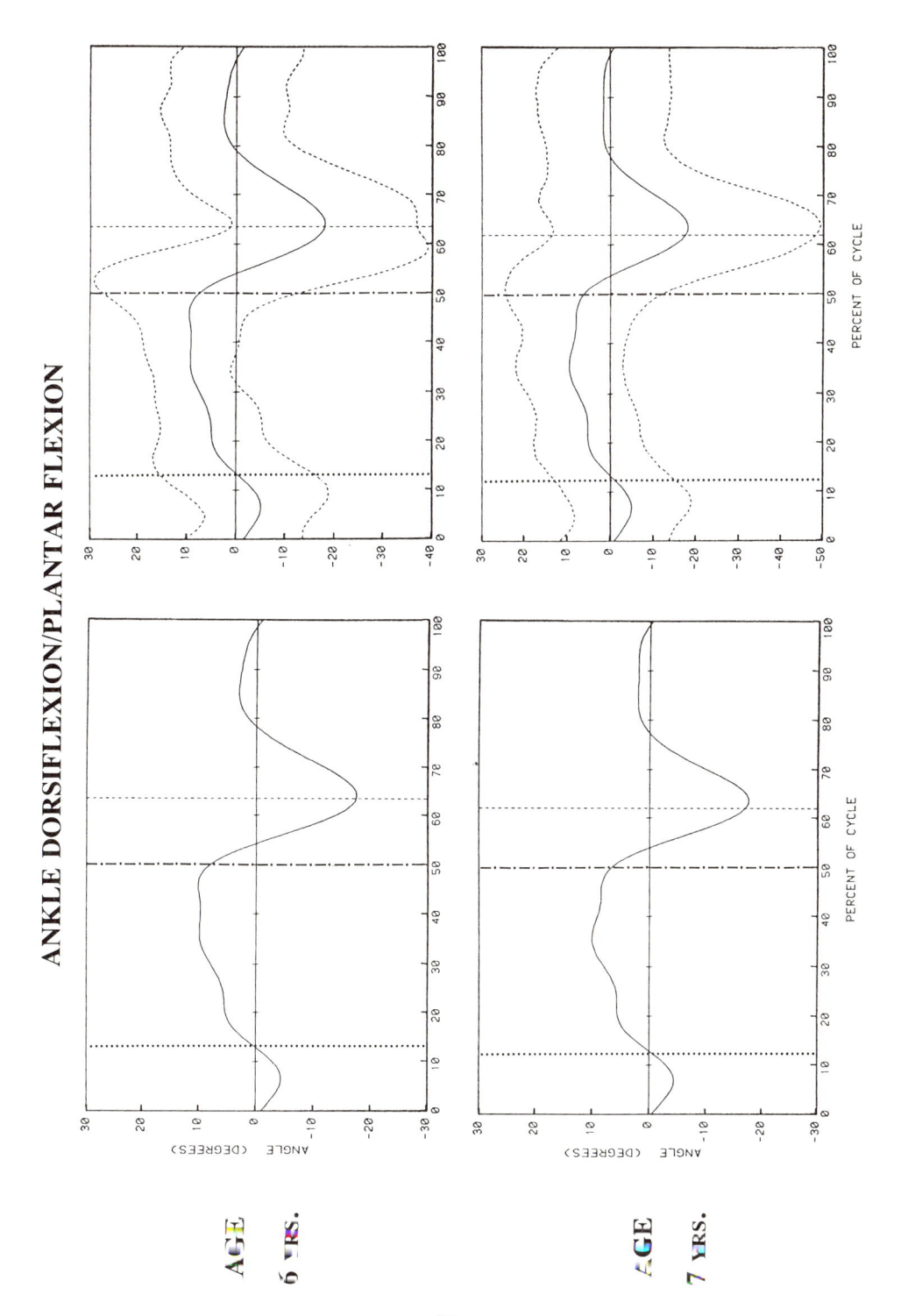

AGE
6 YRS.

AGE
7 YRS.

PELVIC ROTATION

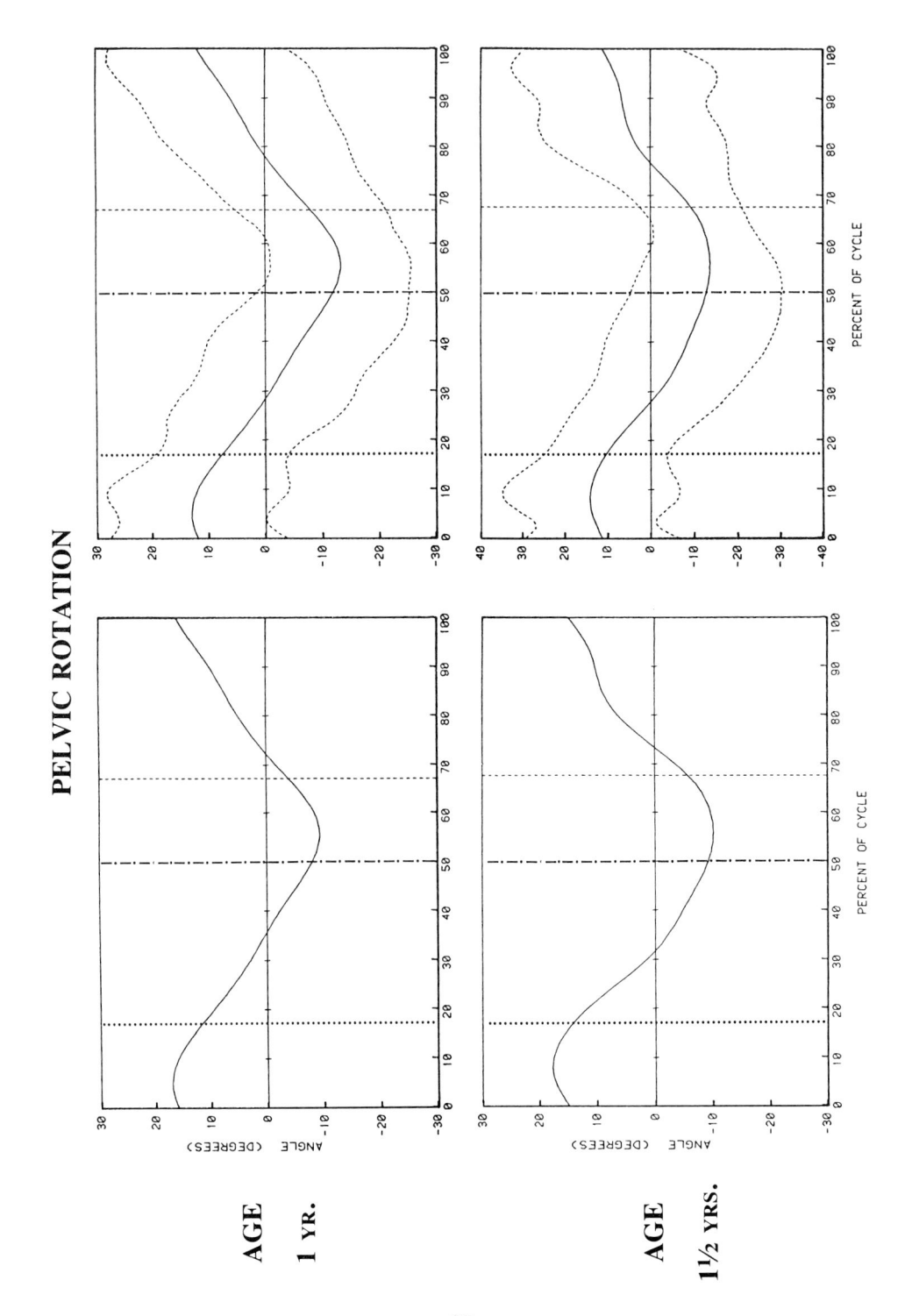

AGE
1 YR.

AGE
1½ YRS.

PELVIC ROTATION

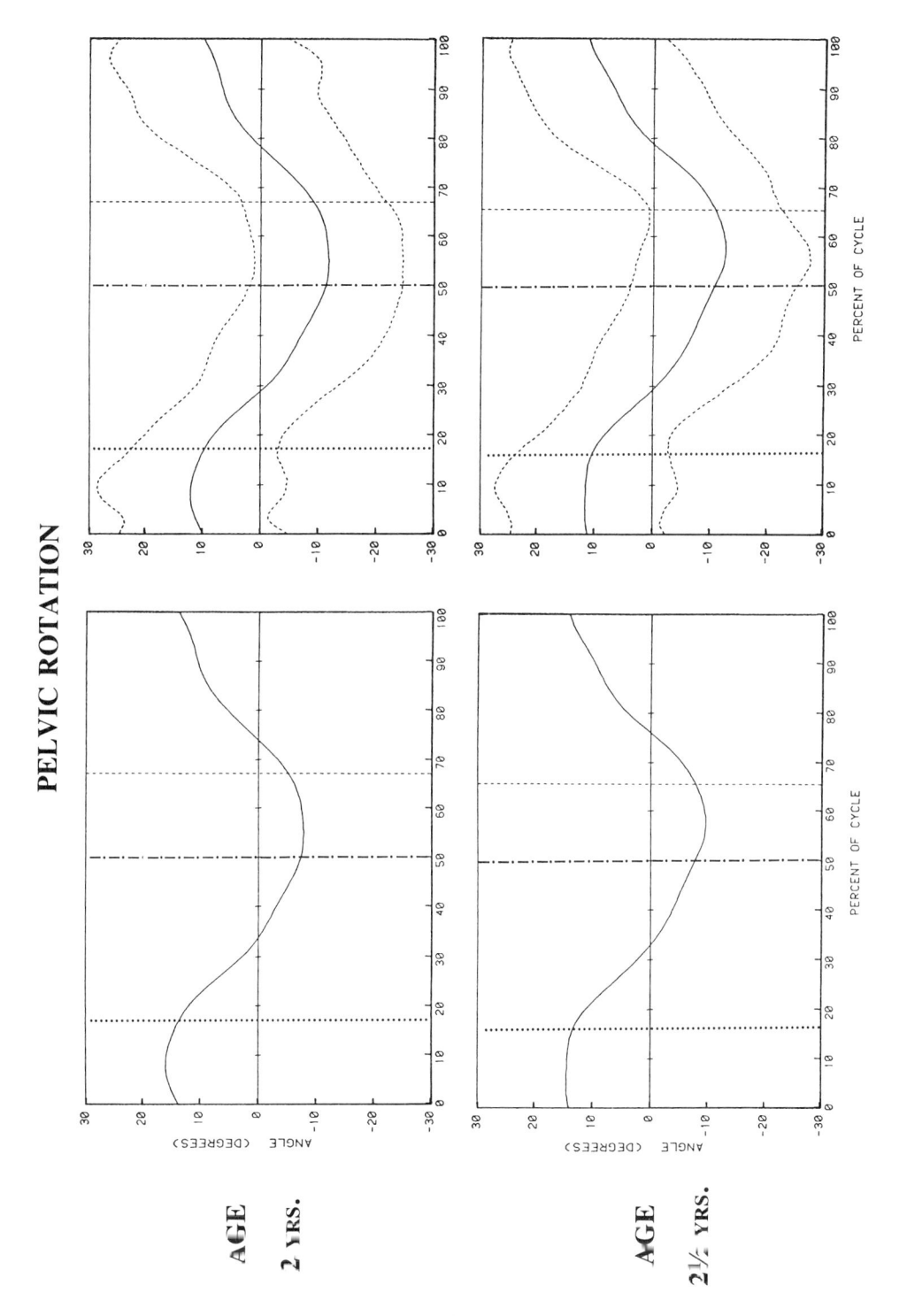

AGE
2 YRS.

AGE
2½ YRS.

PELVIC ROTATION

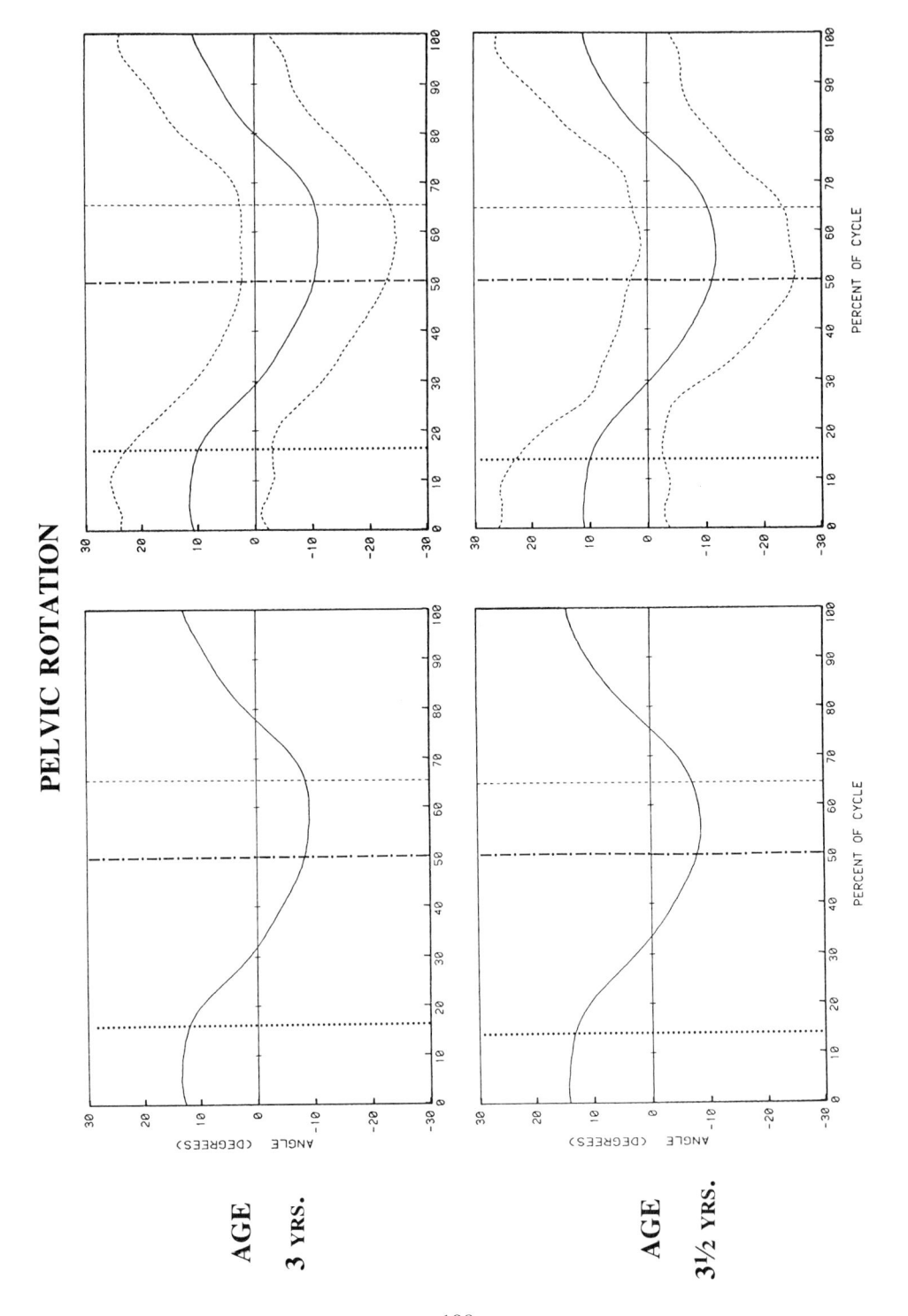

ANGLE (DEGREES)

PERCENT OF CYCLE

**AGE
3 YRS.**

**AGE
3½ YRS.**

PELVIC ROTATION

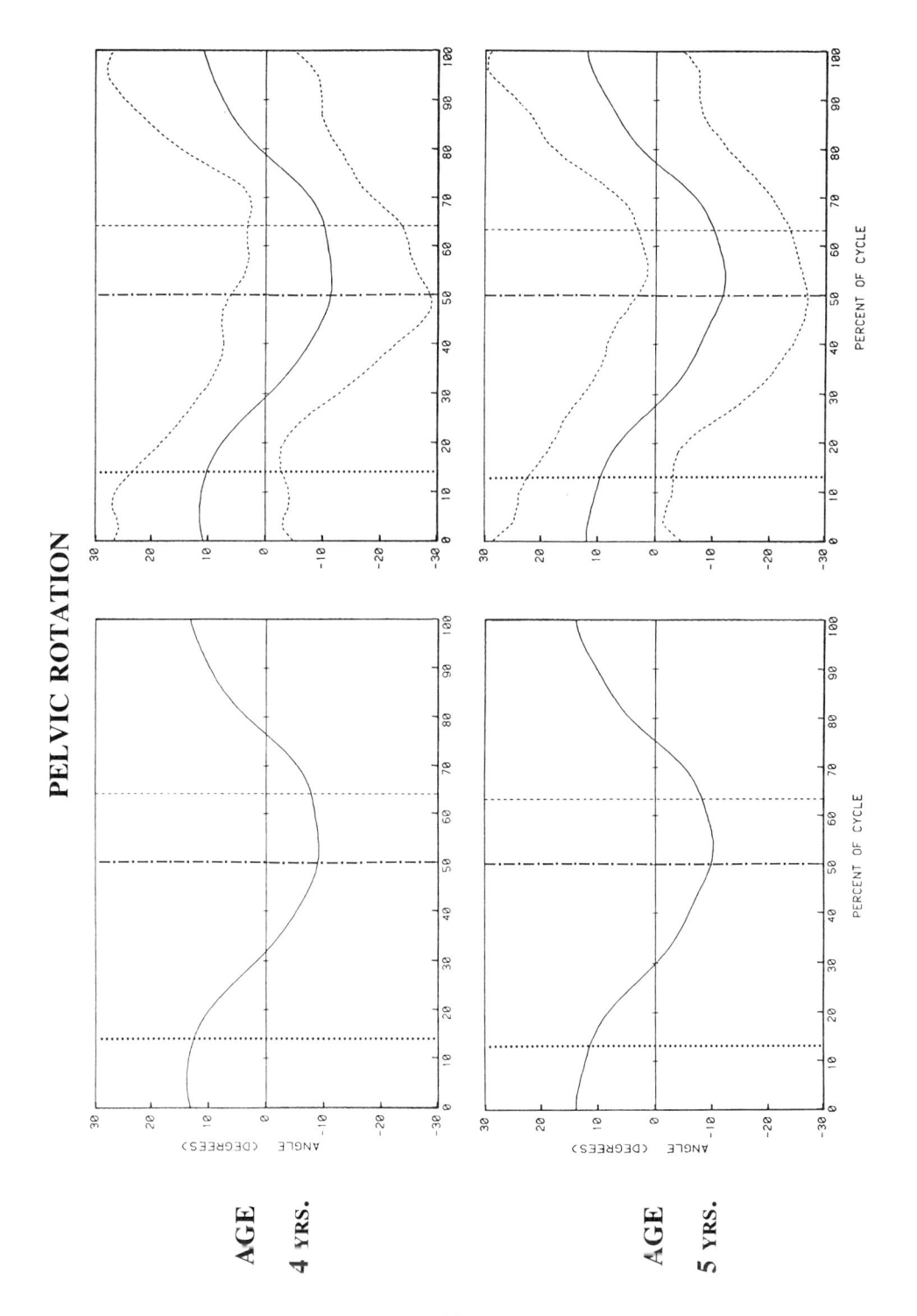

AGE 4 YRS.

AGE 5 YRS.

101

PELVIC ROTATION

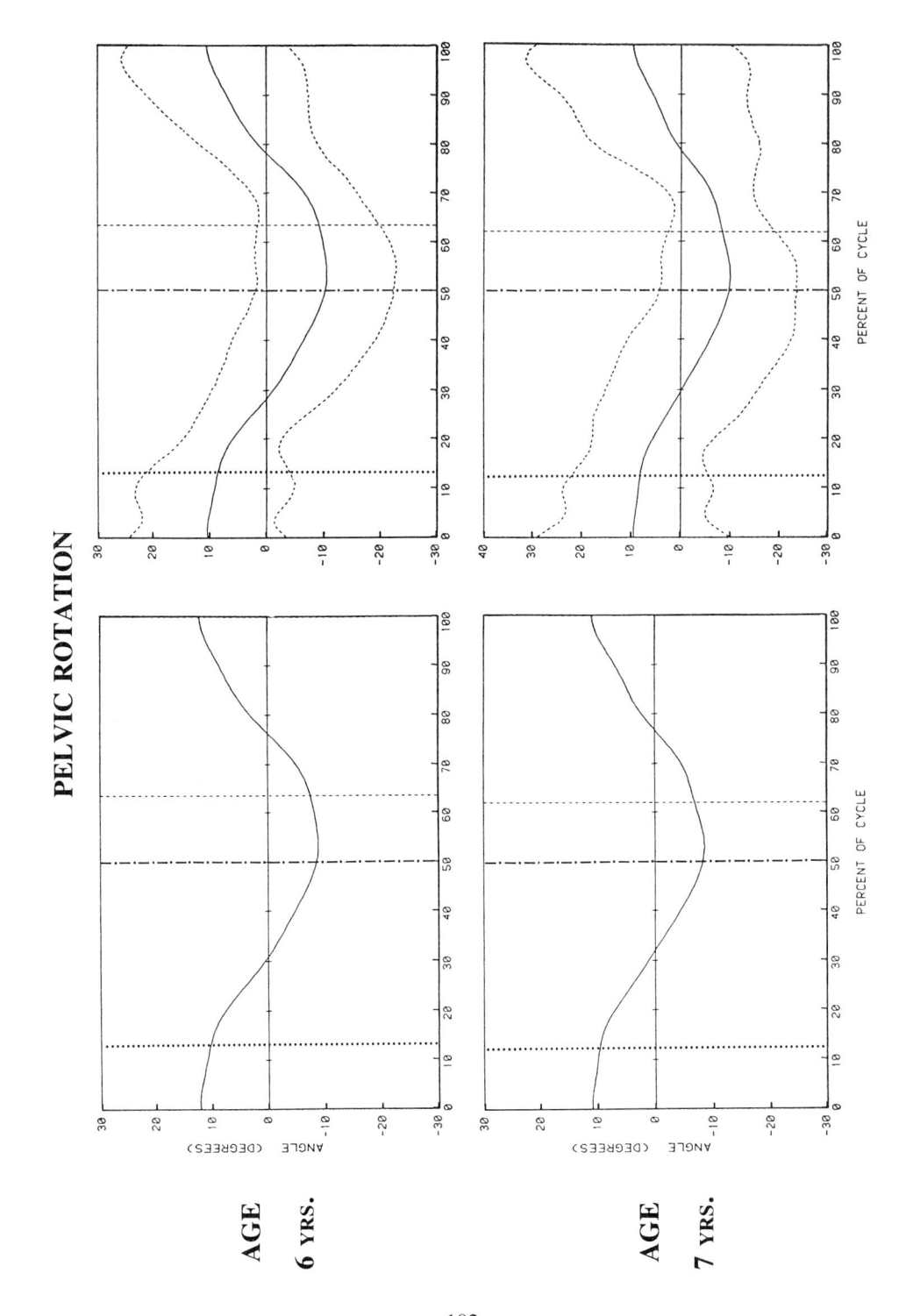

AGE 6 YRS.

AGE 7 YRS.

FEMORAL ROTATION

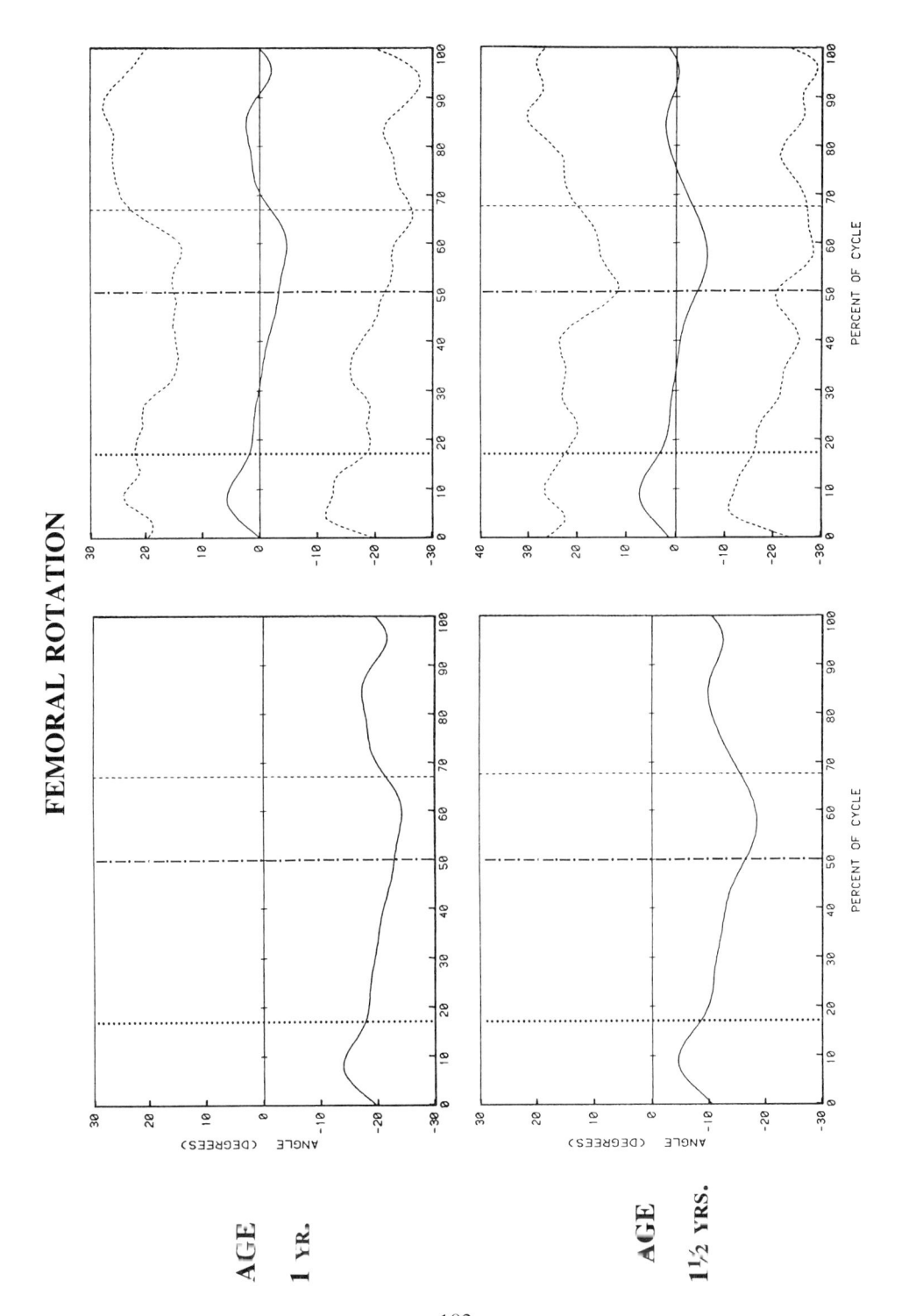

AGE
1 YR.

AGE
1½ YRS.

FEMORAL ROTATION

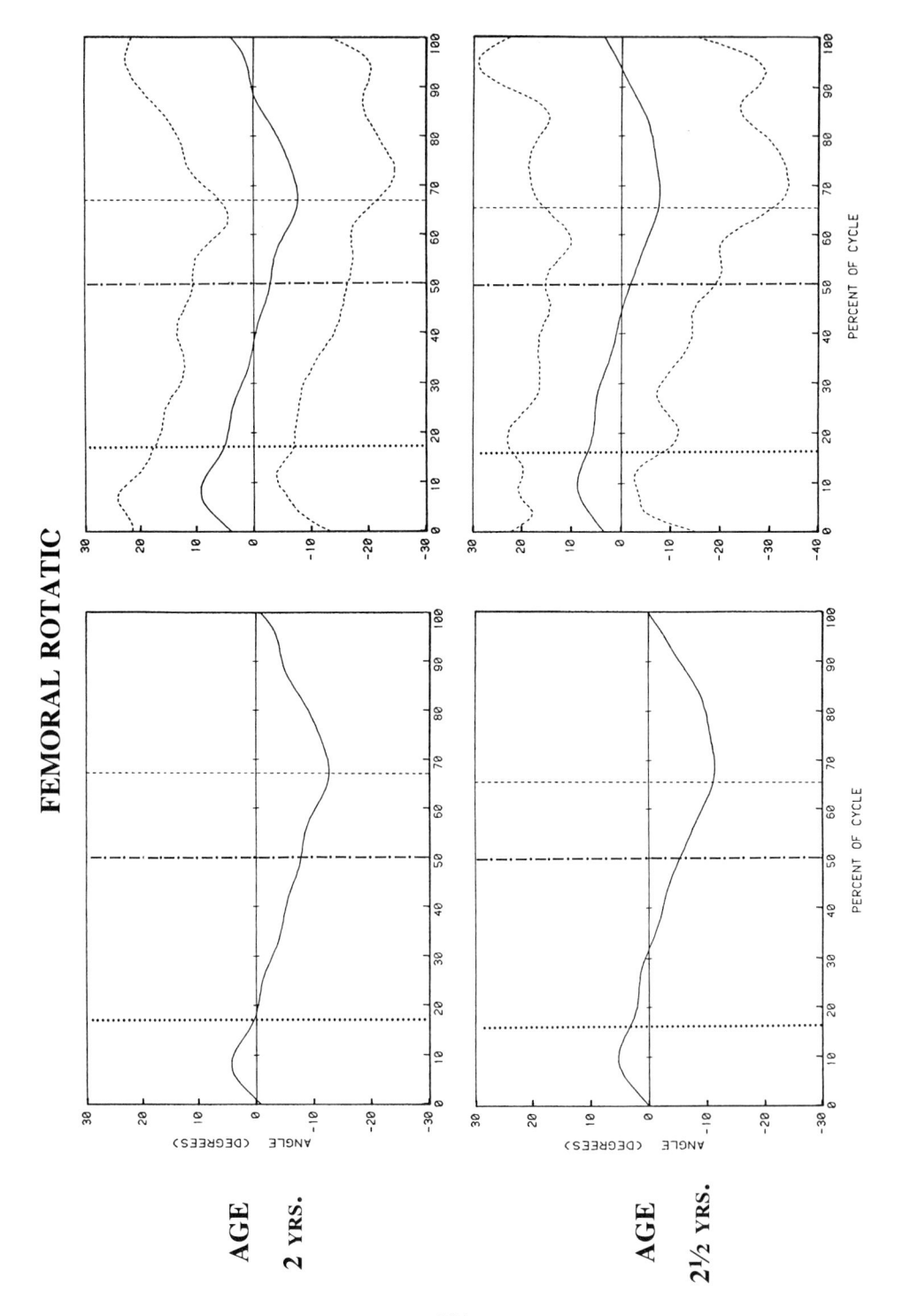

AGE 2 YRS.

AGE 2½ YRS.

104

FEMORAL ROTATION

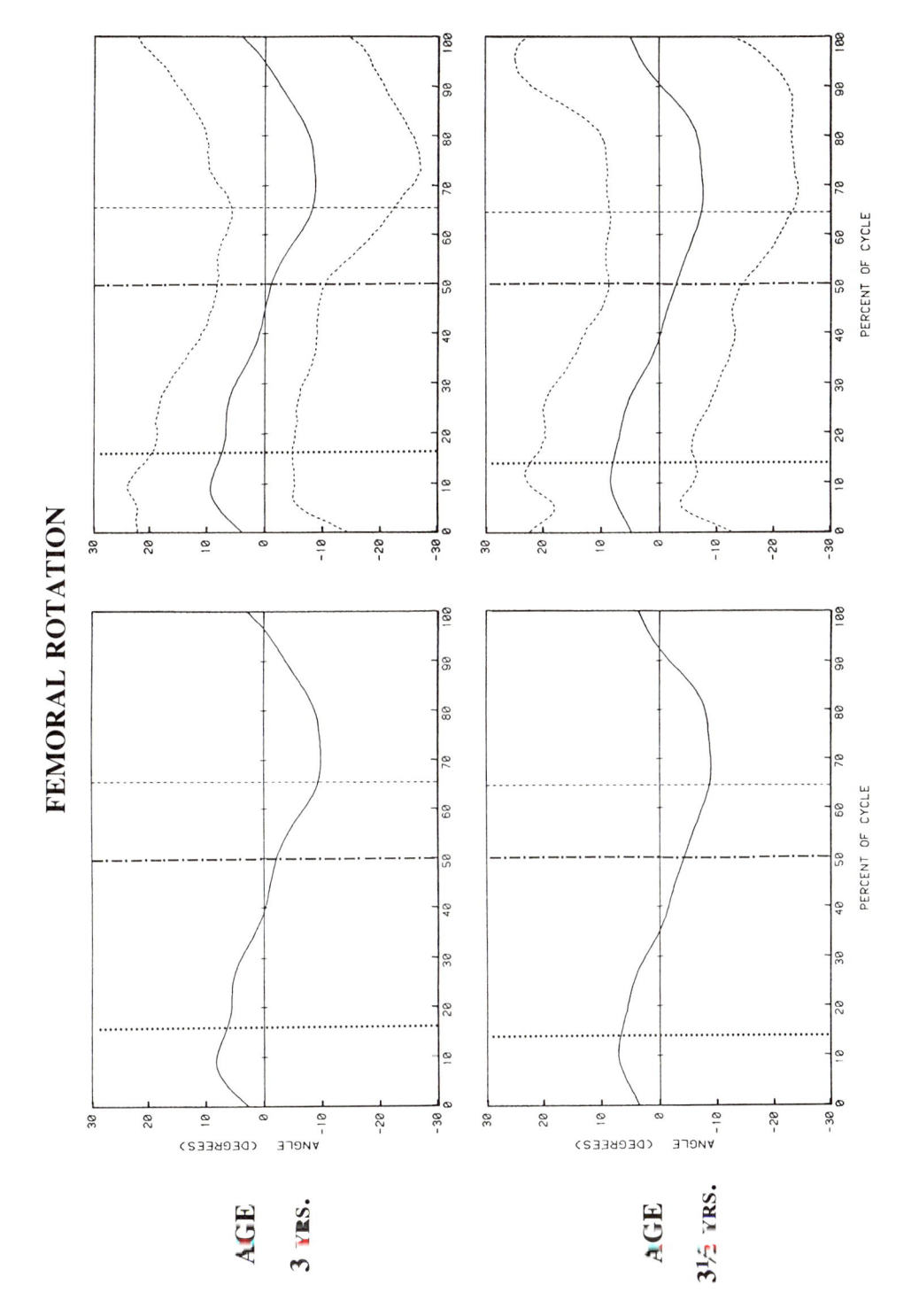

AGE 3 YRS.

AGE 3½ YRS.

FEMORAL ROTATION

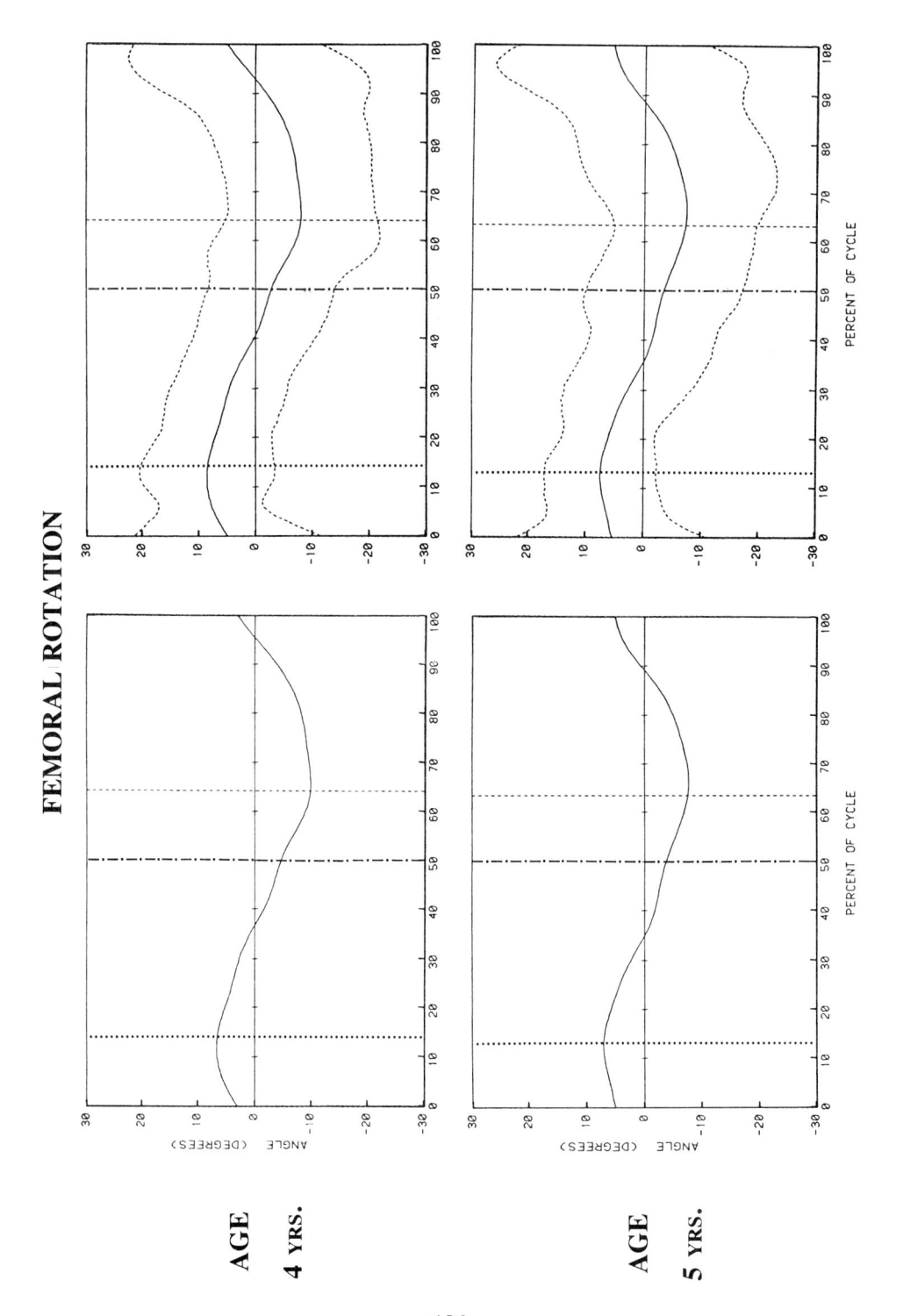

AGE 4 YRS.

AGE 5 YRS.

FEMORAL ROTATION

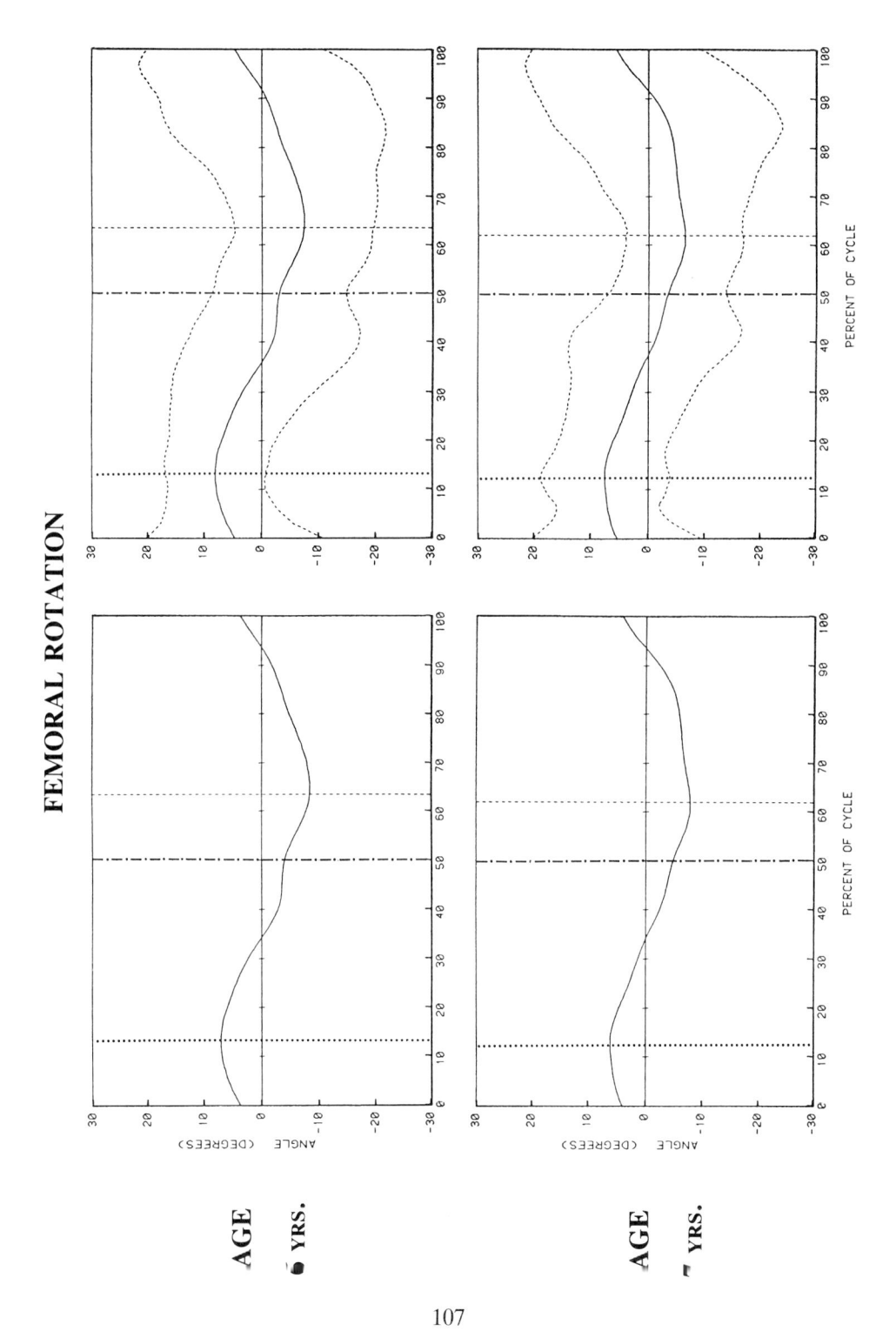

HIP ROTATION

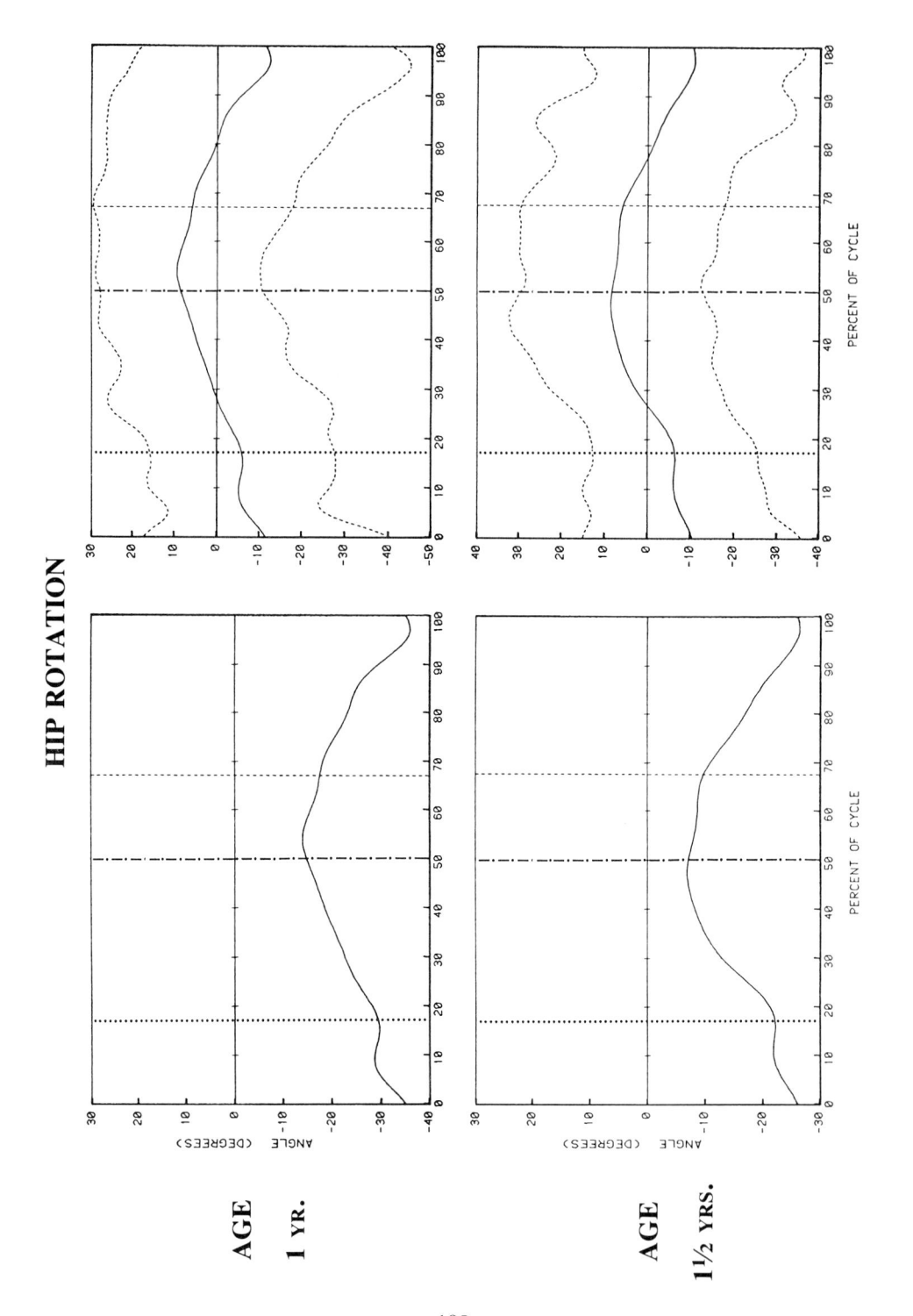

AGE 1 YR.

AGE 1½ YRS.

HIP ROTATION

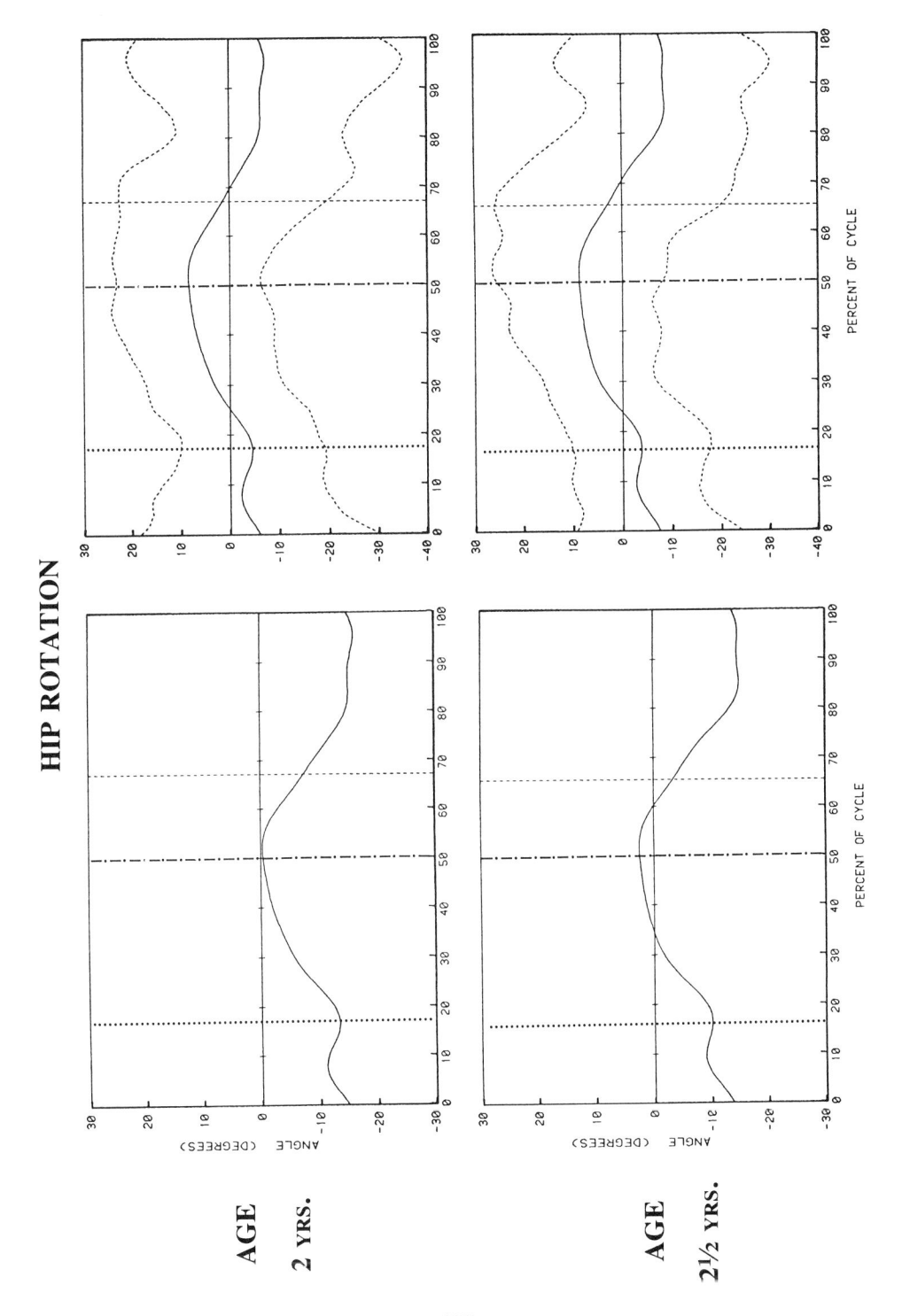

AGE 2 YRS.

AGE 2½ YRS.

109

HIP ROTATION

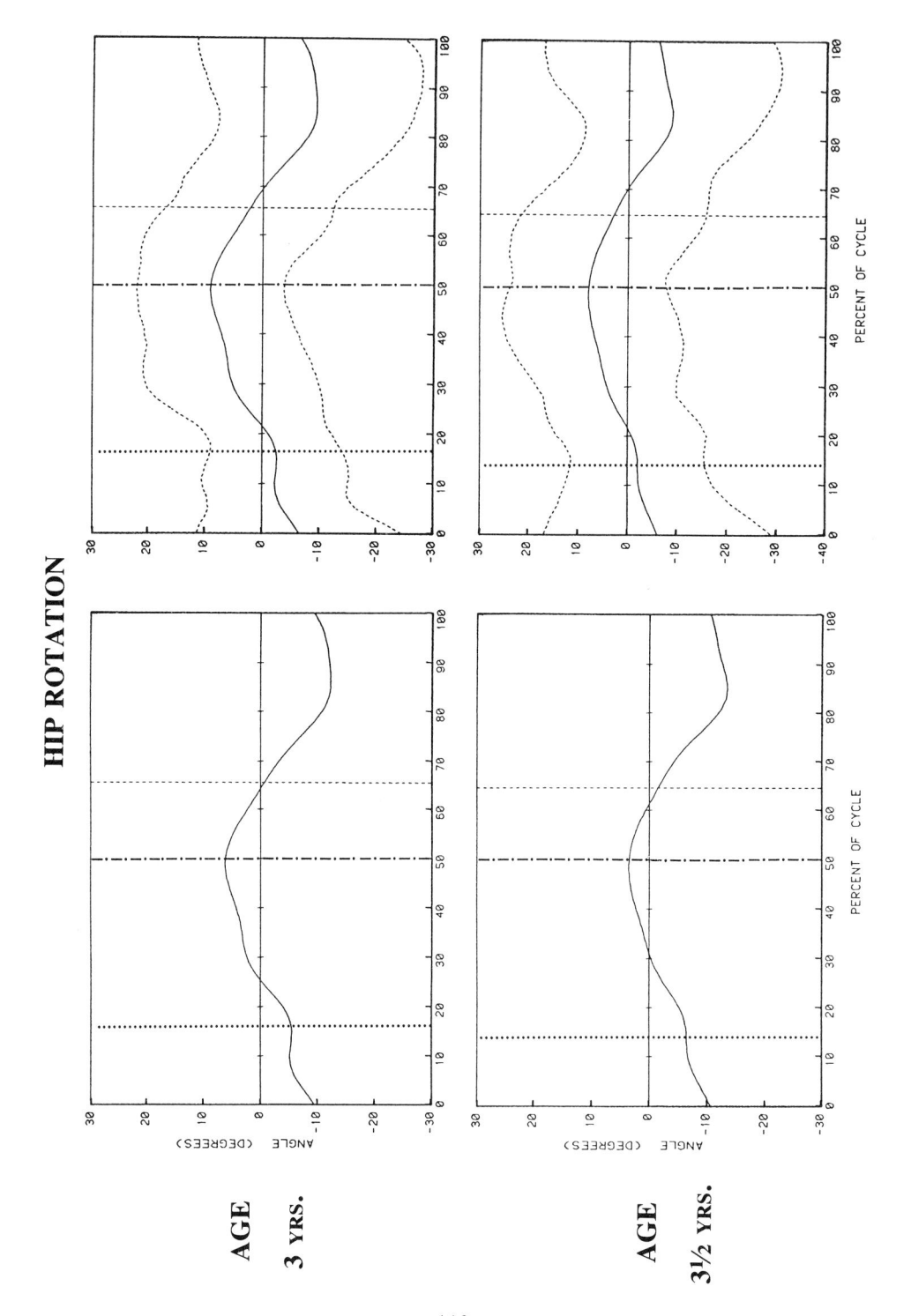

AGE 3 YRS.

AGE 3½ YRS.

HIP ROTATION

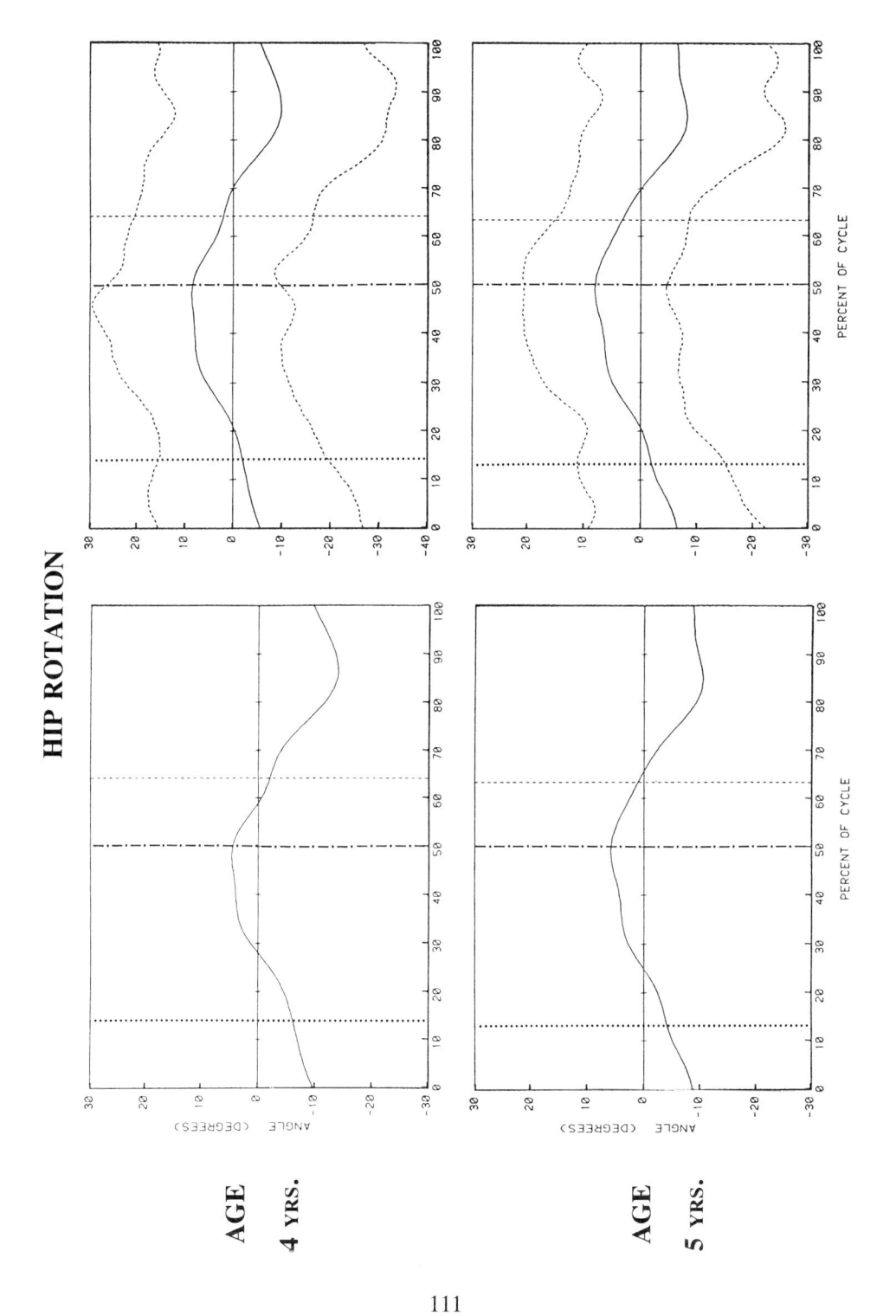

AGE 4 YRS.

AGE 5 YRS.

111

HIP ROTATION

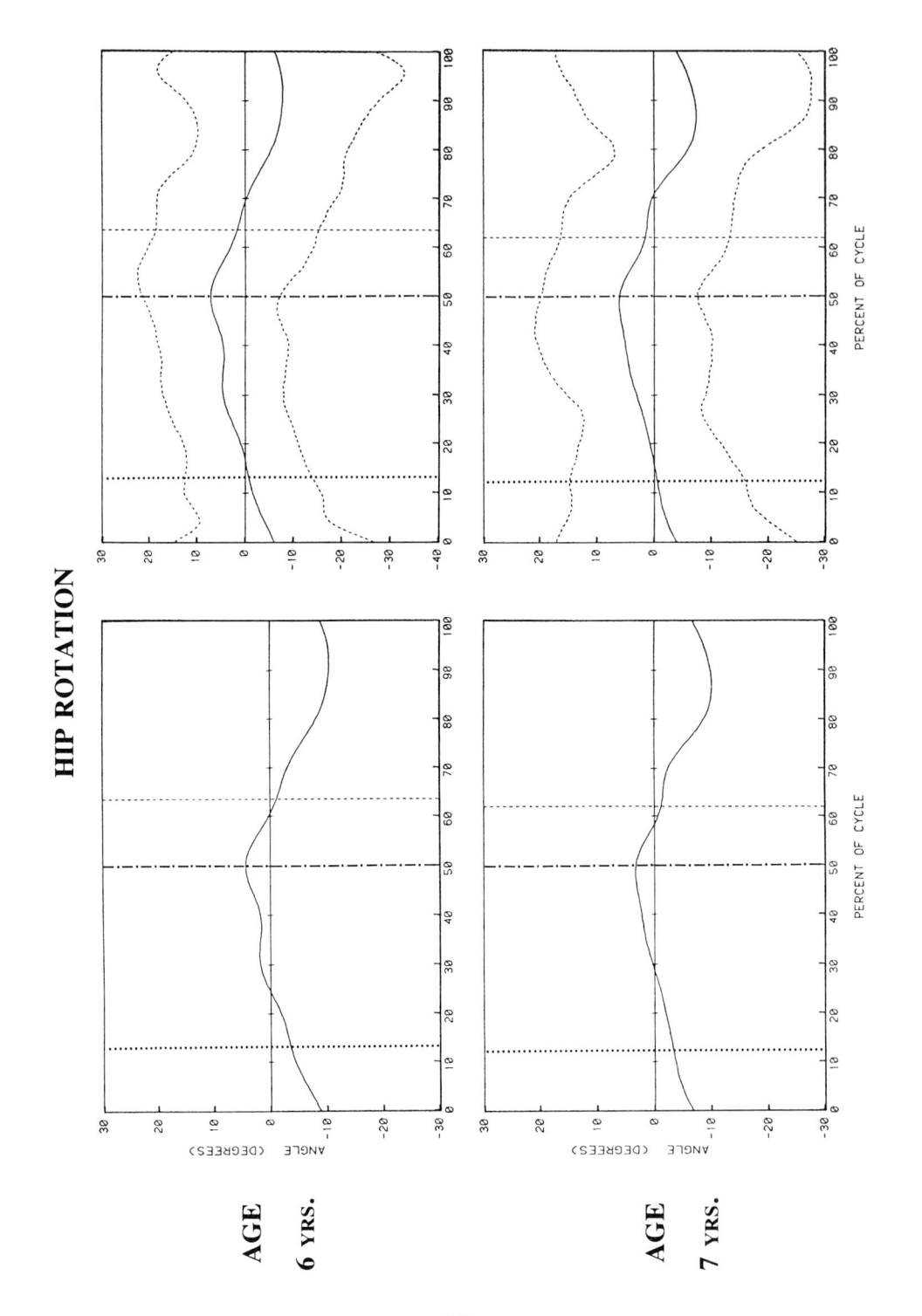

**AGE
6 YRS.**

**AGE
7 YRS.**

TIBIAL ROTATION

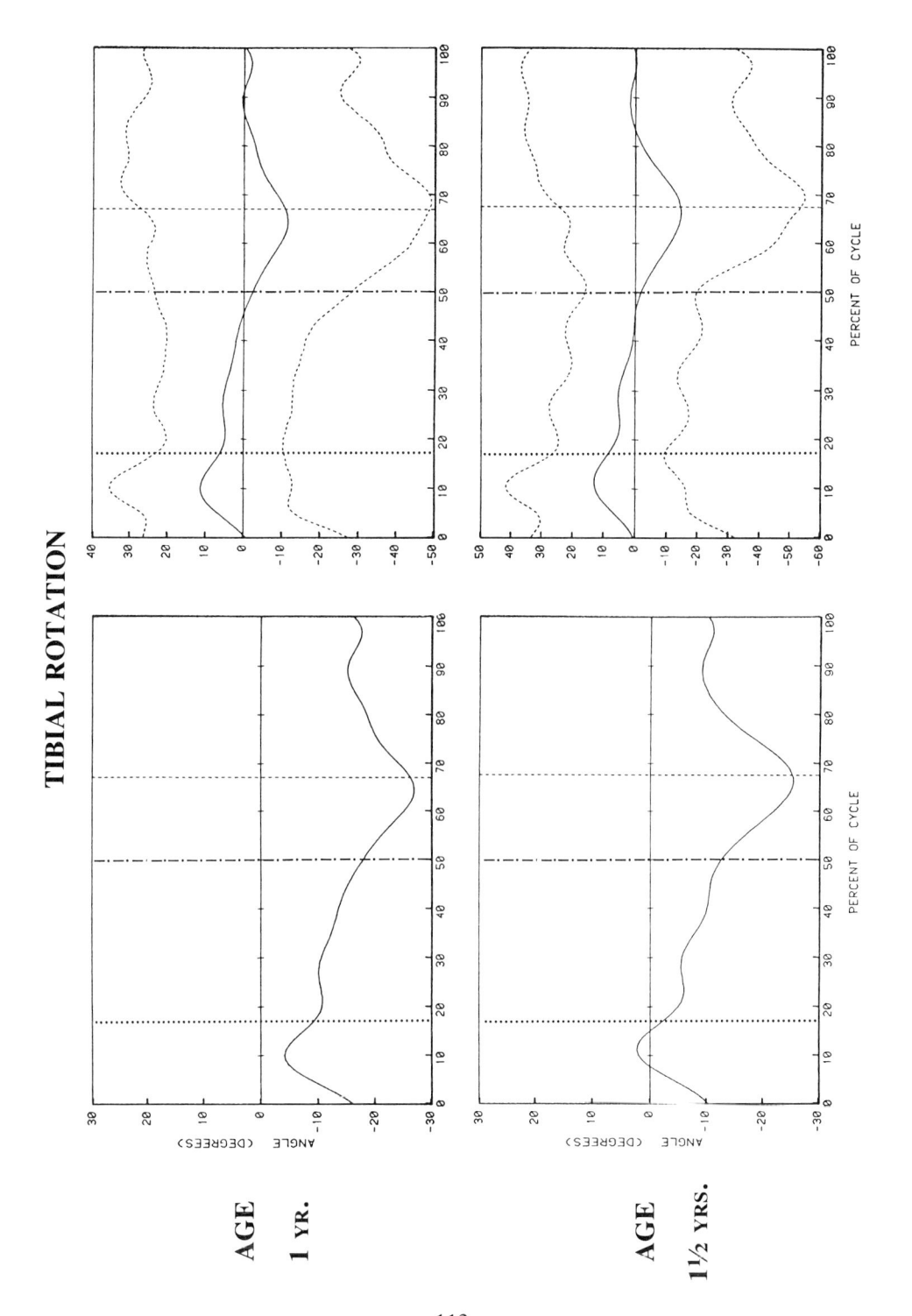

AGE
1 YR.

AGE
1½ YRS.

TIBIAL ROTATION

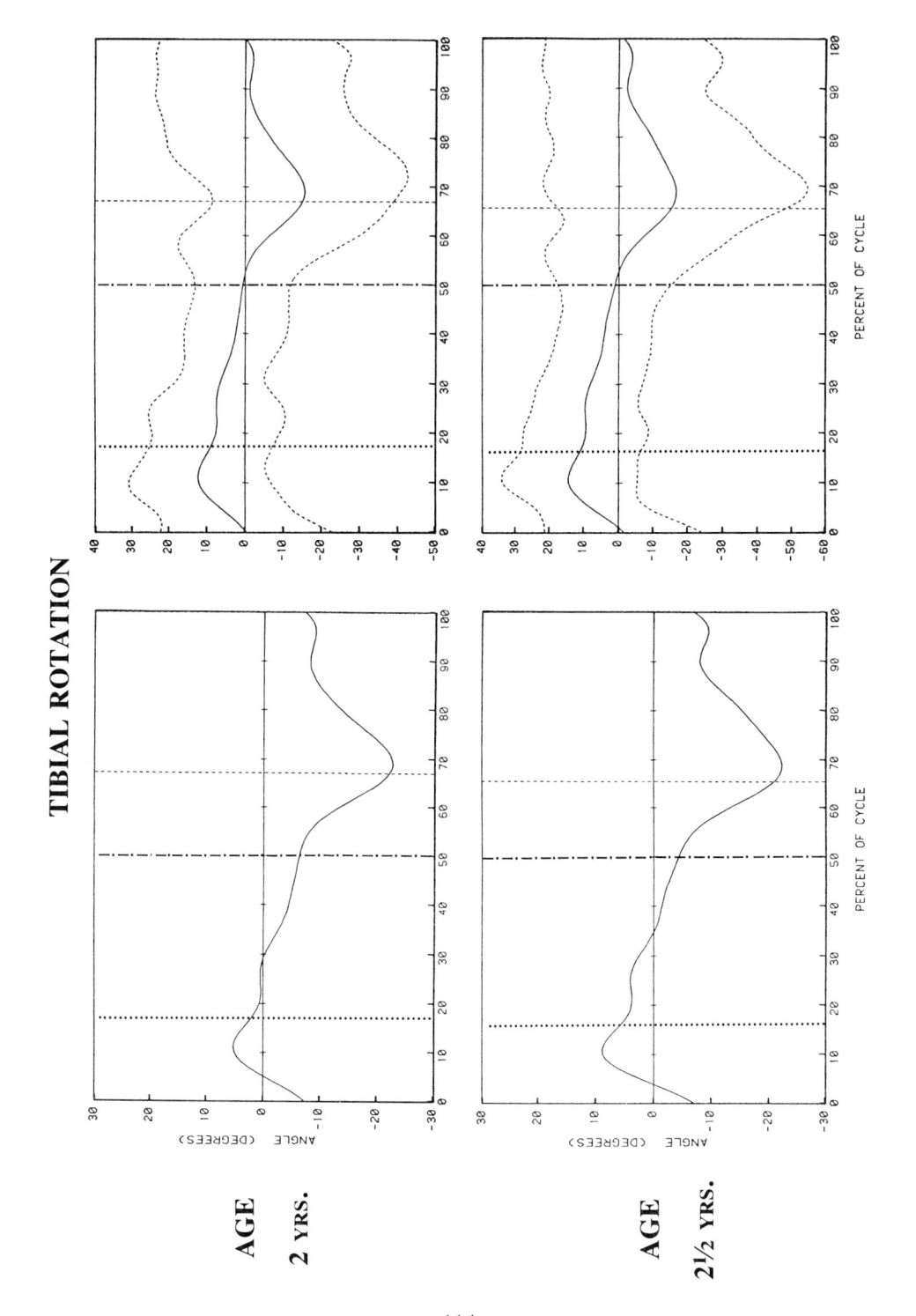

**AGE
2 YRS.**

**AGE
2½ YRS.**

TIBIAL ROTATION

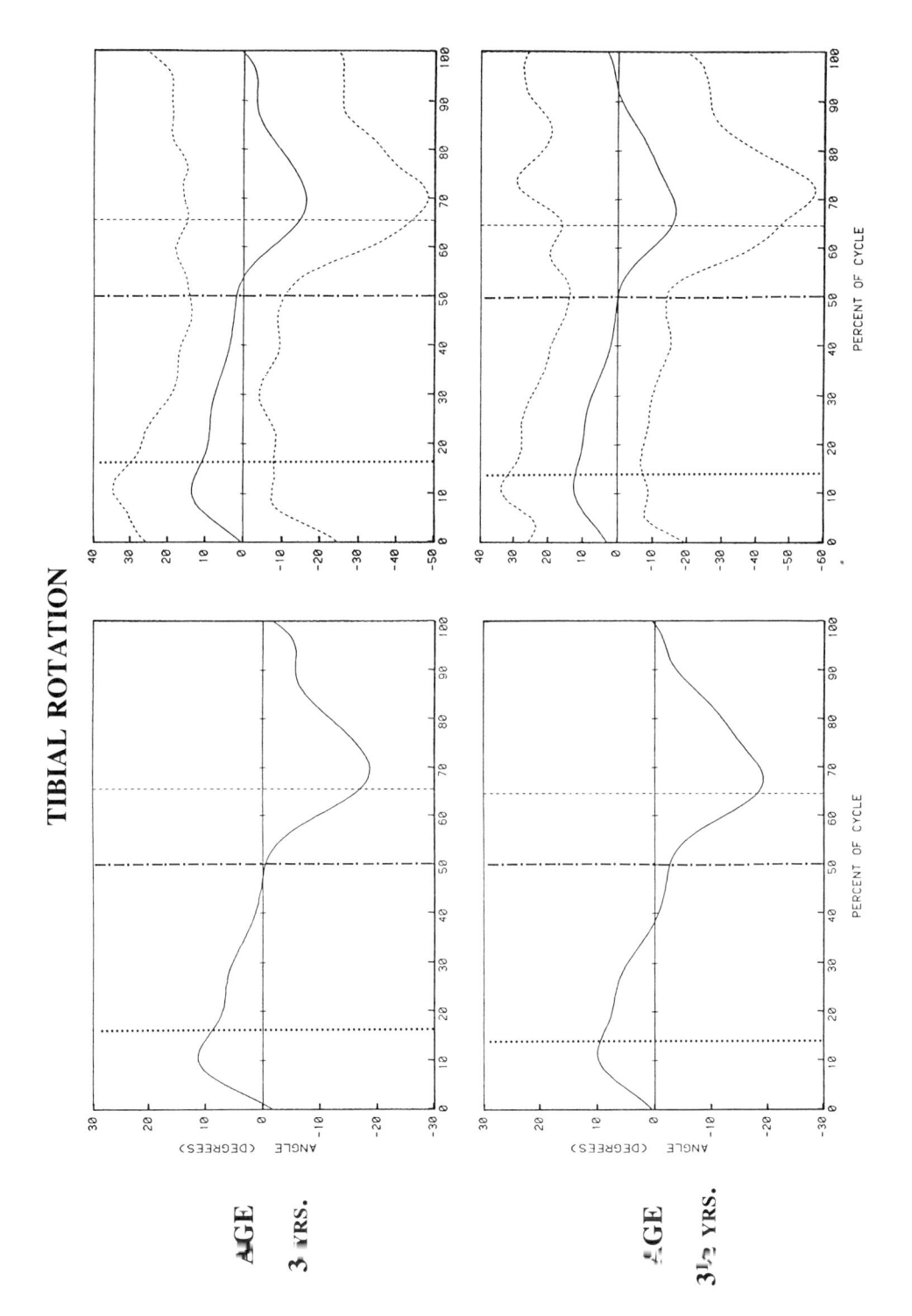

AGE
3 YRS.

AGE
3½ YRS.

TIBIAL ROTATION

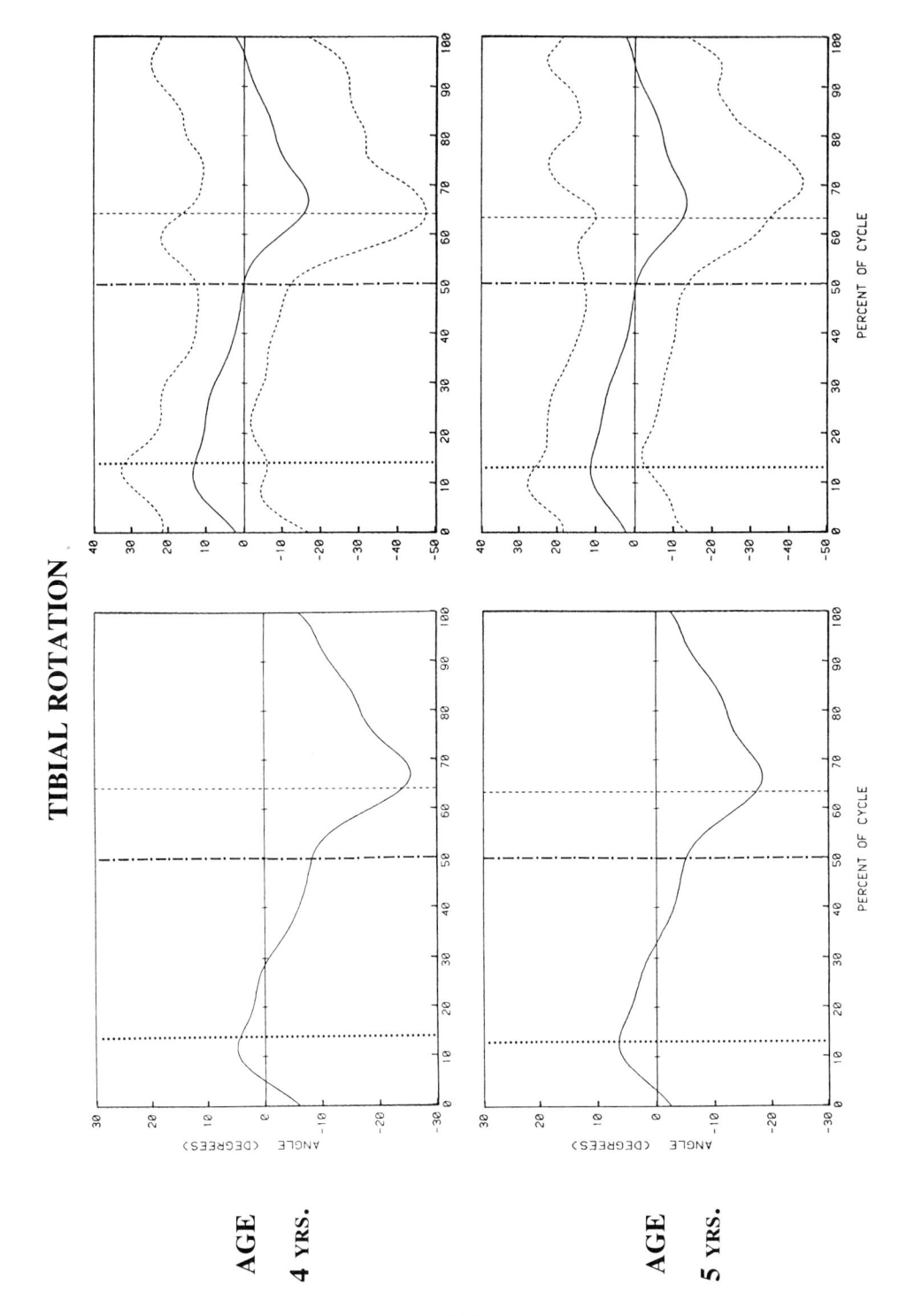

AGE 4 YRS.

AGE 5 YRS.

TIBIAL ROTATION

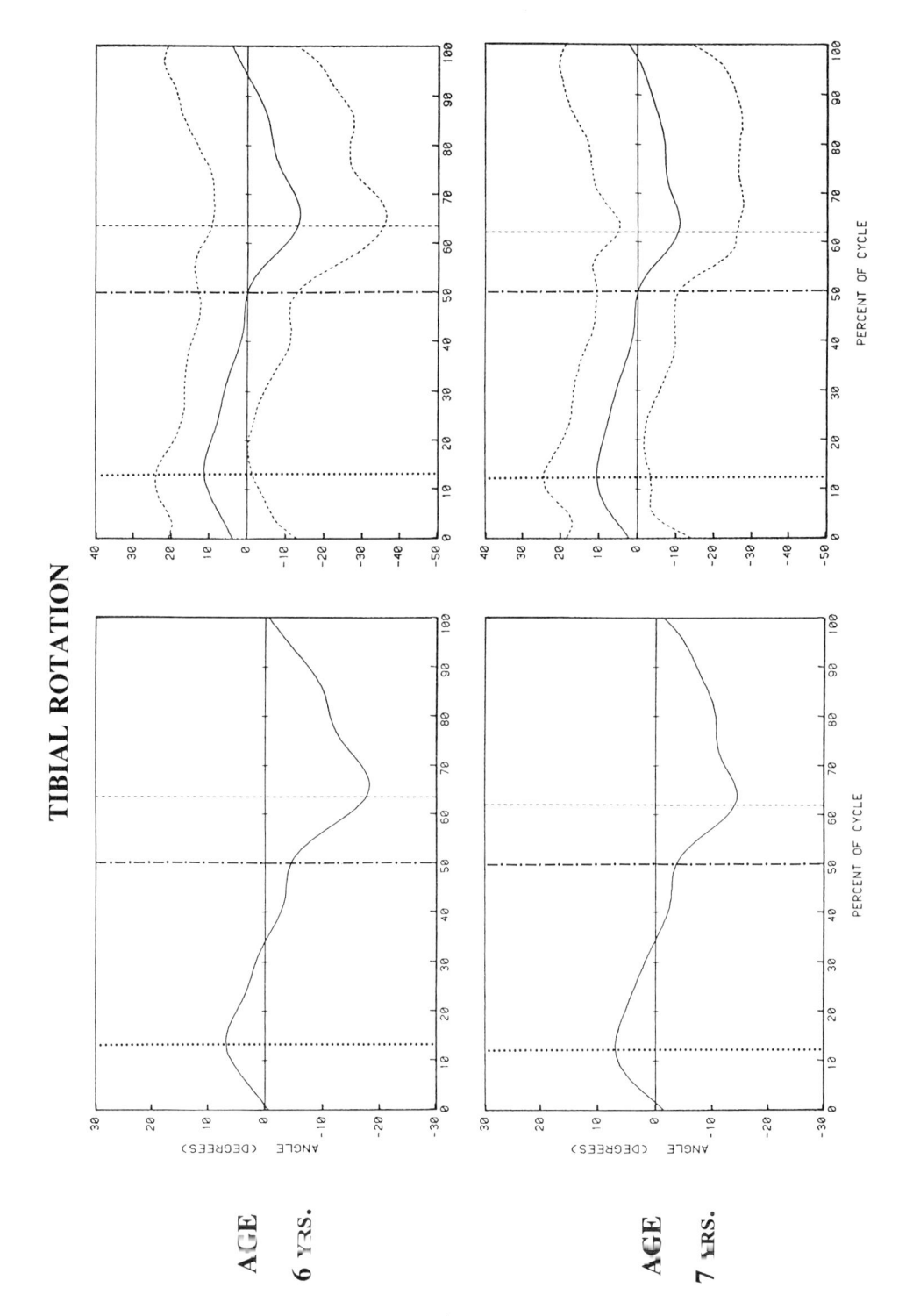

AGE 6 YRS.

AGE 7 YRS.

KNEE ROTATION

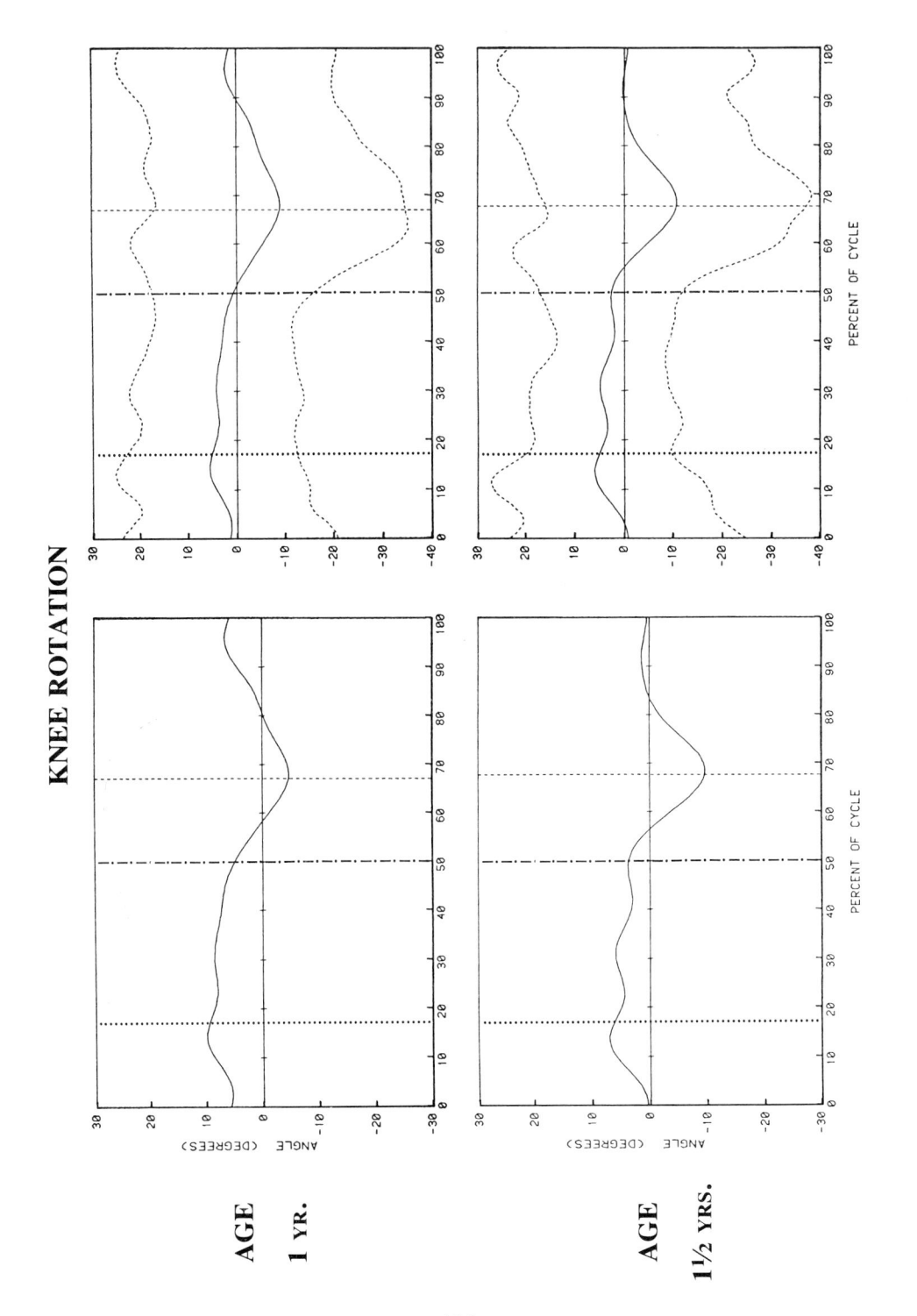

AGE 1 YR.

AGE 1½ YRS.

KNEE ROTATION

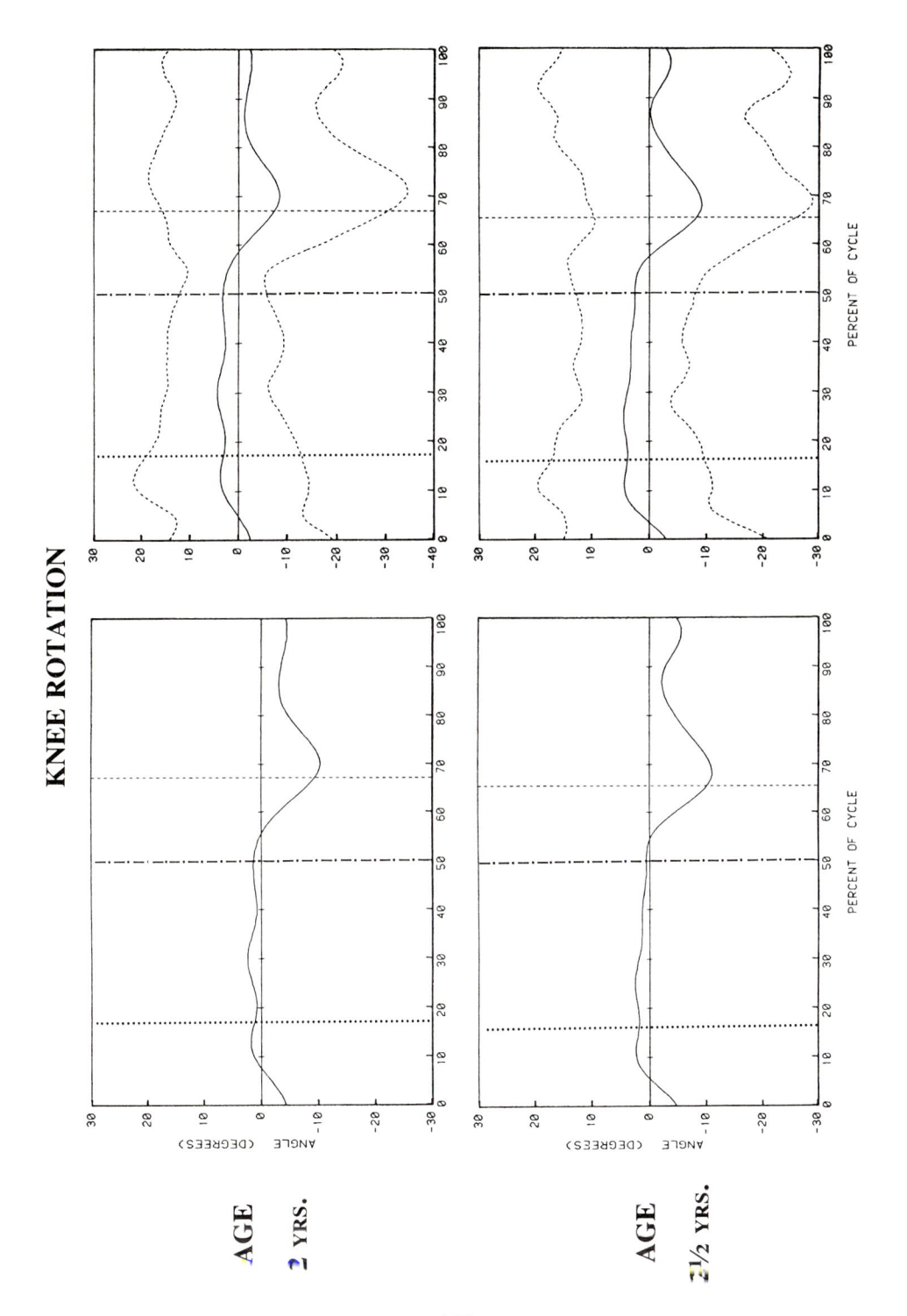

ANGLE (DEGREES)

PERCENT OF CYCLE

AGE
2 YRS.

AGE
2½ YRS.

KNEE ROTATION

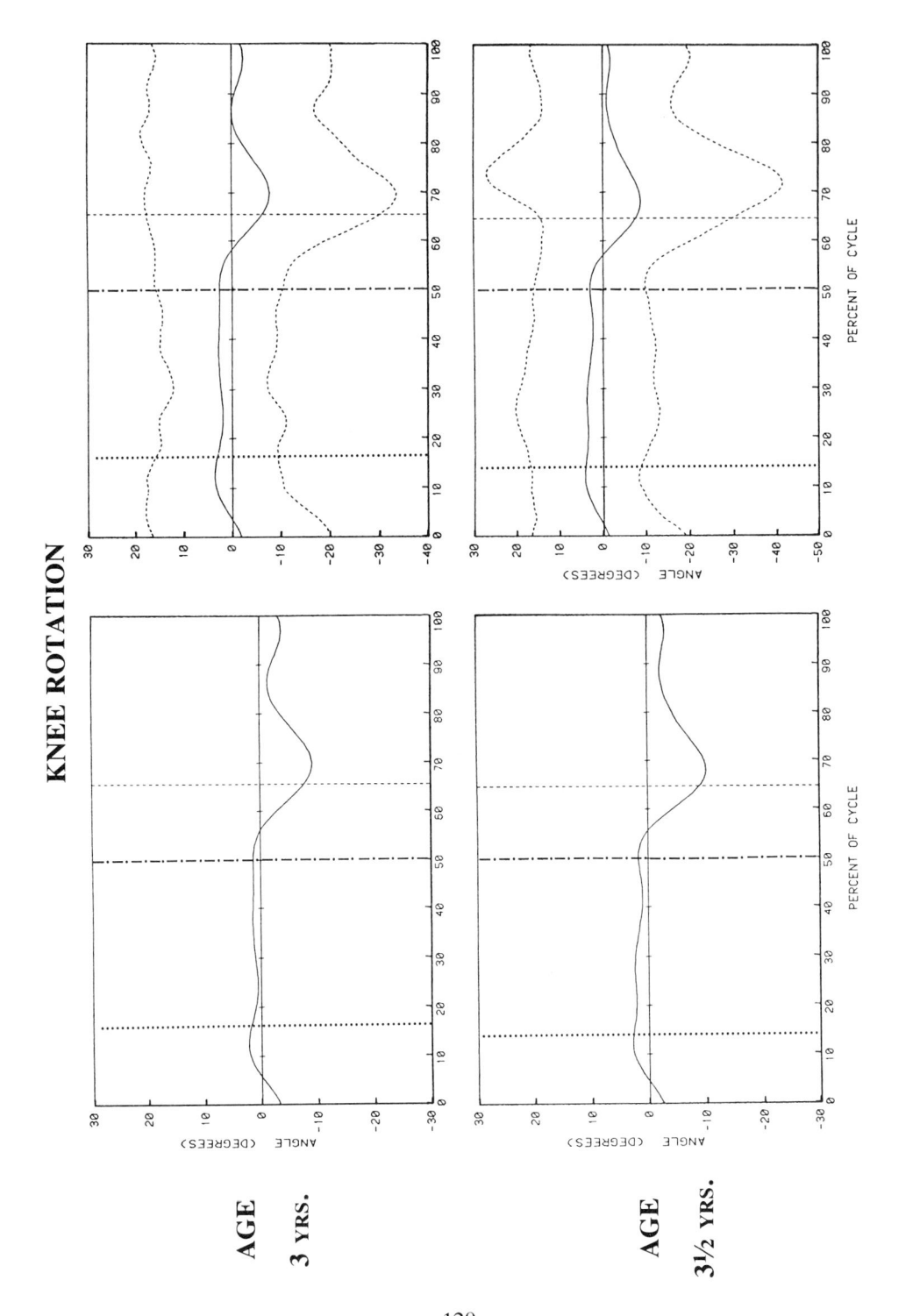

AGE 3 YRS.

AGE 3½ YRS.

KNEE ROTATION

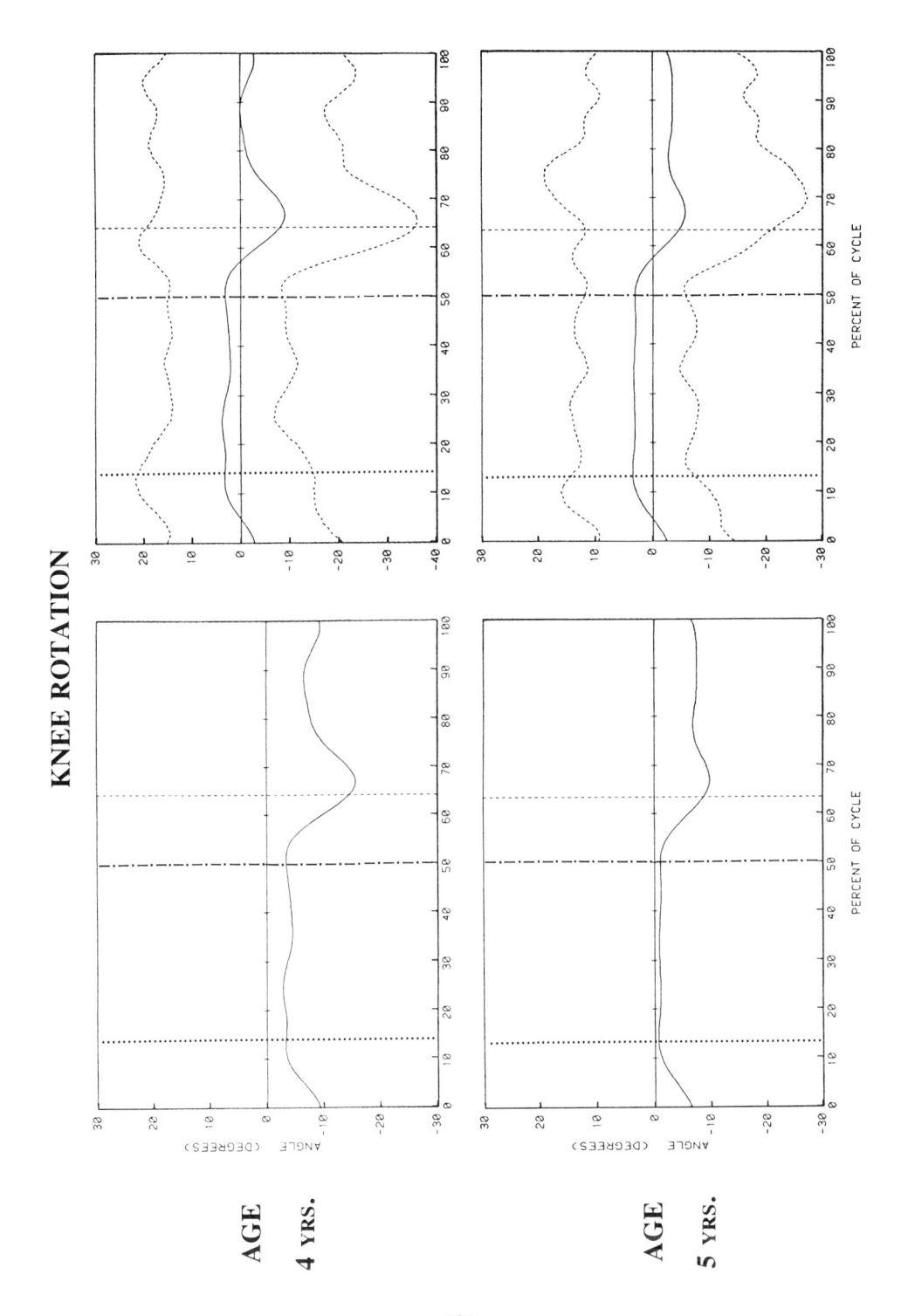

AGE 4 YRS.

AGE 5 YRS.

121

KNEE ROTATION

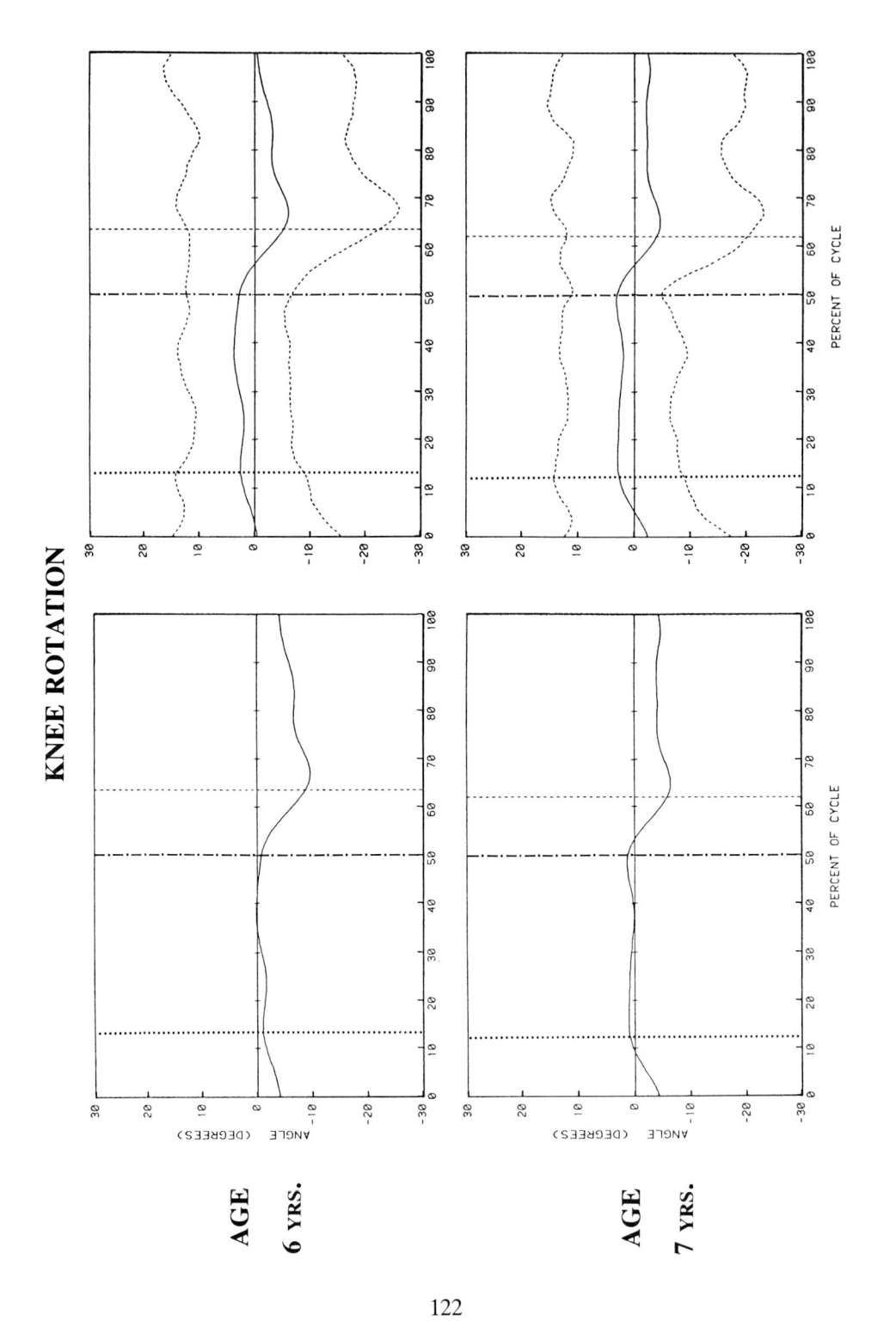

AGE 6 YRS.

AGE 7 YRS.

FOOT ROTATION

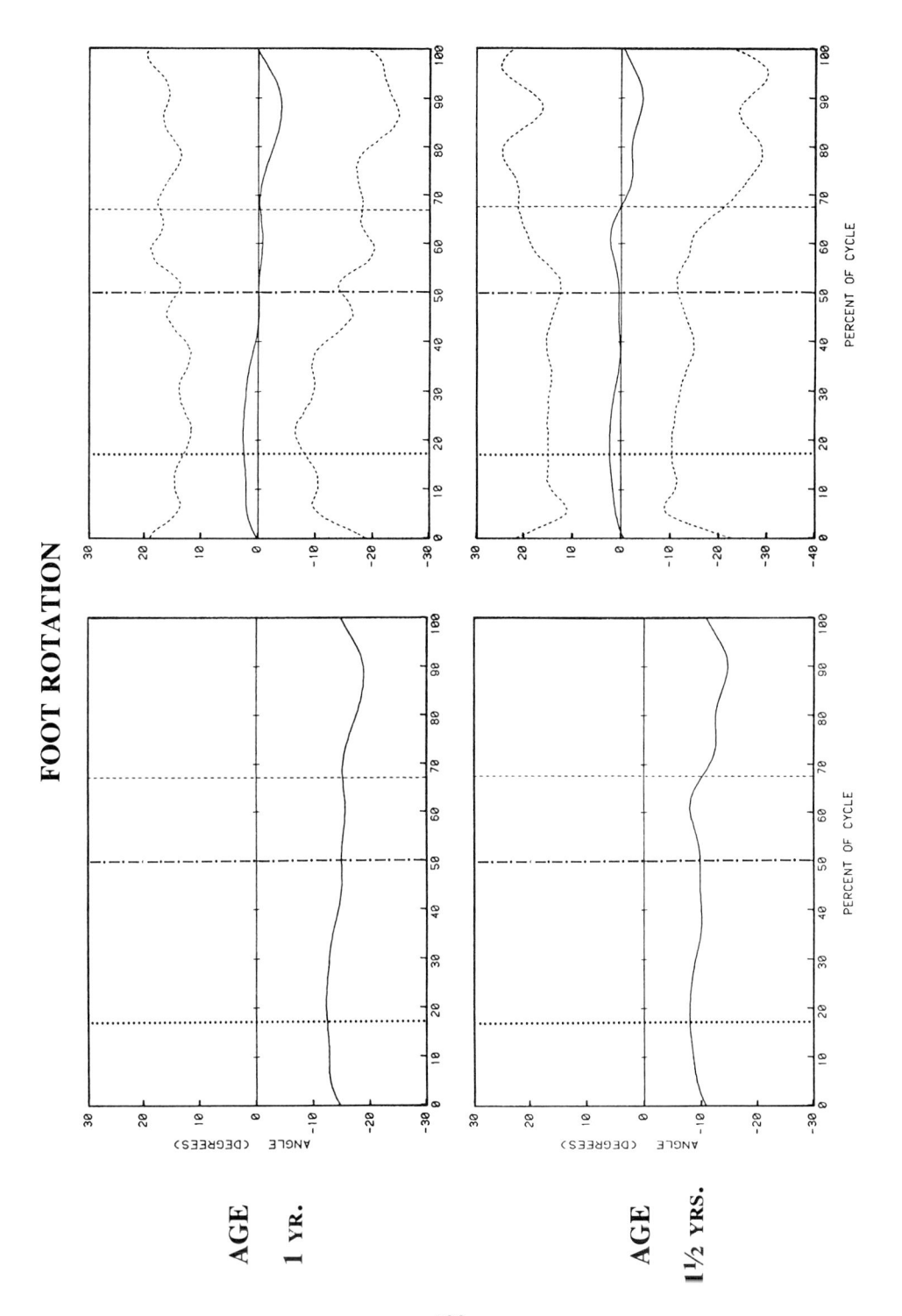

AGE
1 YR.

AGE
1½ YRS.

FOOT ROTATION

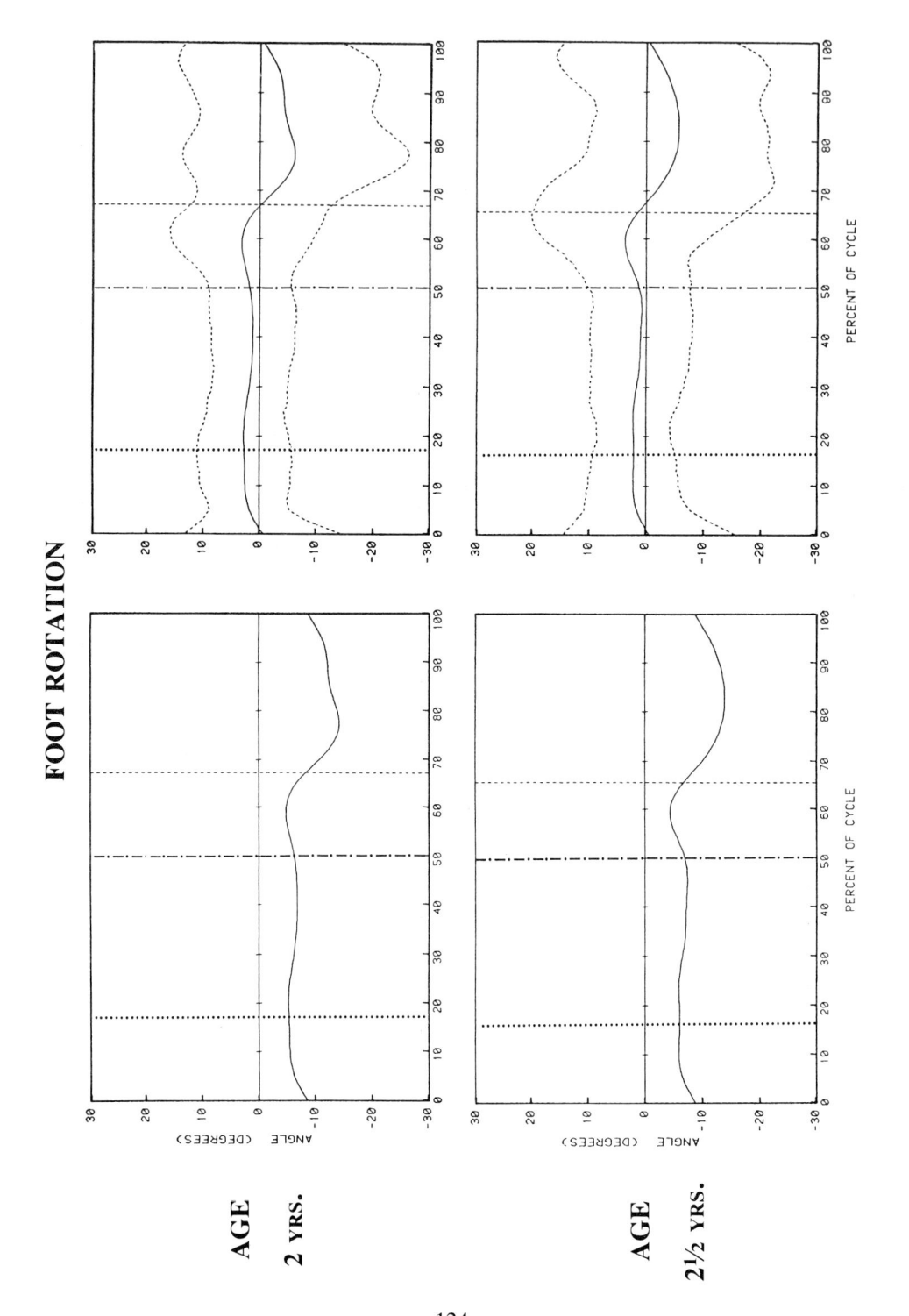

AGE 2 YRS.

AGE 2½ YRS.

124

FOOT ROTATION

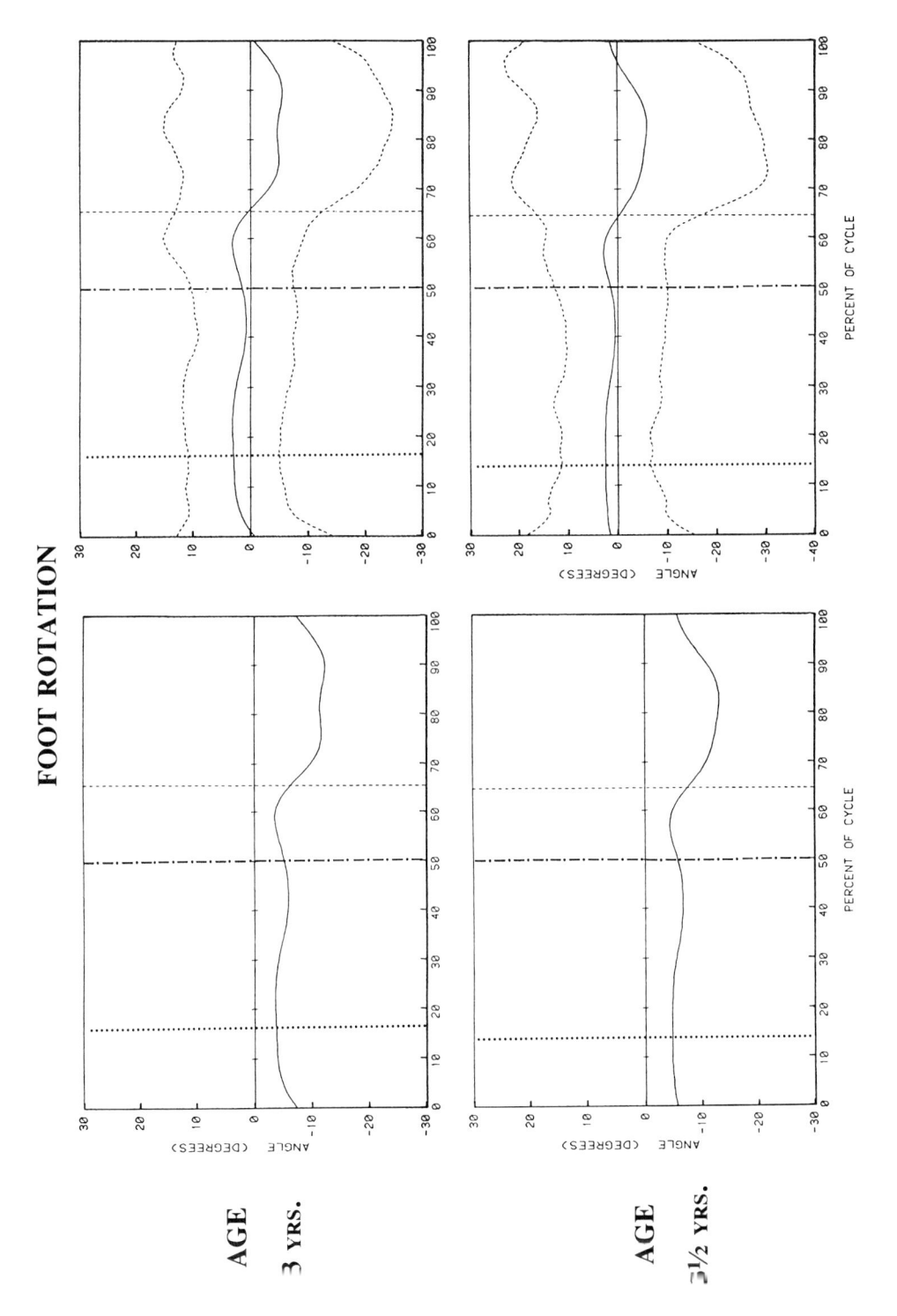

AGE
3 YRS.

AGE
3½ YRS.

FOOT ROTATION

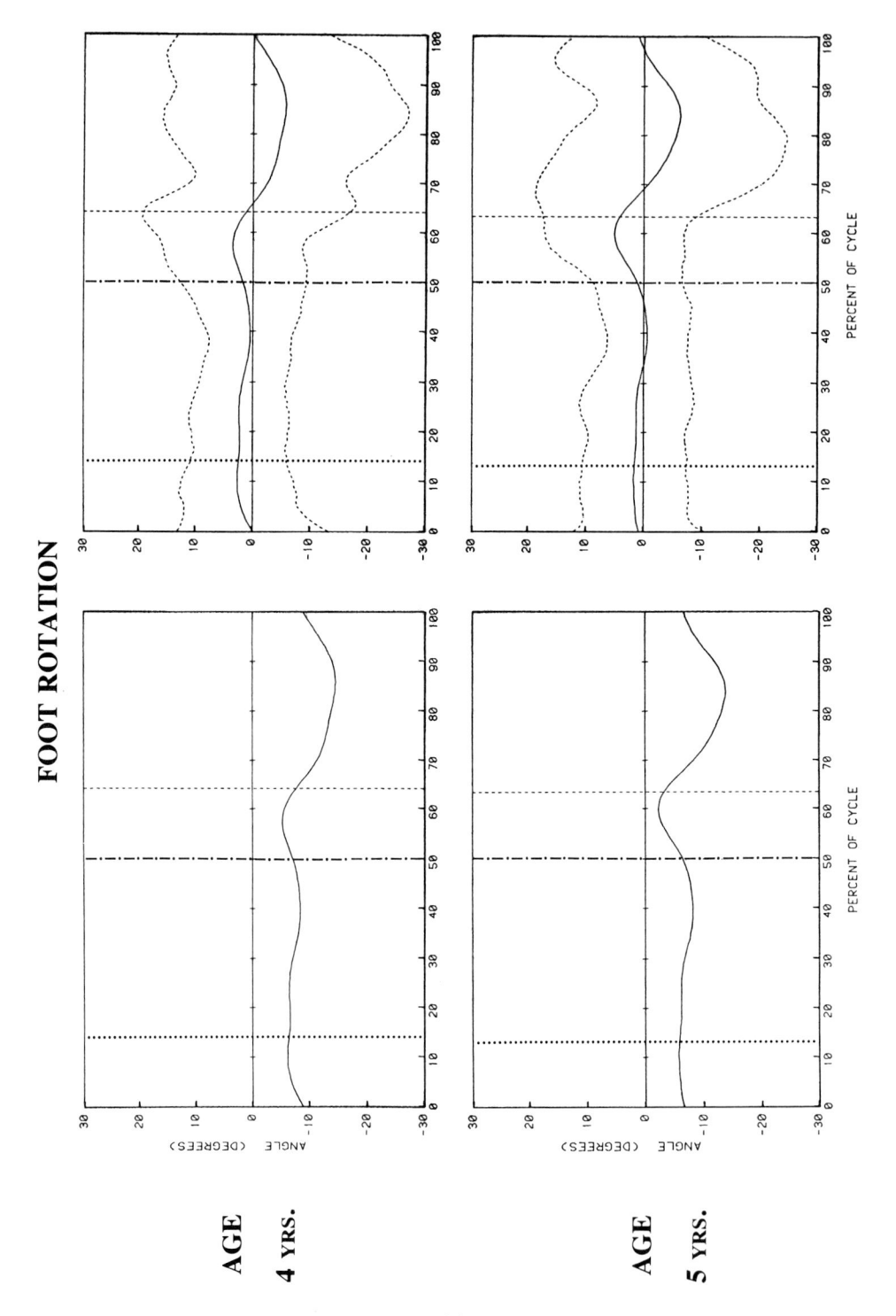

AGE 4 YRS.

AGE 5 YRS.

FOOT ROTATION

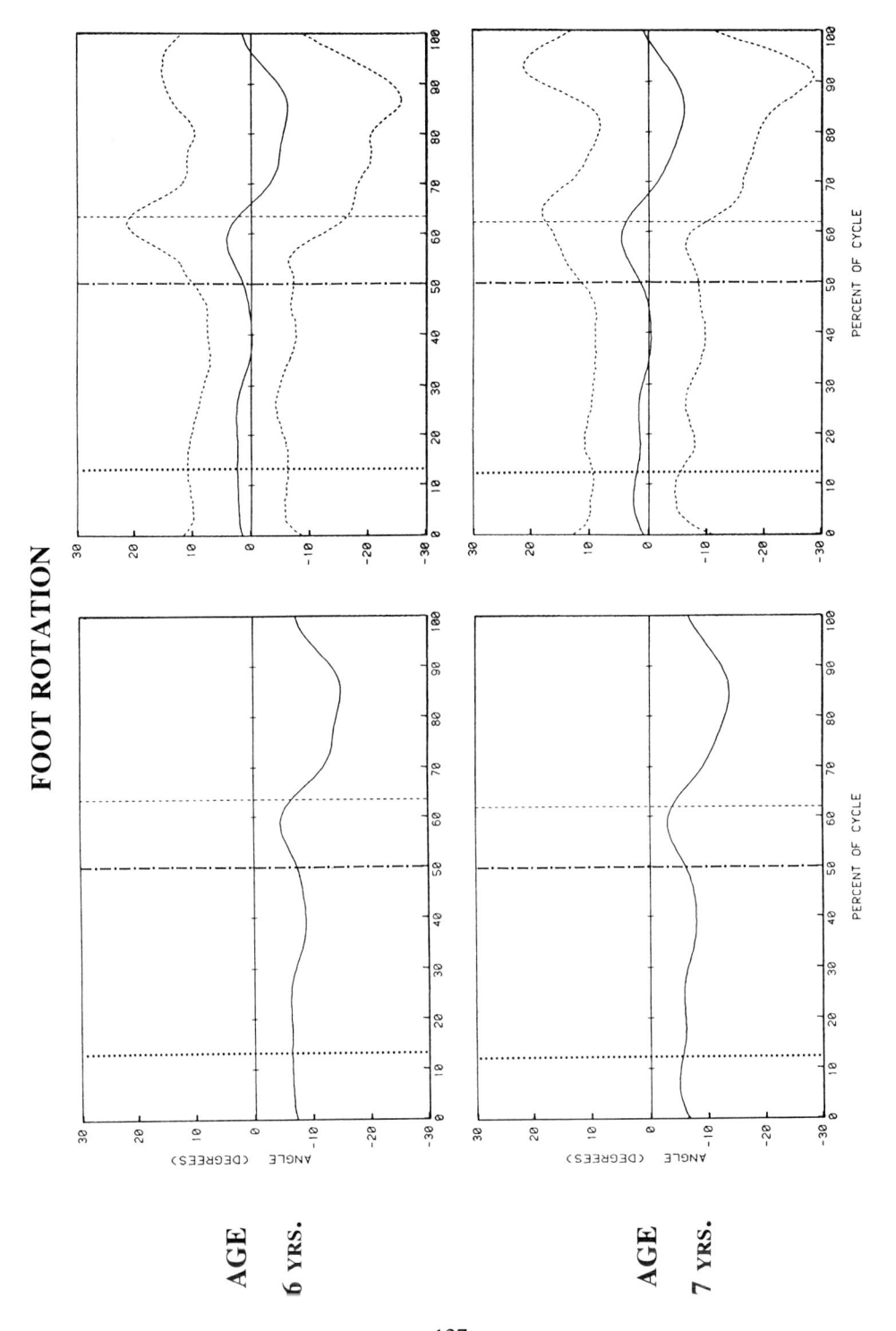

AGE
6 YRS.

AGE
7 YRS.

128

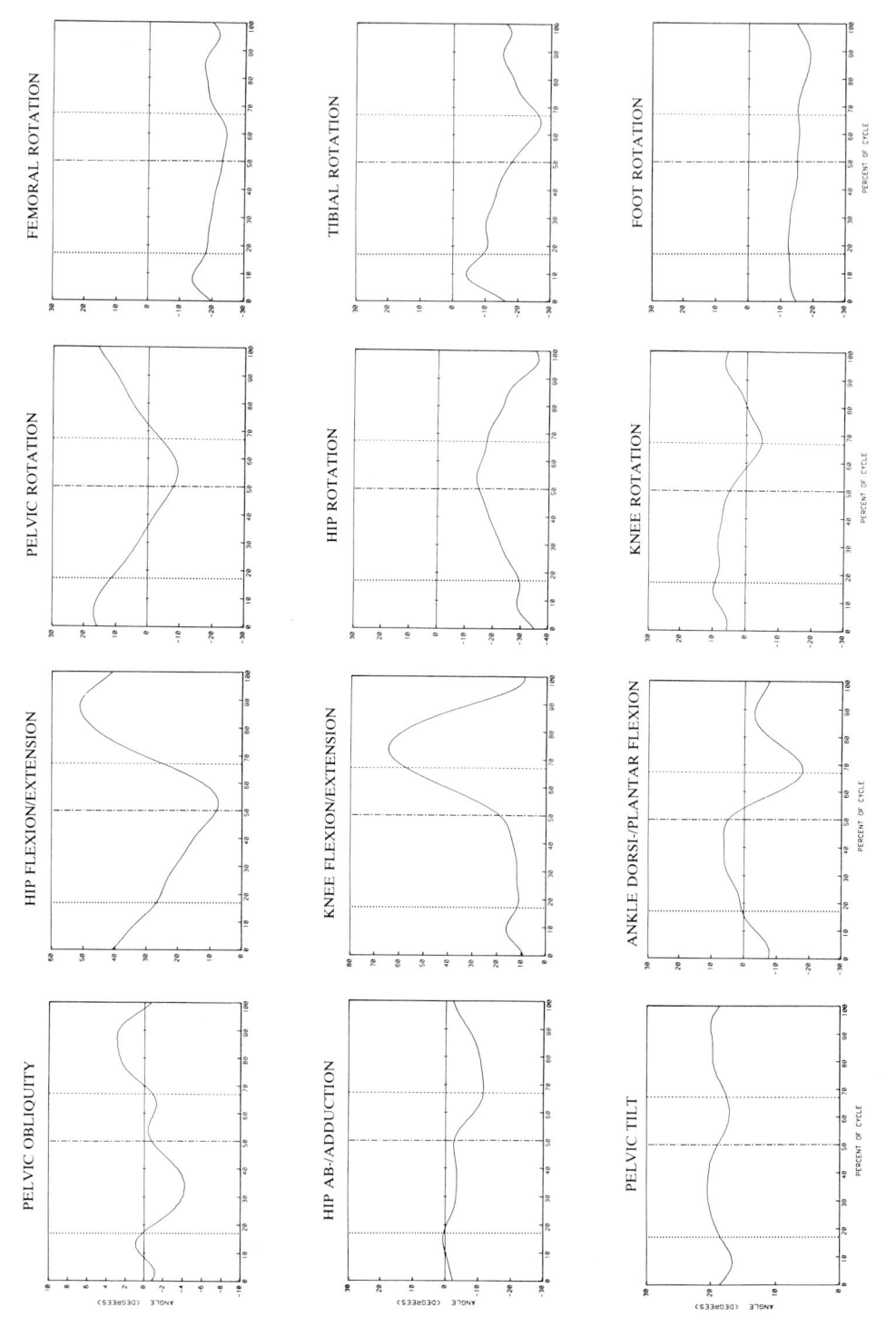

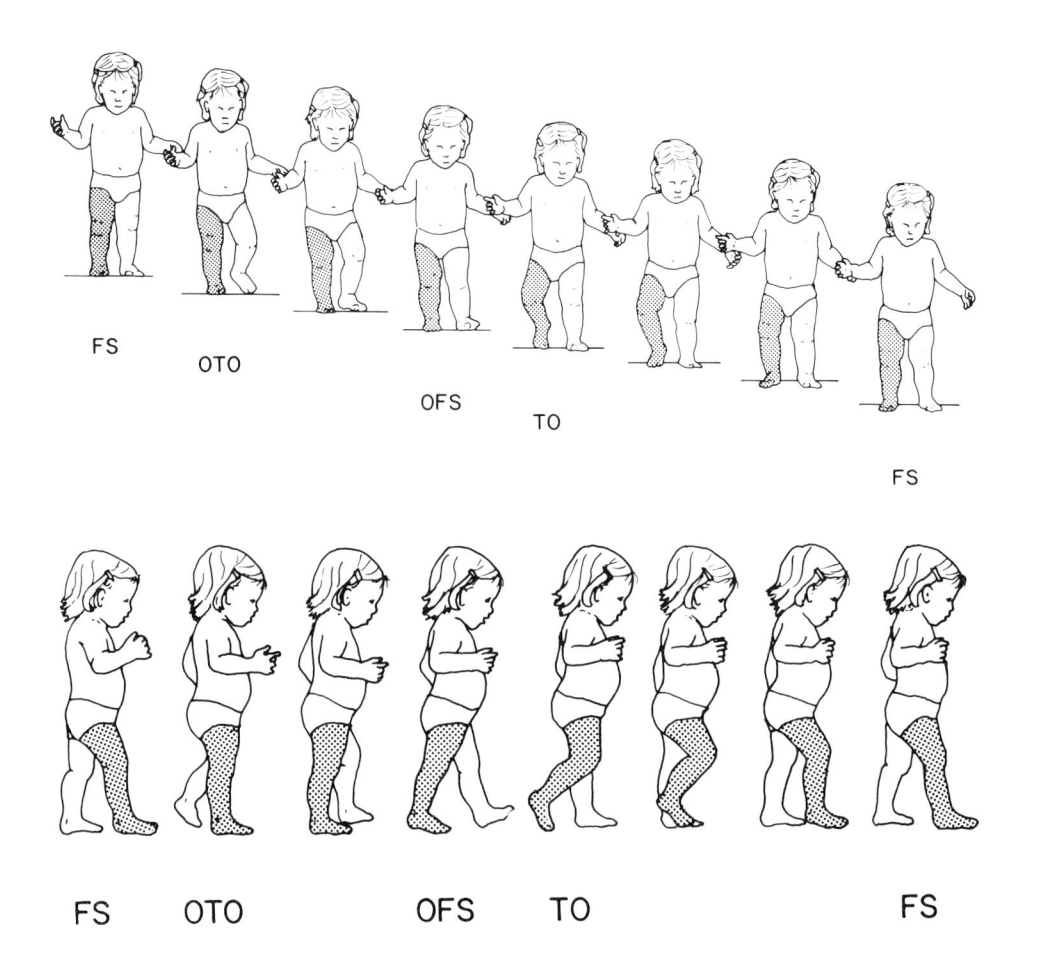

Time/distance parameters*	
Opp. toe-off (% cycle)	17
Opp. foot-strike (% cycle)	49
Single stance (% cycle)	32
Toe-off (% cycle)	67
Step length (cm)	22
Stride length (cm)	43
Cycle time (secs.)	0.68
Cadence (steps/min.)	176
Walking velocity (cm/sec.)	64
(m/min.)	38.4

*N = 31.

Fig. 7.2. Mean time/distance parameters and composite graphs of mean joint angles (right side) for 1-year-old normal subjects, plus cine-film tracings (front and right-side views) of the gait cycle of a representative 1-year-old. (FS = foot-strike; OTO = opposite toe-off; OFS = opposite foot-strike; TO = toe-off.)

Note wide base of support, outstretched arms, lack of reciprocal arm-swing, and flat foot-strike.

130

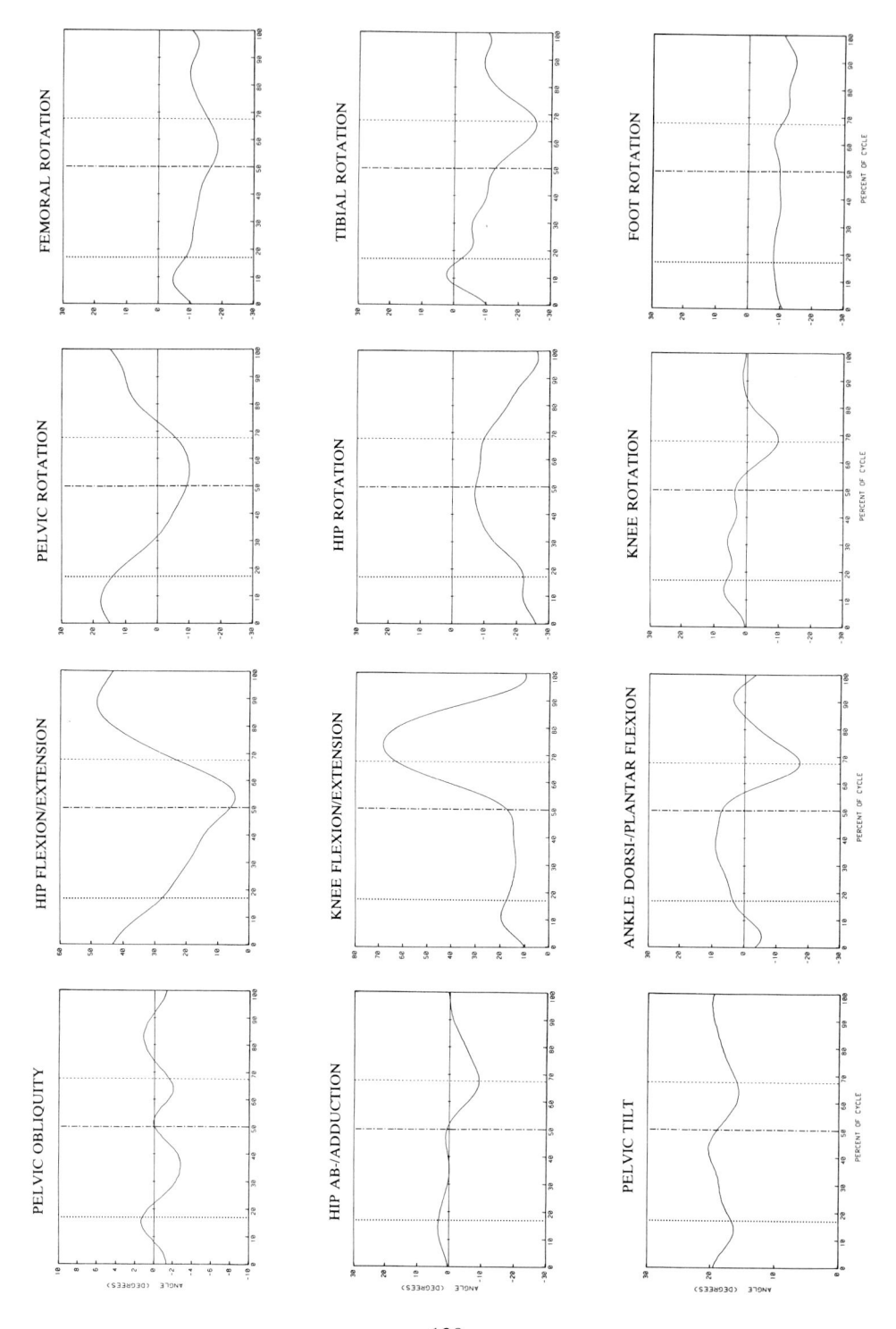

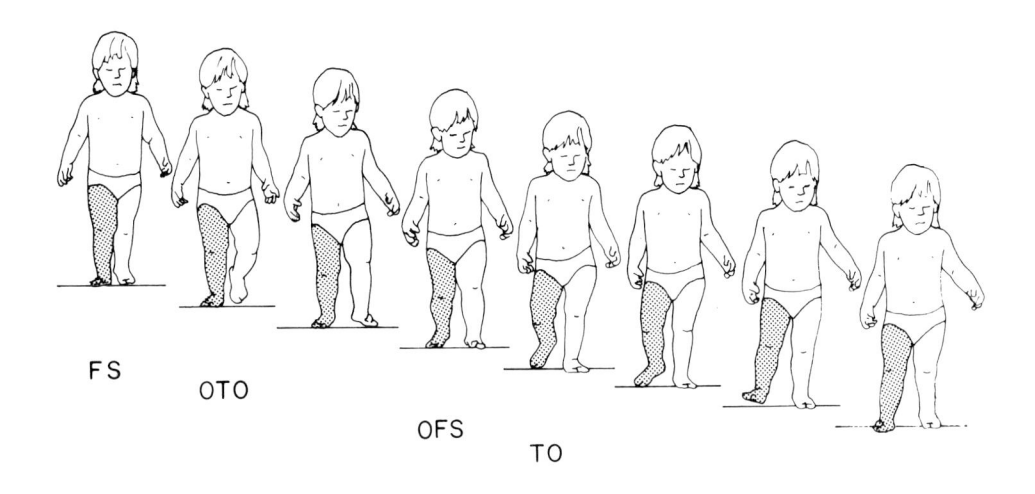

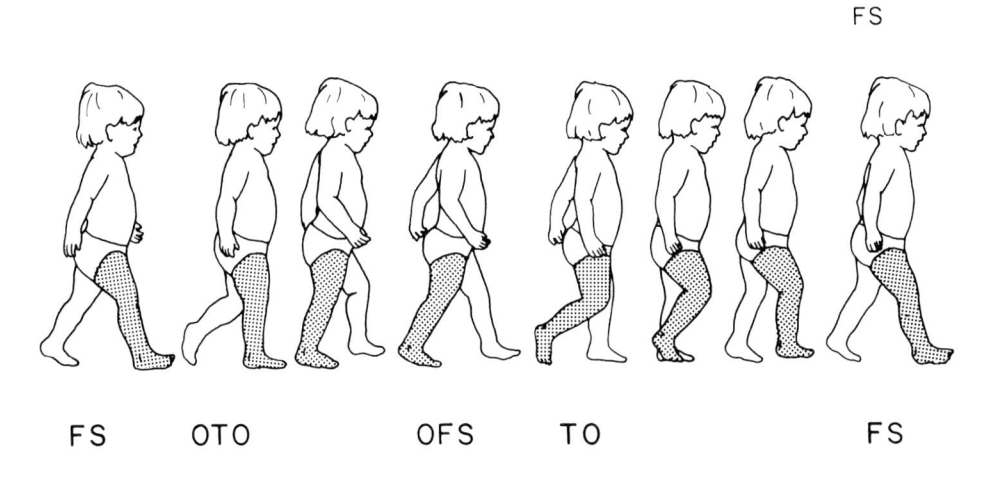

Time/distance parameters*	
Opp. toe-off (% cycle)	18
Opp. foot-strike (% cycle)	50
Single stance (% cycle)	32
Toe-off (% cycle)	68
Step length (cm)	25
Stride length (cm)	50
Cycle time (secs.)	0.70
Cadence (steps/min.)	171
Walking velocity (cm/sec.)	71
(m/min.)	42.6

*N — 40.

Fig. 7.3. Mean time/distance parameters and composite graphs of mean joint angles for 1½-year-old normal subjects, plus film tracings of representative 1½-year-old.

Note that there is much less plantar flexion at foot-strike than at age 1 year. The arms are much lower and reciprocal arm-swing is making an appearance.

132

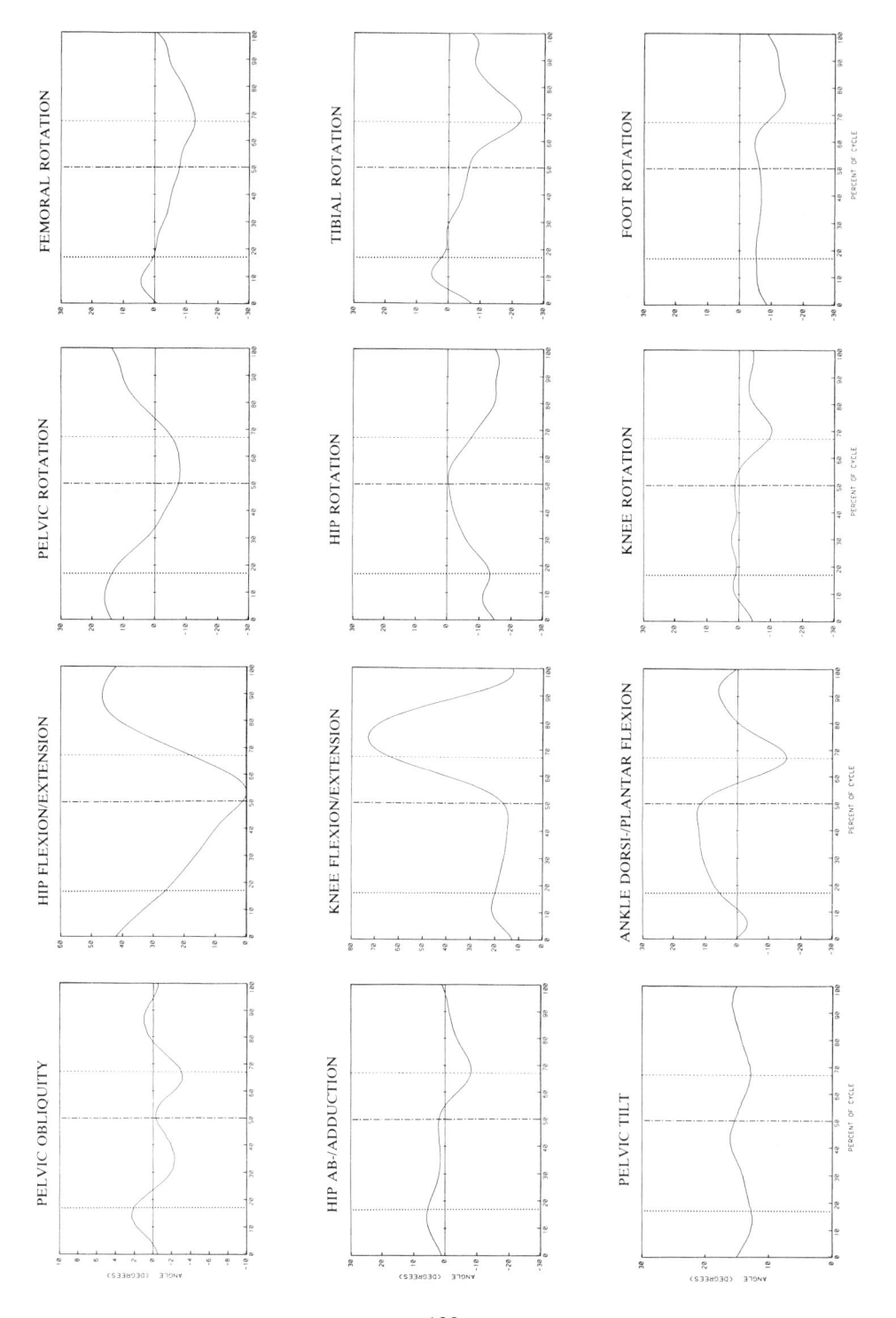

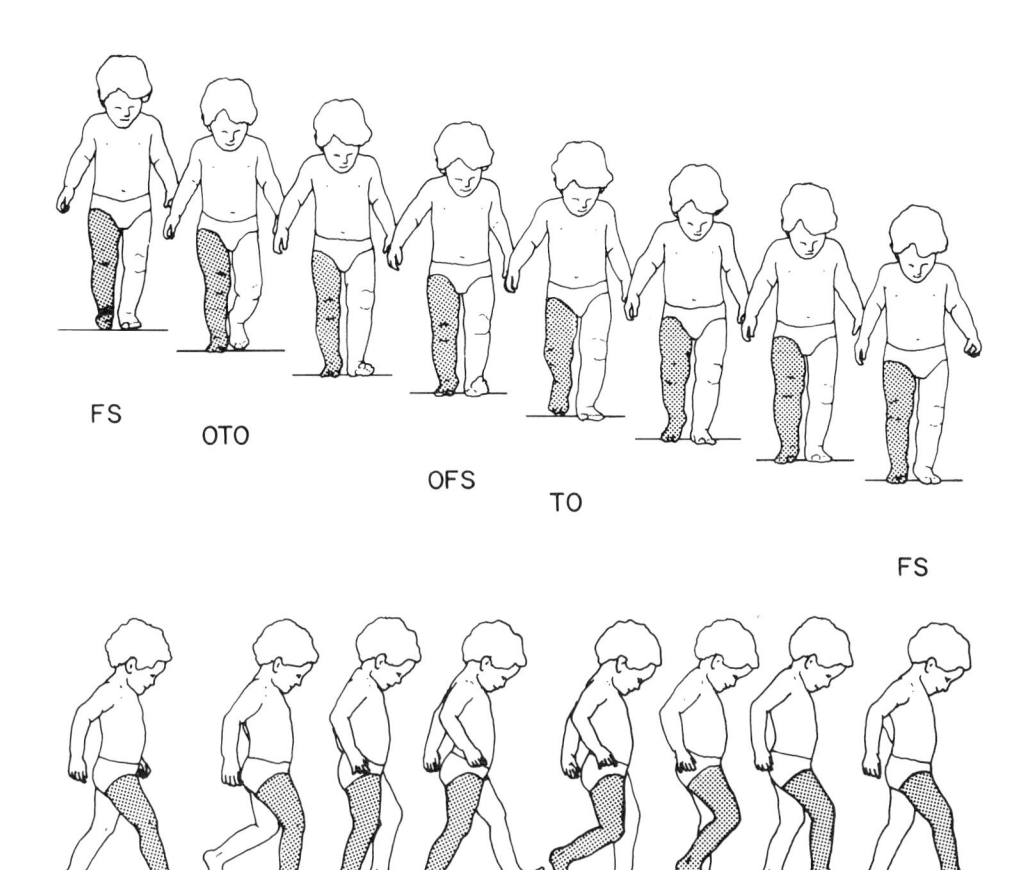

FS   OTO   OFS   TO   FS

FS   OTO   OFS   TO   FS

Time/distance parameters*	
Opp. toe-off (% cycle)	17
Opp. foot-strike (% cycle)	50
Single stance (% cycle)	34
Toe-off (% cycle)	67
Step length (cm)	28
Stride length (cm)	55
Cycle time (secs.)	0.78
Cadence (steps/min.)	156
Walking velocity (cm/sec.)	72
(m/min.)	43.2

¹N = 43.

Fig. 7.4. Mean time/distance parameters and composite graphs of mean joint angles for 2-year-old normal subjects, plus film tracings of representative 2-year-old.

Changes by comparison with the 1½-year-olds include: more clearly defined knee-flexion wave and heel-strike (plantar flexion following foot-strike), increased hip adduction in stance, and decreased external rotation of the hip.

134

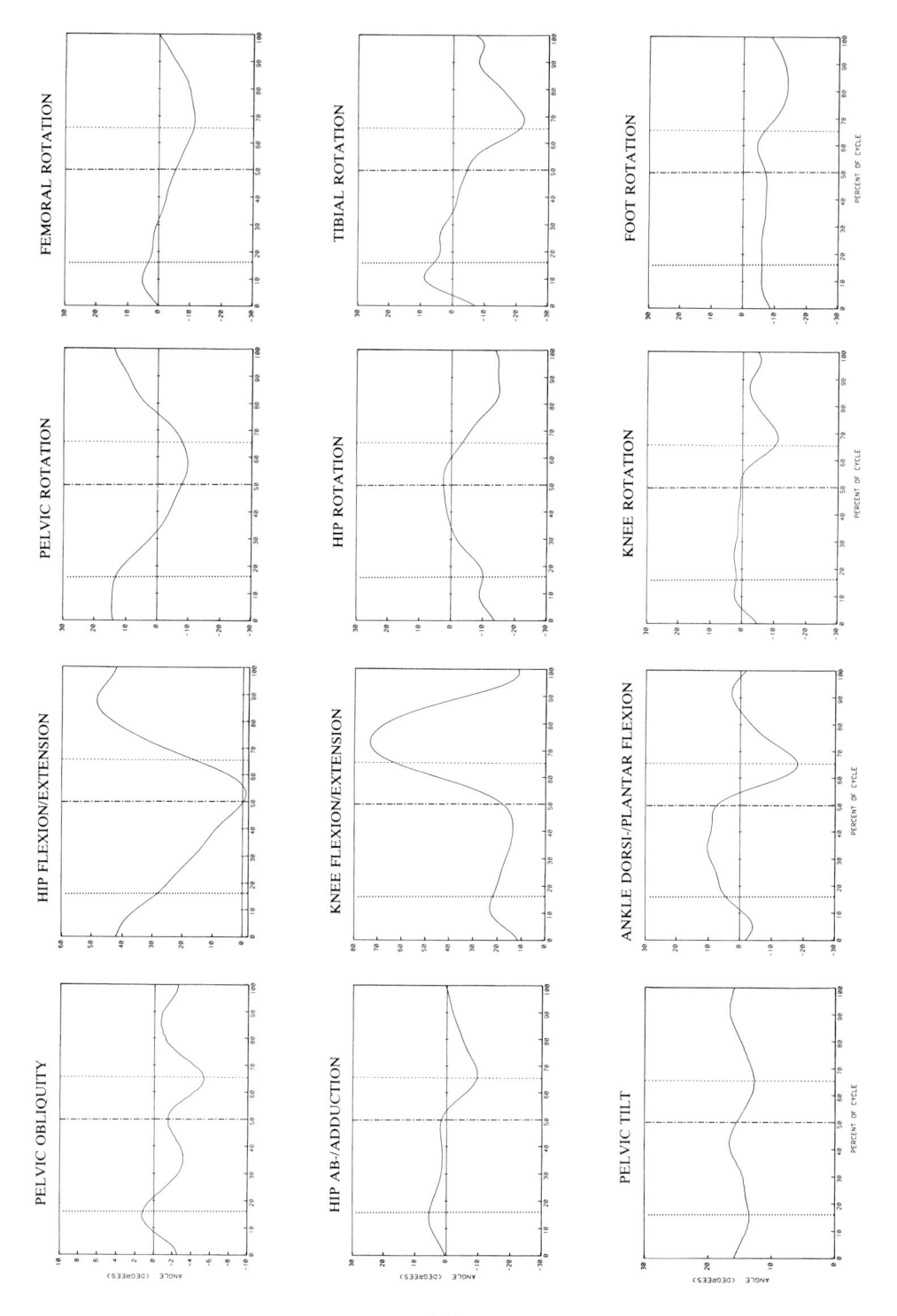

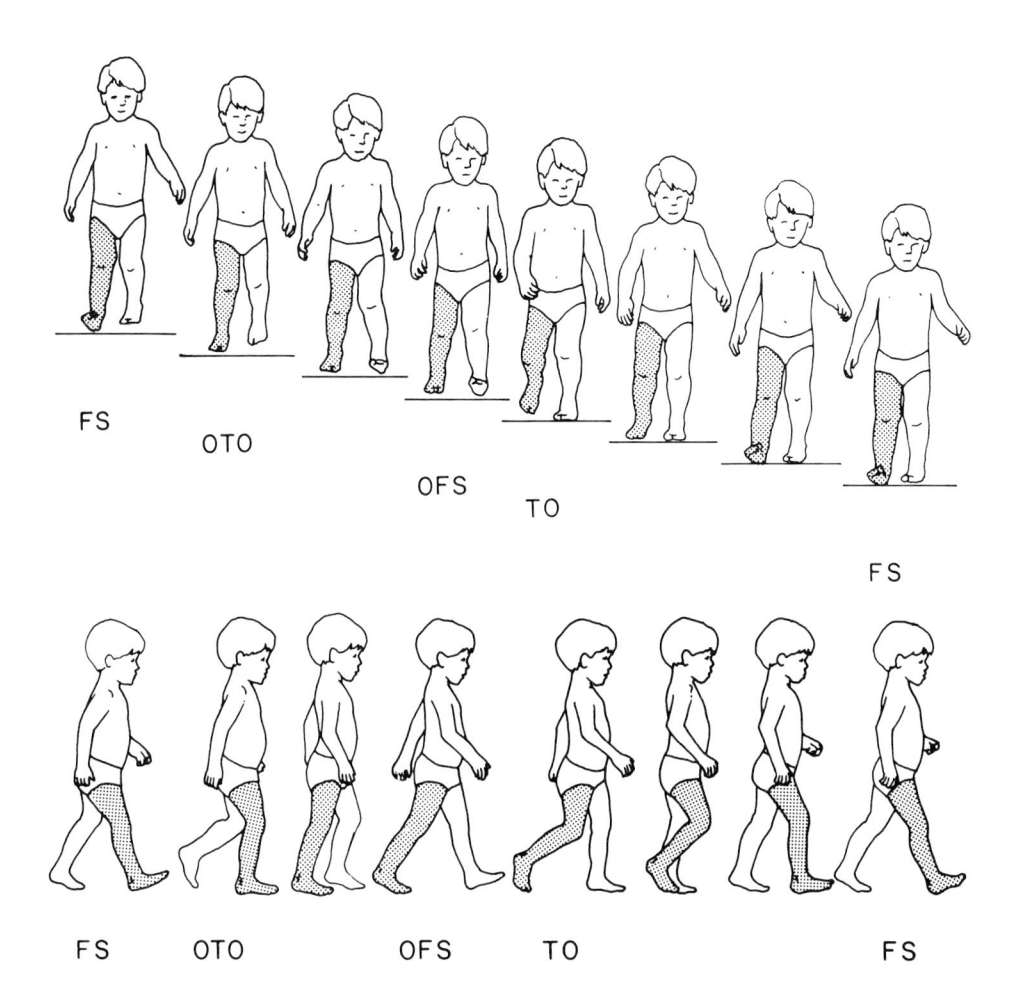

Time/distance parameters*	
Opp. toe-off (% cycle)	16
Opp. foot-strike (% cycle)	50
Single stance (% cycle)	35
Toe-off (% cycle)	66
Step length (cm)	31
Stride length (cm)	62
Cycle time (secs.)	0.77
Cadence (steps/min.)	156
Walking velocity (cm/sec.)	81
(m/min.)	48.6

*N = 36.

Fig. 7.5. Mean time/distance parameters and composite graphs of mean joint angles for 2½-year-old normal subjects, plus film tracings of representative 2½-year-old.

136

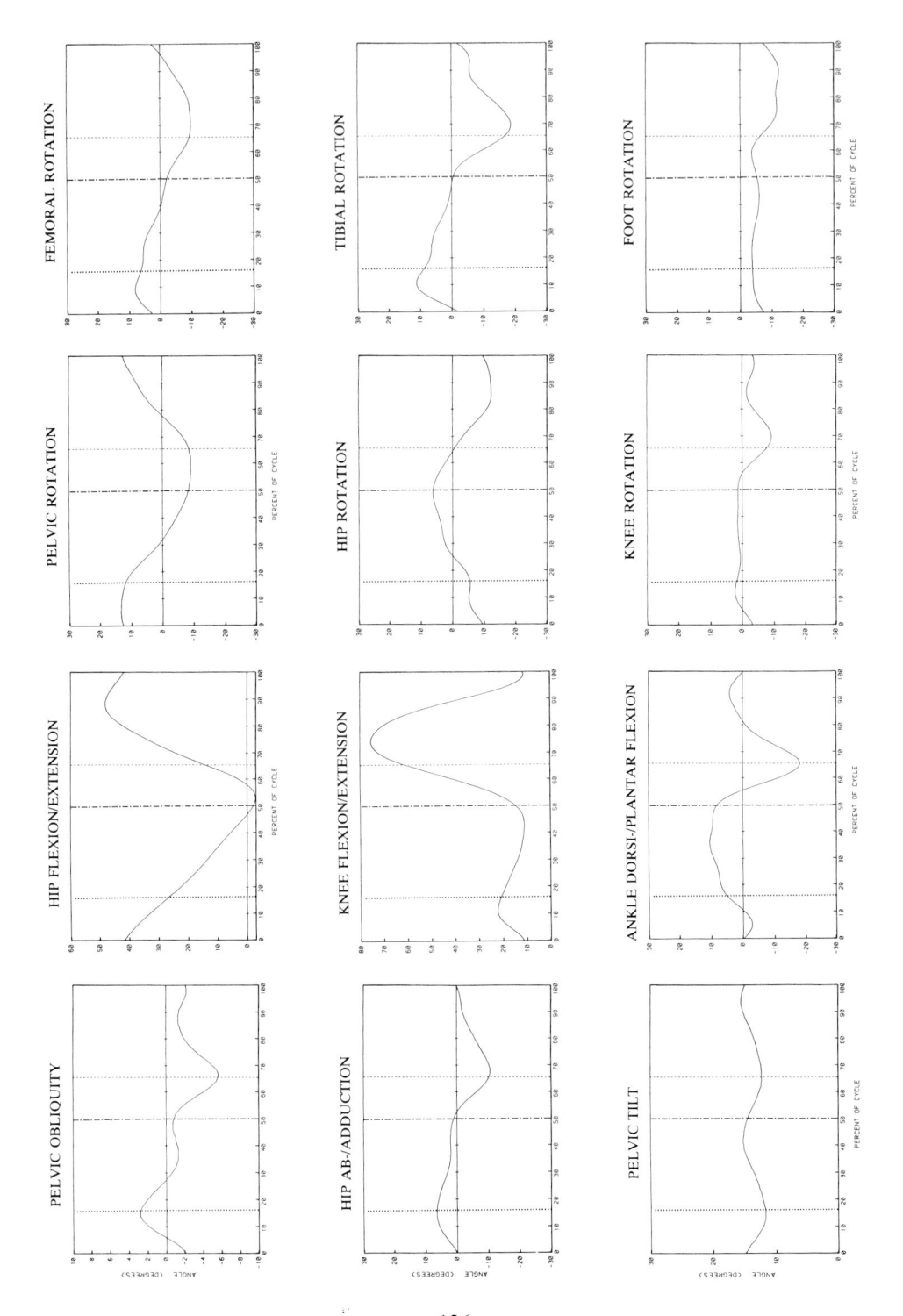

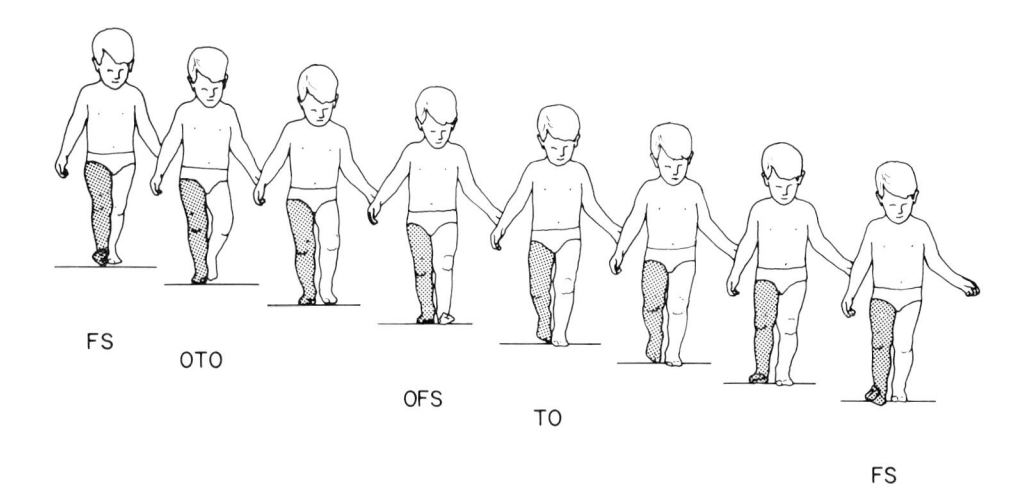

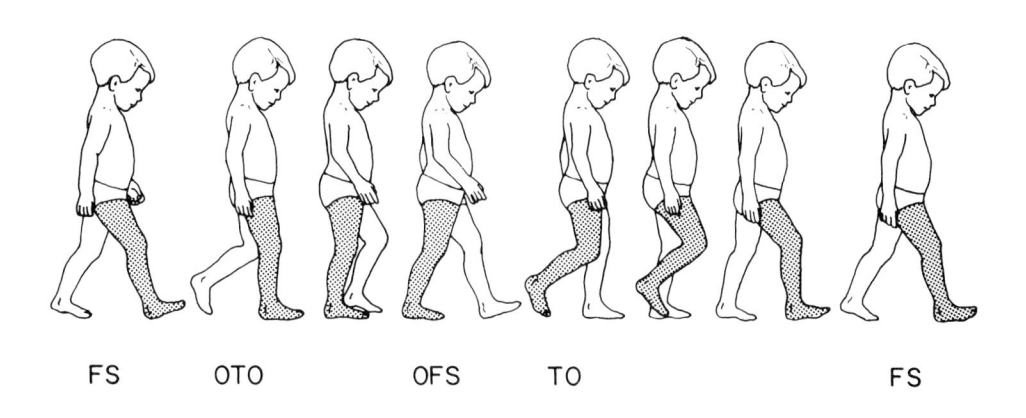

Time/distance parameters*	
Opp. toe-off (% cycle)	16
Opp. foot-strike (% cycle)	50
Single stance (% cycle)	35
Toe-off (% cycle)	66
Step length (cm)	33
Stride length (cm)	67
Cycle time (secs.)	0.77
Cadence (steps/min.)	154
Walking velocity (cm/sec.)	86
(m/min.)	51.6

Fig. 7.6. Mean time/distance parameters and composite graphs of mean joint angles for 3-year-old normal subjects, plus film tracings of representative 3-year-old.

*N = 47.

138

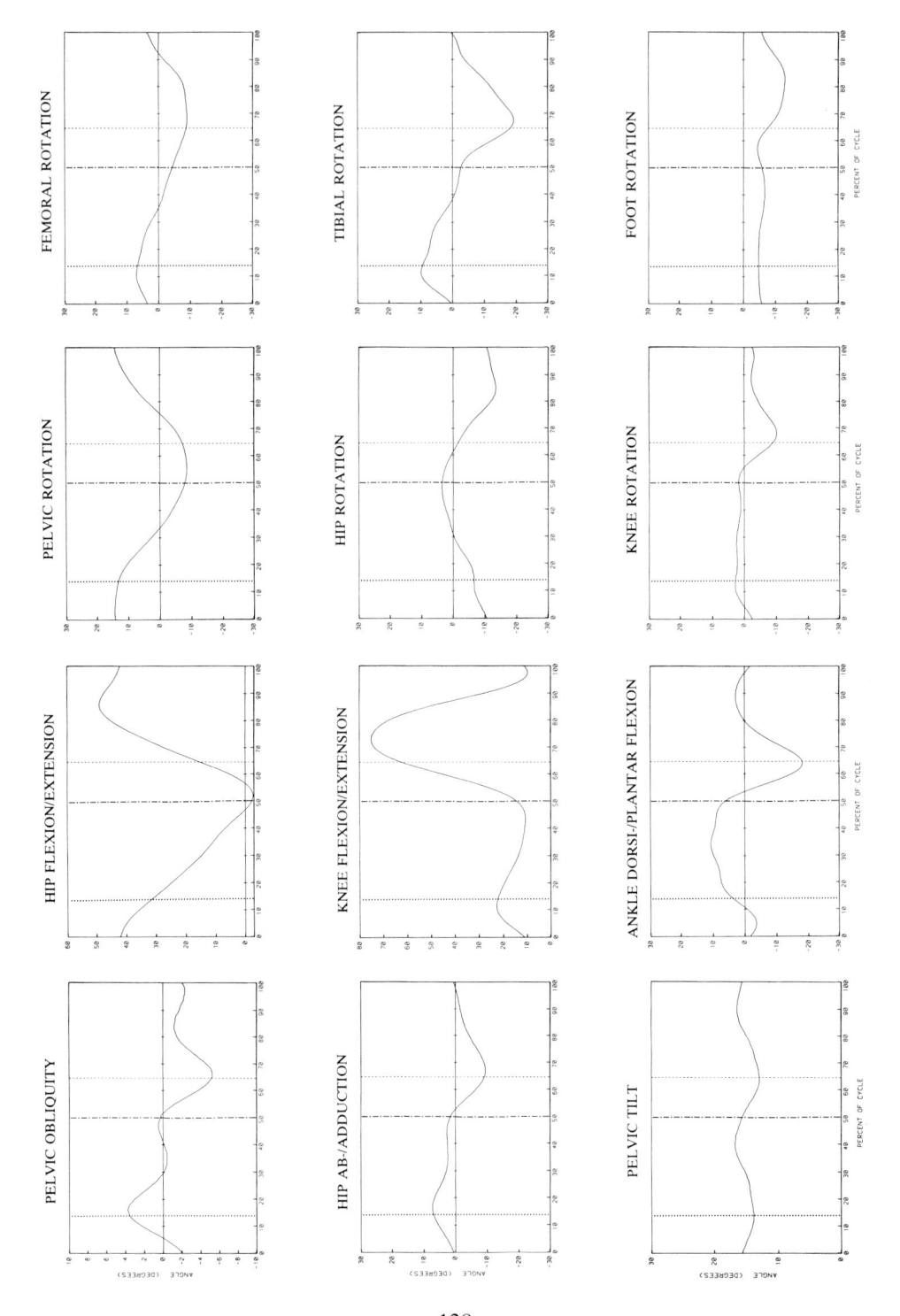

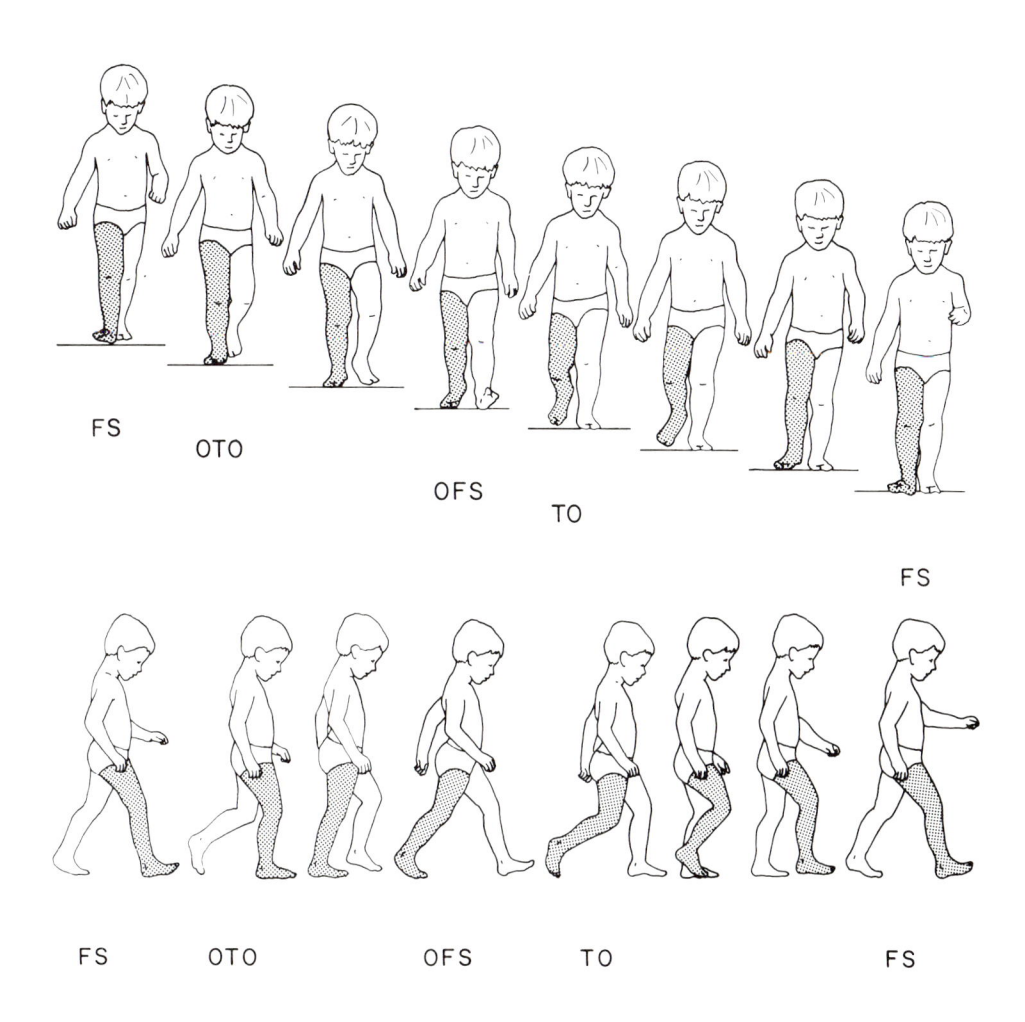

Time/distance parameters*	
Opp. toe-off (% cycle)	14
Opp. foot-strike (% cycle)	50
Single stance (% cycle)	36
Toe-off (% cycle)	65
Step length (cm)	37
Stride length (cm)	74
Cycle time (secs.)	0.74
Cadence (steps/min.)	160
Walking velocity (cm/sec.)	99
(m/min.)	59.4

*N = 40.

Fig. 7.7. Mean time/distance parameters and composite graphs of mean joint angles for 3½-year-old normal subjects, plus film tracings of representative 3½-year-old.

140

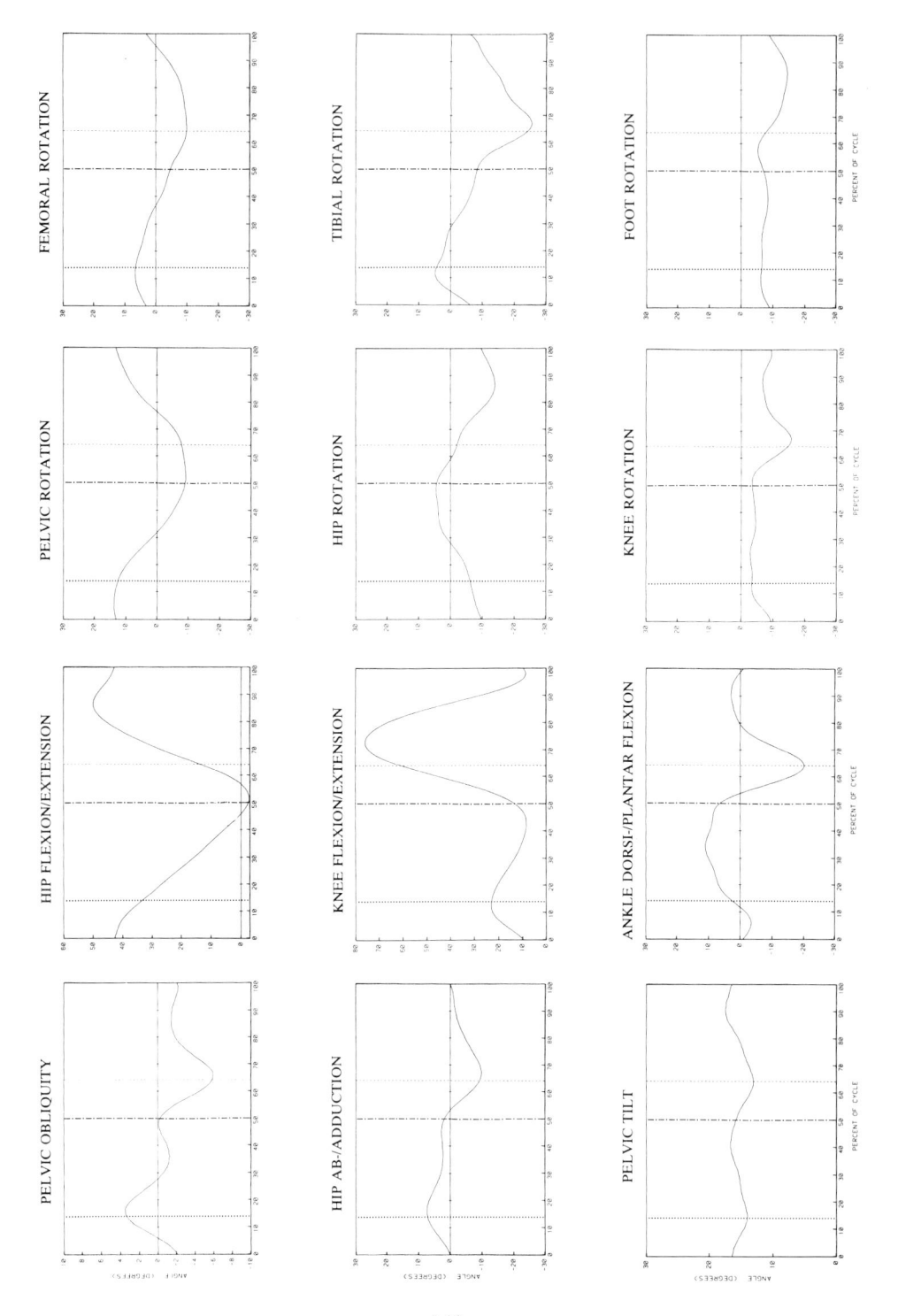

Fig. 7.8. Mean time/distance parameters and composite graphs of mean joint angles for 4-year-old normal subjects, plus film tracings of representative 4-year-old.

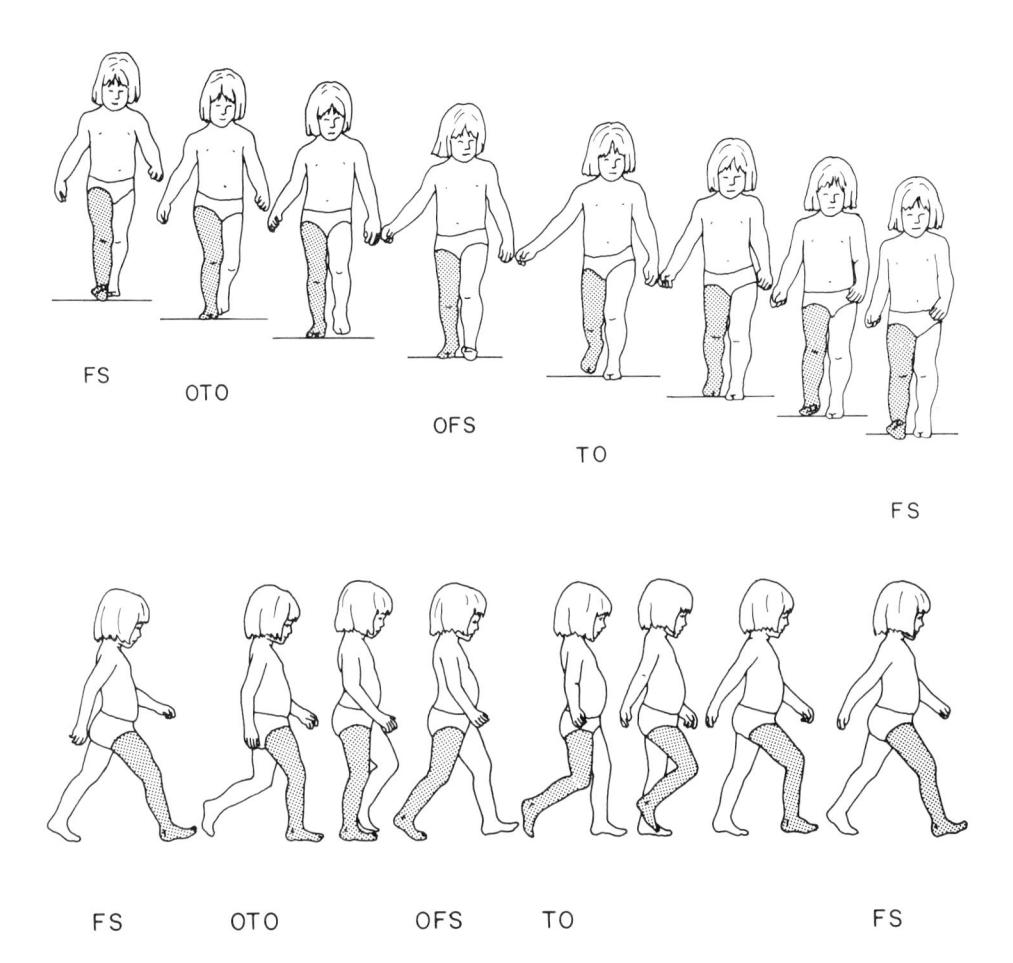

Time/distance parameters*	
Opp. toe-off (% cycle)	14
Opp. foot-strike (% cycle)	50
Single stance (% cycle)	36
Toe-off (% cycle)	64
Step length (cm)	39
Stride length (cm)	78
Cycle time (secs.)	0.78
Cadence (steps/min.)	152
Walking velocity (cm/sec.)	99
(m/min.)	59.4

*N = 39.

142

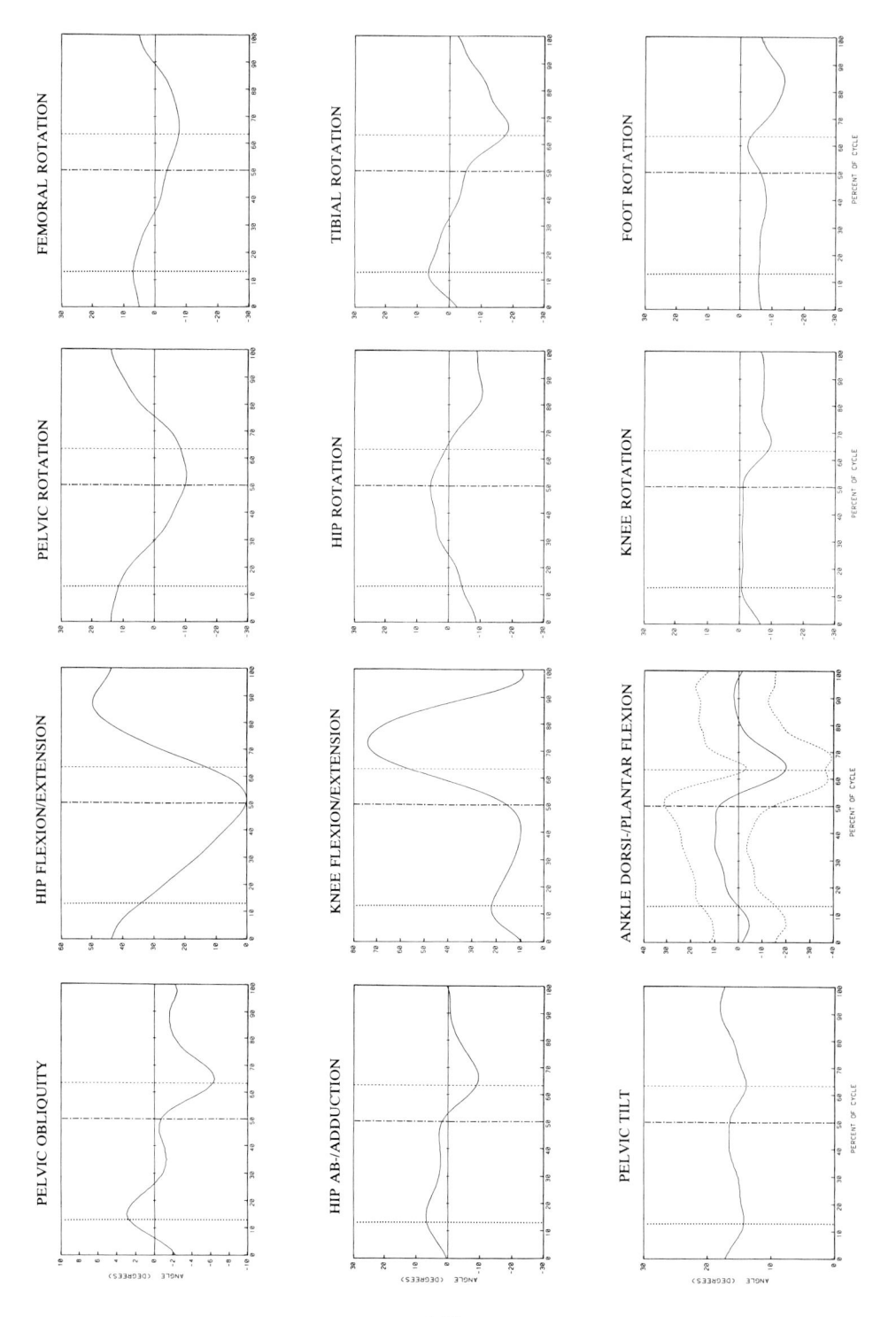

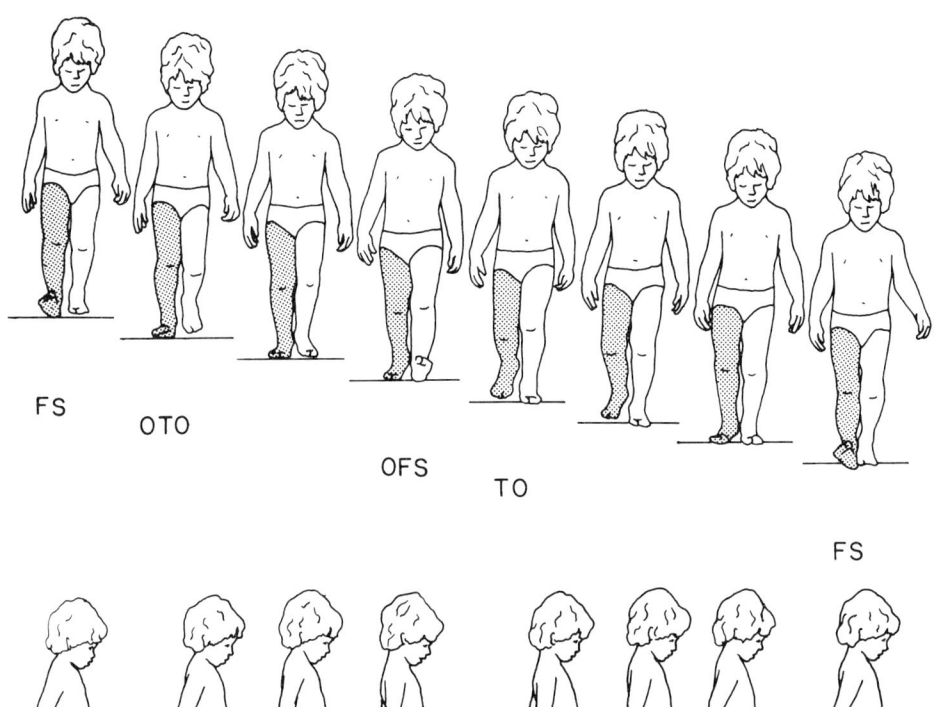

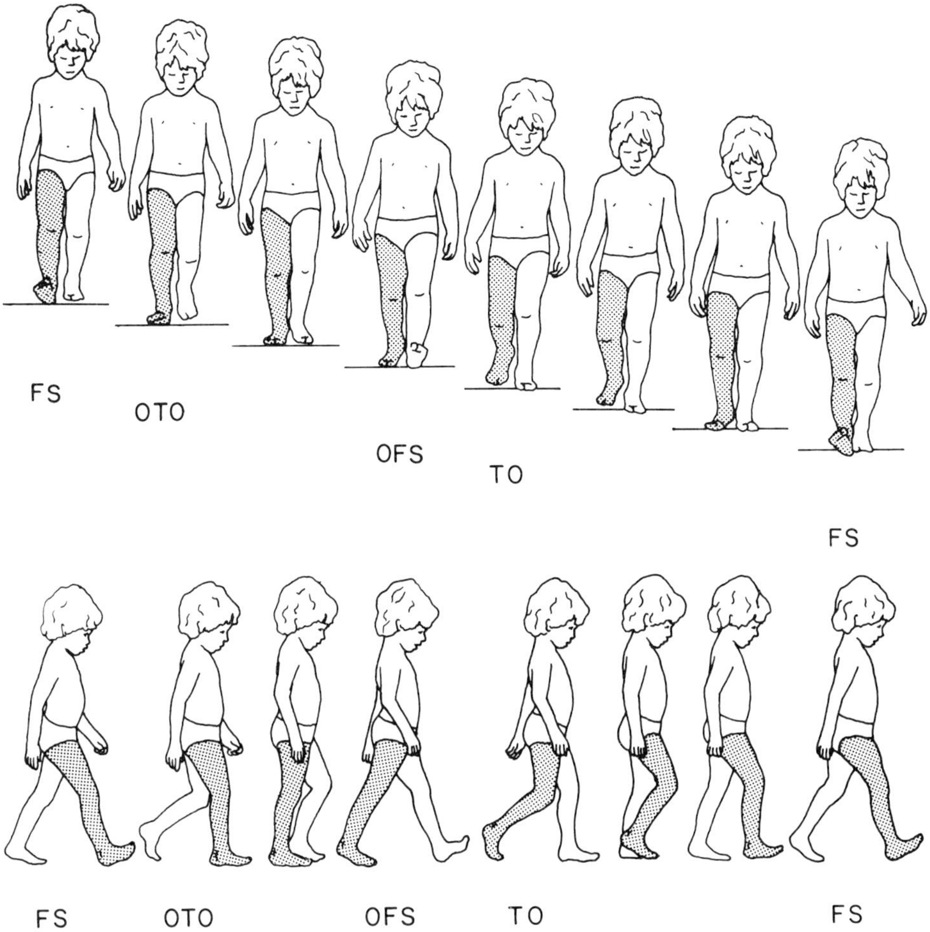

FS OTO OFS TO FS

FS OTO OFS TO FS

Time/distance parameters*	
Opp. toe-off (% cycle)	13
Opp. foot-strike (% cycle)	50
Single stance (% cycle)	37
Toe-off (% cycle)	63
Step length (cm)	42
Stride length (cm)	84
Cycle time (secs.)	0.77
Cadence (steps/min.)	153
Walking velocity (cm/sec.)	108
(m/min.)	64.8

*N = 42.

Fig. 7.9. Mean time/distance parameters and composite graphs of mean joint angles for 5-year-old normal subjects, plus film tracings of representative 5-year-old.

144

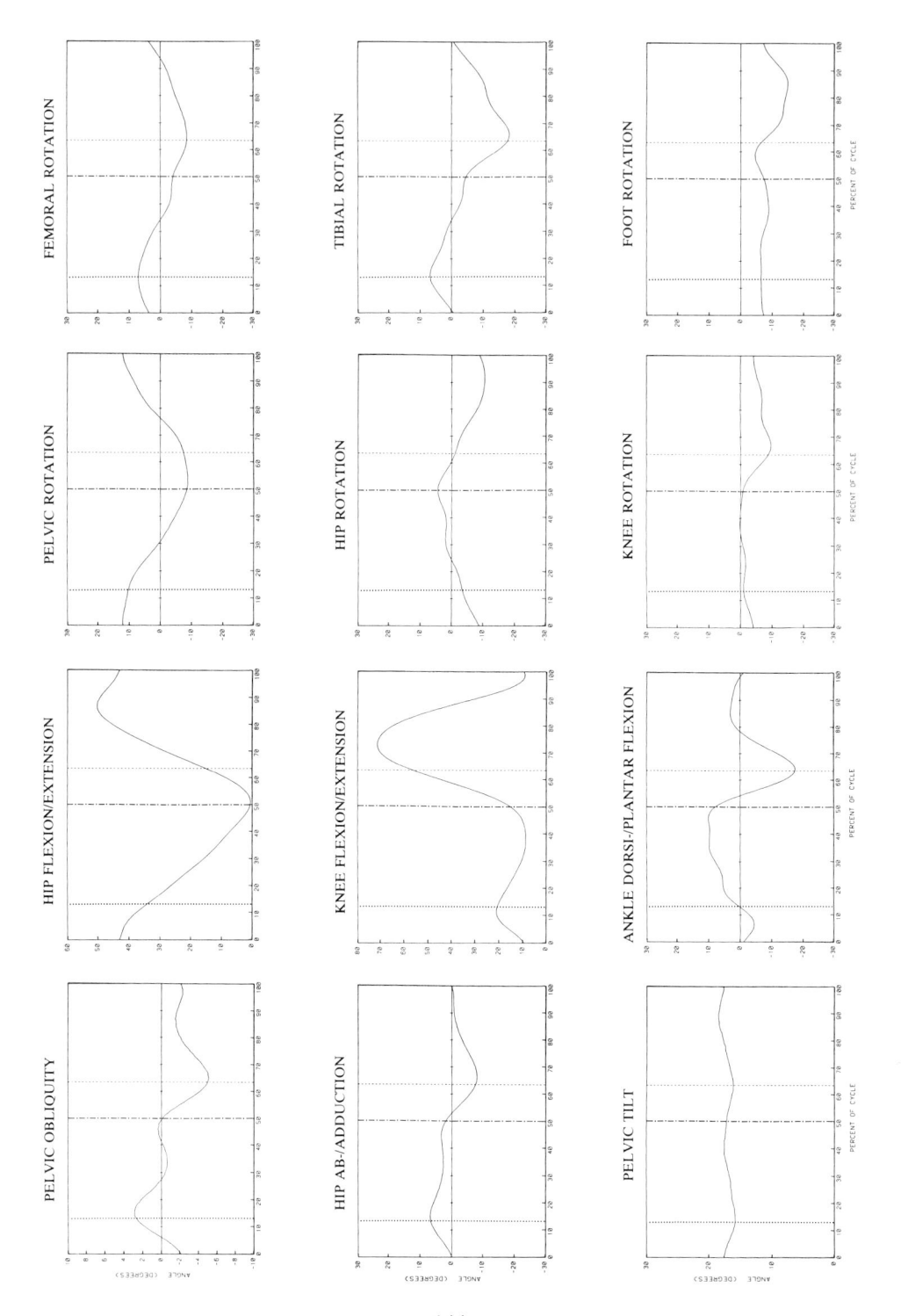

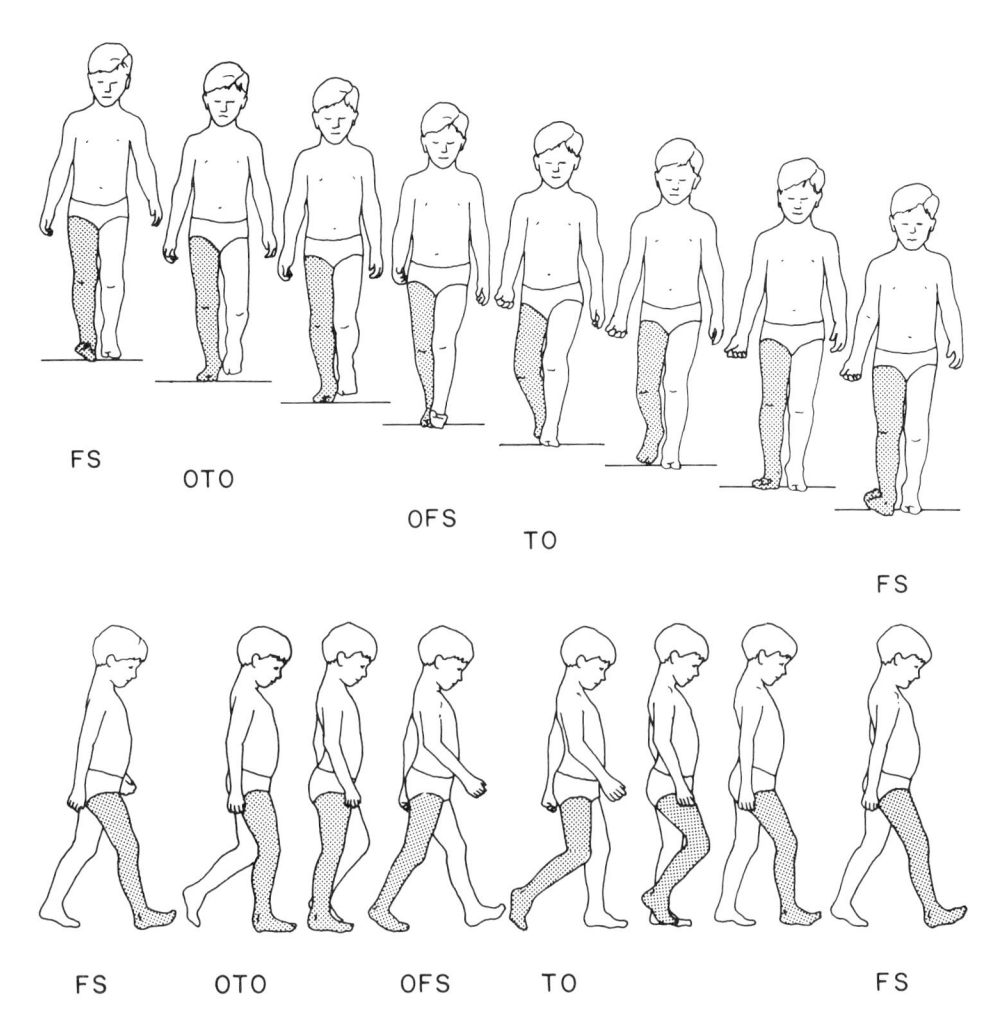

Time/distance parameters*	
Opp. toe-off (% cycle)	13
Opp. foot-strike (% cycle)	50
Single stance (% cycle)	37
Toe-off (% cycle)	64
Step length (cm)	44
Stride length (cm)	89
Cycle time (secs.)	0.82
Cadence (steps/min.)	146
Walking velocity (cm/sec.)	109
(m/min.)	65.4

*N = 44.

Fig. 7.10. Mean time/distance parameters and composite graphs of mean joint angles for 6-year-old normal subjects, plus film tracings of representative 6-year-old.

146

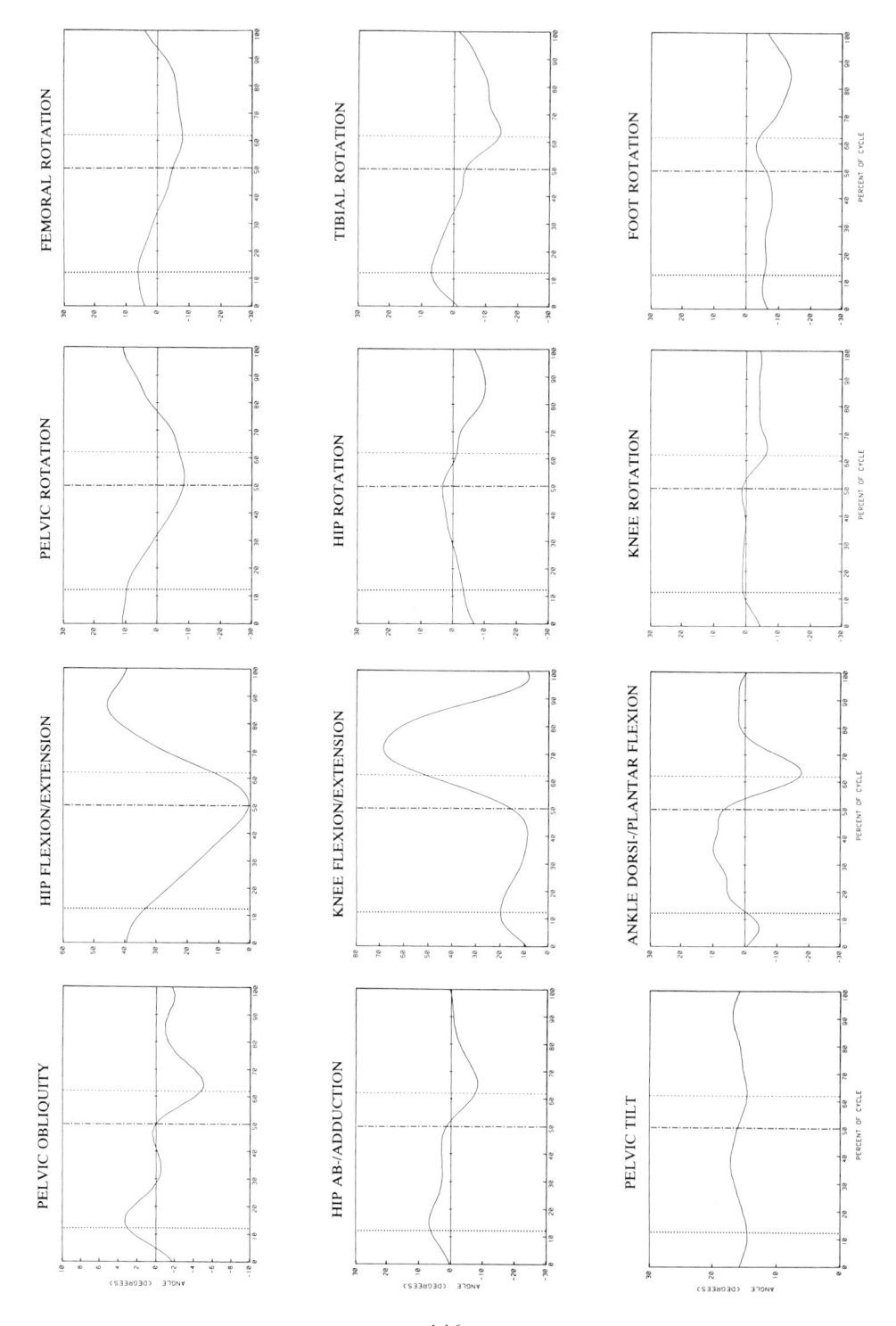

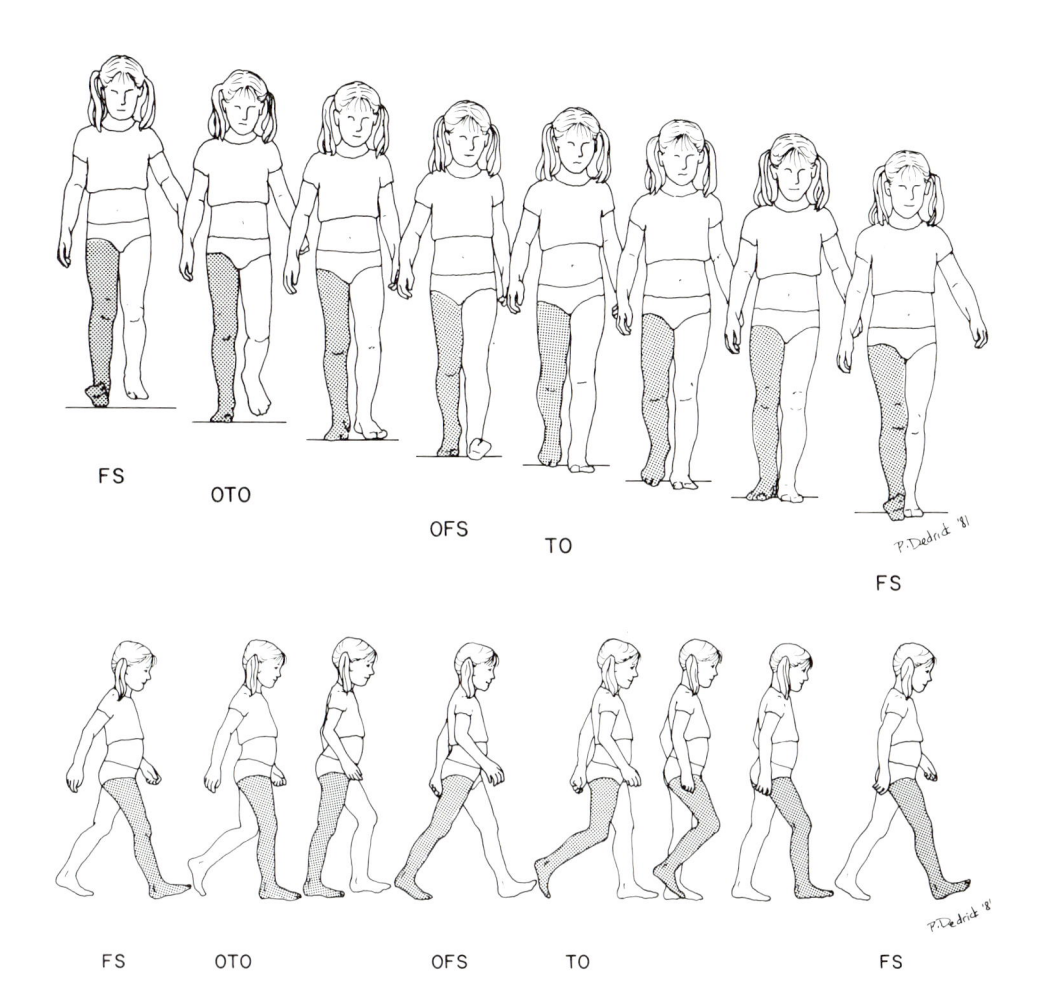

Time/distance parameters*	
Opp. toe-off (% cycle)	12
Opp. foot-strike (% cycle)	50
Single stance (% cycle)	38
Toe-off (% cycle)	62
Step length (cm)	48
Stride length (cm)	97
Cycle time (secs.)	0.83
Cadence (steps/min.)	144
Walking velocity (cm/sec.)	114
(m/min)	68.4

*N = 46.

Fig. 7.11. Mean time/distance parameters and composite graphs of mean joint angles for 7-year-old normal subjects, plus film tracings of representative 7-year-old.

HIP FLEXION/EXTENSION

Sagittal-plane movement of the hip is a very simple progressive flexion during swing phase and extension during stance phase. The change, however, occurs at opposite foot-strike; thus flexion begins during second double support. Peak flexion occurs at 85 per cent of the cycle, diminishing by approximately 5° at foot-strike. Changes with respect to age are rather minor. The dynamic range of motion in the 1, 1½ and 2 year age-groups is 9° less than for the older children.

Hip flexion begins with action of the iliopsoas and rectus femoris muscles. The gluteus maximus and hamstring muscles contribute to hip extension in late swing phase. Both continue to be active for a short period during stance, but this activity does not persist long enough to account for the continuation of hip extension until opposite foot-strike. This, therefore, must be attributed to gravity and inertia.

The line of application of the ground-reaction force falls behind the hip joint at approximately 28 per cent of the gait cycle (Skinner *et al.* 1985). If this time is expressed as a percentage of stance phase rather than of the gait cycle as a whole, it can then be contrasted with the time of cessation of gluteus maximus activity (see Chapter 8). As can be seen in Figure 8.6 (p. 159), this activity ceases at between 40 and 45 per cent of stance phase. This compares with a time for ground-reaction force falling behind the hip of 44 per cent (Skinner *et al.* 1985). Passage of the force line behind the hip best explains the further extension of the hip after cessation of EMG activity in the gluteus maximus.

KNEE FLEXION/EXTENSION

The first knee-flexion wave is the result of an eccentric contraction of the quadriceps during the early part of stance phase. The purpose of this movement is to act as a shock absorber, producing a more gradual elevation of the body's center of mass and reducing the energy requirement for walking (Inman *et al.* 1981). The second and much stronger flexion wave begins well before toe-off in preparation for advancement of the limb.

There is a hint of an initial knee-flexion wave in the 1-year-olds but the motion is not fully developed until the age of 3 or 4 years. The range of flexion can most easily be seen in the graphs with the α_0 terms retained.

In the 1-year-olds the knee is flexed 10° at foot-strike. There is a very small increase in flexion with incomplete return to the foot-strike position. By 1½ years flexion following foot-strike has increased by 4° or 5° and return to the original degree of flexion, though as yet incomplete, has increased. Thus there is a flexion wave, though qualitatively it is immature. At 2 years, children show a further increase in the knee-flexion wave in stance, and in swing it is indistinguishable from the adult form. 3-year-olds demonstrate a slightly greater knee extension following initial flexion, and by 4 years subjects show a totally mature knee-flexion wave in stance phase. No significant change occurs in knee movements from this time on.

ANKLE DORSIFLEXION/PLANTAR FLEXION

Ankle motion in mature walking is represented by a complex curve with two peaks and two valleys. The first valley is produced by ankle plantar flexion immediately following foot-strike. This section of the curve is missing in the 1-year-olds and is only slightly developed in the 1½-year-olds. Plantar flexion is dependent on heel-strike which is missing in the 1-year-olds (who strike flat-footed) and transitory or absent in the 1½-year-olds (Sutherland *et al.* 1980*a*). After the foot-flat position, ankle dorsiflexion proceeds through much of single-limb stance, peaking at around 40 per cent of the cycle. The direction of motion then reverses, ankle-joint acceleration begins, and dorsiflexion slowly diminishes until opposite foot-strike. Rapid plantar flexion follows, reaching a maximum at toe-off. There is no EMG activity in the ankle plantar flexors during this phase, and it seems very likely that the motion is entirely passive. If any muscle activity is contributing to the plantar flexion, it could only arise from the continuation of muscle tension after the cessation of EMG activity.

The dynamic range of motion over the 10 age-groups varies between 23° at age 1 and 31° at age 4. If the 1 and 1½ year age-groups are excluded, the average dynamic range of motion is 29°. Thus there is an increase of approximately 6° in the dynamic range of motion after the age of 1½ years.

Transverse plane
PELVIC ROTATION
The dynamic range of pelvic rotation varies only slightly across the 10 age-groups. As the swinging limb is advanced, the pelvis rotates internally. Peak internal rotation occurs slightly after foot-strike. With load acceptance, the pelvis begins a counter-rotation (external) about the weight-bearing femur, continuing to opposite foot-strike when internal rotation begins again. There is a trend toward a lower dynamic range of motion over the age of 3 years.

FEMORAL ROTATION
Dynamic rotation of the femur in the transverse plane occurs in two phases. From toe-off to opposite toe-off it rotates internally. Then the direction reverses and external rotation occurs until following toe-off.

Average external rotation of the femur at foot-strike (before removal of the α_0 term) is $-20°$ at 1 year, $-10°$ at 1½, neutral at 2 and 2½, $+3°$ at 3 and 3½, $+8°$ at 4 and 5, and $+4°$ at 6 and 7 years. In spite of these changes in the relative position of the femur through the various age-groups, the dynamic range of rotation varies very little throughout. It is slightly less at 1 year and 1½ years: the average for these two groups is 13°, compared with 17.5° across the remaining age-groups. Although there is greater external rotation at ages 1 and 1½, passive internal rotation is comparatively limited in these age-groups.

The influence of toe-off on femoral rotation is obvious. Peak external rotation occurs at toe-off in all age-groups except the 1-year-olds, in whom external rotation peaks slightly before toe-off.

HIP ROTATION
The walk cycle begins with the hip in external rotation. Progressive internal rotation follows, peaking at opposite foot-strike. The direction then changes and

external rotation continues through roughly half of swing phase until internal rotation begins again.

The dynamic range of motion across all age-groups is approximately 15°. External rotation in stance phase is much greater between the ages of 1 and 2 years. At 1 year the right hip is externally rotated about 35° at foot-strike; at age 1½, 25°; at 2, 15°; at 2½, 13°; thereafter there is very little change. As with femoral rotation, the range of hip external rotation is greater in the younger age-groups. This correlates with the changes seen in the passive range of motion of the hip (see Chapter 5, pp. 37–38). Passive external rotation of the hip exceeds internal rotation at birth, and a progressive decrease in the range of external rotation occurs between 1 and 3 years of age. This could be explained by either acetabular retroversion or soft-tissue constraints which limit internal rotation in the younger age-groups. Femoral retroversion cannot be a cause, however, because the femur is maximally anteverted in the earliest years of life.

After removal of the α_0 term the motion curves for all age-groups are remarkably similar.

TIBIAL ROTATION

During the loading phase of initial double-limb support the tibia rotates internally. This, coupled with the unique 'miter hinge' relationship of the tibia to the subtalar joint, produces pronation in early stance (Inman *et al.* 1981). Following loading, the tibia externally rotates until toe-off, then internally rotates until foot-strike. As with femoral rotation, there are two phases of motion during a gait cycle: internal rotation from toe-off through swing phase into initial double support (approximately 10 to 13 per cent of the gait cycle), then external rotation until following toe-off.

The range of motion is remarkably constant across all age-groups in terms of total dynamic range of movement, peak internal rotation and peak external rotation.

External rotation is greater in the three youngest age-groups. This tendency can be seen in the curves without prediction regions. There is a similar tendency with regard to hip external rotation in these age-groups. This correlation suggests that external tibial rotation arises in the hip. (Evidence of exaggerated hip external rotation has been discussed in Chapter 5.)

KNEE ROTATION

Knee rotation occurs in two phases, with an intervening period of minimal movement. Internal rotation begins at around toe-off and ends at around opposite toe-off. There is then a plateau of little movement until opposite foot-strike, when external rotation begins, continuing to around following toe-off. The pattern of movement is similar at all ages, with a dynamic range of motion of approximately 10°.

FOOT ROTATION

Foot-strike normally occurs with the foot in external rotation. During initial double support this external rotation diminishes slightly as weight is distributed over the entire foot. No appreciable change occurs then until heel-off, when external rotation again decreases. Foot rotation subsequently follows a sinusoidal pattern, moving into external rotation through the first half of swing phase and turning inward again until foot-strike.

The average dynamic range of foot rotation in the transverse plane is about 10° for nearly all age-groups. The only exceptions are at 1 year (8°) and 6 years (12°). Since these two groups are virtually at opposite ends of the age-range, we are unable to attach any significance to their slight deviation.

There are several qualitative changes in the pattern of movement which permit descriptions of a 'mature' and an 'immature' pattern: (1) at age 1 only, there is no internal rotation during second double support; (2) there is irregularity during swing phase up to the age of 2½; (3) greater external rotation is evident at 1 year, diminishing gradually until age 2; (4) up to 1½ years the prediction regions are quite broad, emphasizing the greater variability in foot rotation in the youngest children.

Relationship of gait events to joint-angle changes

There are a number of constant relationships between gait-cycle events and joint angles which should be appreciated. Toe-off comes at maximum plantar flexion. Opposite foot-strike always occurs at 50 per cent of the cycle, coinciding closely with maximum hip extension, maximum external rotation of the pelvis and maximum internal rotation of the hip. Maximum hip abduction is at toe-off, and maximum hip adduction is closely related to opposite toe-off.

The greatest correlations between events and motion curves appear to be in: (1) the abrupt change from ankle plantar flexion to ankle dorsiflexion at toe-off; (2) the peaks of hip adduction at opposite toe-off and opposite foot-strike; and (3) peak abduction of the hip at toe-off. Opposite toe-off appears to exert less effect on joint-angle changes than opposite foot-strike and toe-off. Hip extension is complete at opposite foot-strike but there is a flat area in the curve for a time after this.

We conclude from these observations that gait events impose motions which are resisted by muscles. The sequence of joint flexion or muscle shortening to advance the limb is: knee—hip—ankle. By concentrating on the movements linked to gait events we can use the insights gained from these studies to understand the effect of inappropriate muscle control in children with gait impairment.

Indicators of gait maturation

It would be convenient if there were signs of gait maturity that could be observed easily without resort to sophisticated gait analysis. The presence of heel-strike, knee-flexion wave and reciprocal arm-swing have sometimes been used as a gauge of maturity, but because all these indicators appear very early they are of only limited value (Sutherland *et al.* 1980*a*). Their presence does not necessarily indicate maturation; however, persistent absence of any of these features in a child of 2 years or older may be a highly significant pointer to pathological gait.

Five important determinants of mature gait are: duration of single-limb stance, walking velocity, cadence, step length, and the ratio of pelvic span to ankle spread (Sutherland *et al.* 1980*a*). All require the use of measurement techniques. We give

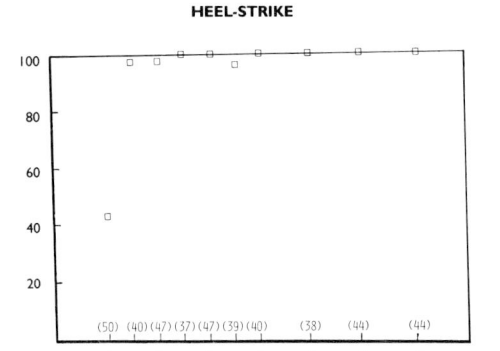

HEEL-STRIKE

KNEE-FLEXION WAVE

Fig. 7.12. Percentage of subjects showing right heel-strike in each of the 10 age-groups studied. Numbers of subjects in each age-group are given in parentheses along the horizontal axis.

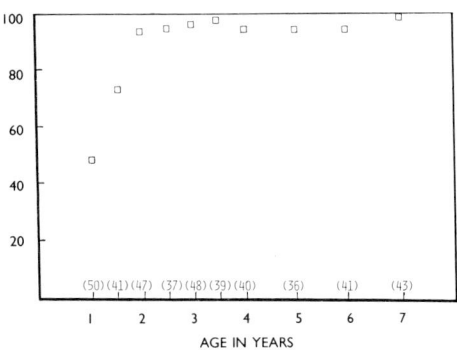

Fig. 7.13. Percentage of subjects showing a knee-flexion wave in each of the 10 age-groups studied. Numbers of subjects in each age-group are given in parentheses along the horizontal axis.

here the results of our tests for the presence of heel-strike, knee-flexion wave and reciprocal arm-swing, and for the ratio of pelvic span to ankle spread. In Chapter 10 we will re-examine the question of gait maturity, aided by a larger data base and by newly developed statistical techniques.

Heel-strike
Less than one-half of the 1-year-olds demonstrated heel-strike, but by 1½ years it was present in nearly all subjects (Fig. 7.12).

Knee-flexion wave
Slightly less than one-half of the 1-year-olds demonstrated a knee-flexion wave; by 1½ years the proportion had risen to approximately 75 per cent. A knee-flexion wave was established in most subjects of 2 years and older (Fig. 7.13).

Reciprocal arm-swing
In mature gait, the leg and contralateral arm move forward in synchrony. None of our 1-year-olds had yet developed this feature. By 1½ years it was demonstrated by approximately 65 per cent of subjects. Between 2 and 3½ years the proportion rose from around 92 to 98 per cent, and the feature was universal from 4 years upwards (Fig. 7.14).

Pelvic-span/ankle-spread ratio
Pelvic span is the body width, in the coronal plane, at the level of the anterior superior iliac spines. Ankle spread is the distance, in the coronal plane, between the left and right ankle centers during double-limb support. Figure 7.15 clearly shows a maturation process, with the ratio increasing roughly linearly from 1 to 3 years and thereafter remaining constant.

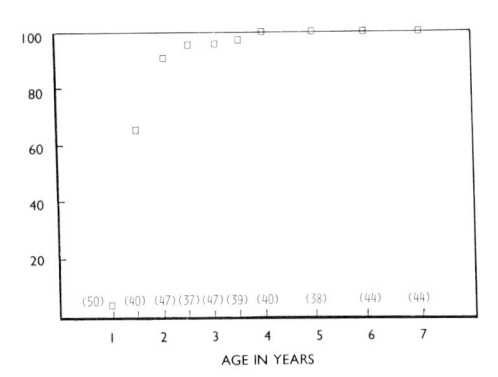

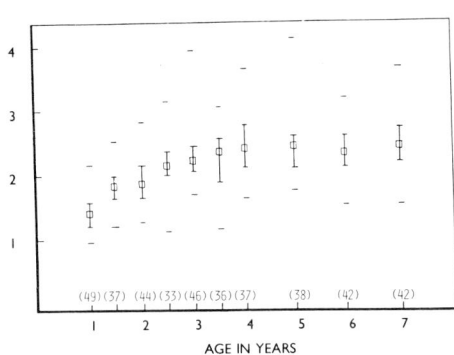

Fig. 7.14. Percentage of subjects showing reciprocal arm-swing in each of the 10 age-groups studied. Numbers of subjects in each age-group are given in parentheses along the horizontal axis.

Fig. 7.15. Pelvic-span/ankle-spread ratio in each of the 10 age-groups studied. The square indicates the median value, the vertical bar encompasses the middle 50 per cent of subjects, and the upper and lower marks respectively indicate the greatest and least values recorded.

The pelvic-span/ankle-spread (P/A) ratio is an important barometer of mature gait. It is possible that the ratio is influenced in a negative direction by the wearing of diapers. Virtually all of our 1- and 1½-year-old subjects wore diapers. In a recent study of the P/A ratio in 49 2-year-olds (32 with diapers and 17 without) we found (by two sample t-tests) that the p-value in a test of the null hypothesis* that P/A was identical for the two groups was less than 0.02 (*unpublished data*). However, since the diapered children were not studied without diapers, we cannot know if they were less mature (with a resultant 10 per cent lower P/A ratio), or whether the diapers hampered adduction (a possibility that did not occur to us until after the study was closed).

Null hypothesis is the term given to an assumption that two proportions do not differ by more than might readily be due to chance. If a subsequent t-test shows a non-significant probability, the null hypothesis is shown to be still tenable, but if the result is significant then it is unlikely that the assumption is valid.

8
DYNAMIC ELECTROMYOGRAPHY BY AGE

Introduction
Knowledge of the changes in the activity of muscles with age is essential to our comprehension of the maturation process. Publications concerning muscle activity in children during the walking cycle have been few and infrequent. Changing movement, of necessity, requires changes in the timing and/or intensity of muscle action. We have chosen in this study to consider only the *timing* of muscle activity.

The intensity of muscle action, as measured by quantification of the EMG signal, is not directly related to muscle tension except under limited conditions (Ralston *et al.* 1947, 1949; Inman 1973; Solomonow *et al.* 1986). Inman (1973) noted a direct relationship of the integrated EMG to muscle tension under the condition of isometric contraction (constant length); however, during walking muscle activity takes place under conditions of changing length and changing load.

We can with confidence draw one of three conclusions from dynamic EMG and related movement: (1) the muscle is contributing to a movement (muscle shortening, *i.e.* concentric action); (2) the muscle is resisting a movement (muscle lengthening, *i.e.* eccentric action); or (3) the muscle has no active influence on the movement (EMG silence). The actions of all the muscles that might affect the movement plus the contributions of gravity and inertia must be considered before arriving at a complete understanding of the forces responsible. We have used movement measurements, force studies and EMG studies to arrive at the conclusions about muscle function which follow in this chapter. We have also drawn on the work of other investigators who have used dynamic gait studies to revitalize the subject of functional anatomy (Perry 1974; Simon *et al.* 1978; Winter 1979, 1980, 1983; Inman *et al.* 1981; Basmajian and DeLuca 1985).

Using surface electrodes, EMGs of seven muscles in one lower extremity were obtained for each child who would co-operate, for a total of 369 studies. In using surface electrodes one must be content with less precise muscle identification than is possible with indwelling electrodes. For this reason we selected relatively large muscles close to the surface such as the vastus medialis and gluteus maximus, or muscle groups such as the medial and lateral hamstrings.

In previous publications our plots of muscle phasic activity have been prepared on the basis of percentages of gait cycle (Sutherland 1966, 1984; Sutherland *et al.* 1960, 1980*a*). This method of plotting is advantageous when comparing muscle phasic activity with joint-angle rotations, since both can be placed on the same scale. Our studies of pathological gait have usually been prepared in this manner. However, in spite of the convenience of this method of plotting, there is also some advantage in normalizing stance and swing phases across the different age-groups. Because stance is more prolonged in the younger age-groups than in the more mature walkers, we have chosen to present muscle phasic activity times as

TIBIALIS ANTERIOR

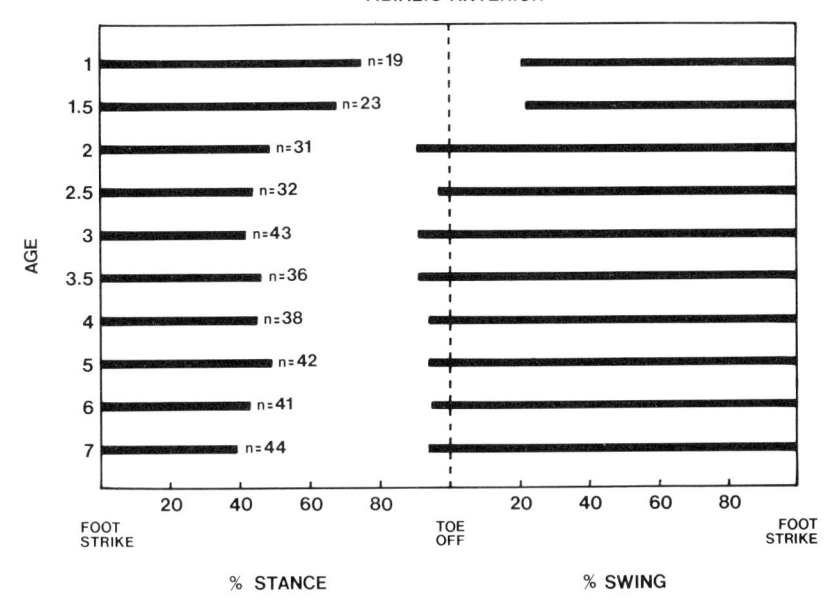

Fig. 8.1. Mean times of onset and cessation of EMG activity in the tibialis anterior in each of the 10 age-groups.

In this and the following figures in this chapter, the 'on' and 'off' times are expressed as percentages of stance and swing phases. All measurements were made using surface electrodes. In each case, the number of subjects in each age-group is noted following the point of cessation of stance-phase activity.

percentages of the stance or swing phase (rather than of the gait cycle as a whole). This method of data display simplifies comparisons of the changes in phasic activity across the different age-groups.

The muscles studied are discussed individually, and graphs of their timing with respect to the stance and swing phases of the gait cycle are presented.

Tibialis anterior
The function of the tibialis anterior consists of swing-phase activity to lift the foot (concentric contraction), followed by eccentric action to decelerate the foot from heel-strike to the foot-flat position.

This activity was strikingly different in the 1- and 1½-year-old subjects compared to the remaining age-groups (Fig. 8.1). The 1-year-olds lacked initial heel-strike, landing foot-flat; stance-phase activity of the tibialis anterior was prolonged and there was a delay in the onset of swing-phase activity, demonstrating an immature pattern. Activity in the 1½-year-olds was similar, but with somewhat less stance-phase prolongation. From 2 to 7 years the EMG phasic activity was nearly constant, demonstrating a mature pattern with onset just before toe-off and full swing-phase activity continuing to approximately the 40 per cent point of stance phase.

Vastus medialis
The function of the vastus medialis (quadriceps) in normal, level walking is to prepare the limb for load acceptance in swing phase and to act as a shock absorber in early stance phase (eccentric action).

Once again, the differences with age were evident primarily in the 1 and 1½ year age-groups (Fig. 8.2). At these ages there was prolonged activity in swing phase. EMG activity was present throughout swing phase in the 1-year-olds and was of only slightly shorter duration in the 1½-year-olds. A slight prolongation of activity during stance phase also was evident in the 1- to 2½-year-old subjects in comparison with the older children.

These differences are probably related to delayed maturation of the control system, resulting in some lack of precision in movement. By the age of 4 years a mature pattern had emerged, with onset of muscle activity in late swing (at around the 60 per cent point), continuing into stance phase to approximately 35 per cent.

Gluteus medius
The most important function of the gluteus medius is to stabilize the hip. Its decelerating (eccentric) action prevents excessive drop of the opposite pelvis during single-limb stance. Swing-phase activity is also present, indicating that limb placement in preparation for load acceptance is also important.

There was little change in the stance-phase dynamic EMG across the 10 age-groups (Fig. 8.3). There was a trend toward reduction of activity in swing phase after 4 years. The mature pattern consists of onset at approximately 60 per cent of swing, continuing to approximately 60 per cent of stance.

Medial hamstrings
In level walking the hamstrings contract in swing phase to decelerate the swinging limb (eccentric action) and act in the early portion of stance phase to stabilize the hip.

In the 1-year-olds, stance-phase activity was prolonged (immature pattern). The most likely explanation for this is that the control system is poorly developed, resulting in less precision and control of movements. Alternatively, it could be that balance is so precarious that increased muscle firing is required to maintain an upright posture. If the latter explanation is valid, then the muscle phasic prolongation is in response to dynamic postural demands. By age 2 a mature pattern was present, with activity commencing at approximately 50 per cent of swing and continuing to approximately 55 per cent of stance (Fig. 8.4).

Lateral hamstrings
The dynamic phasic activity of the lateral hamstrings was very similar to that of the medial hamstrings (Fig. 8.5). The two youngest age-groups showed slightly more prolonged activity in stance phase, again demonstrating an immature pattern. There was no late-stance/early-swing activity in the lateral hamstrings. The mature pattern, first seen at 2 years, consists of onset at about 55 per cent of swing, continuing to around 60 per cent of stance.

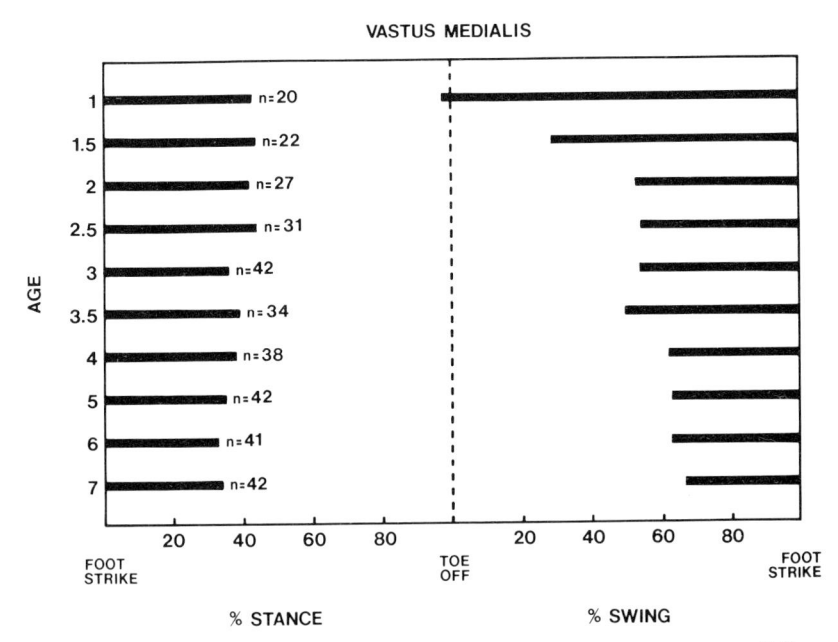

Fig. 8.2. Mean times of onset and cessation of EMG activity in the vastus medialis.

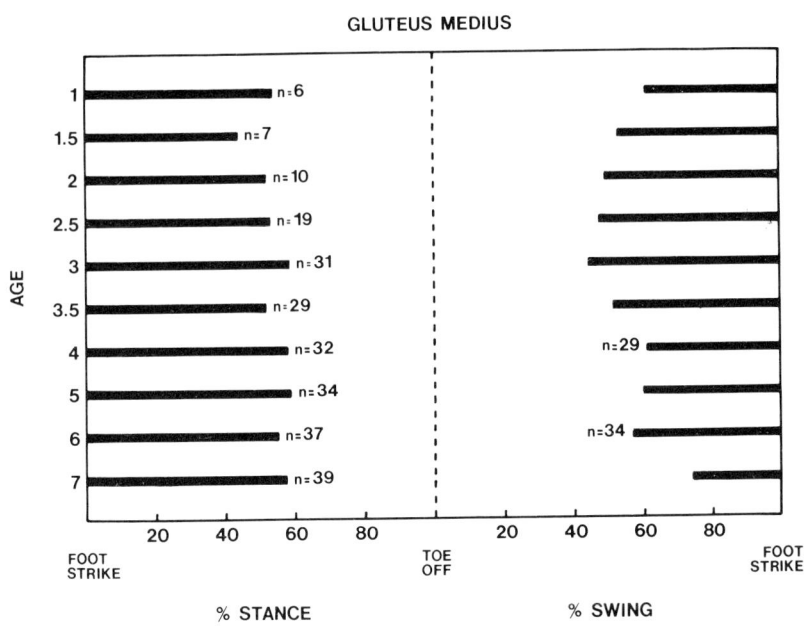

Fig. 8.3. Mean times of onset and cessation of EMG activity in the gluteus medius. (As indicated, no swing-phase activity was recorded in three 4-year-olds and three 6-year-olds.)

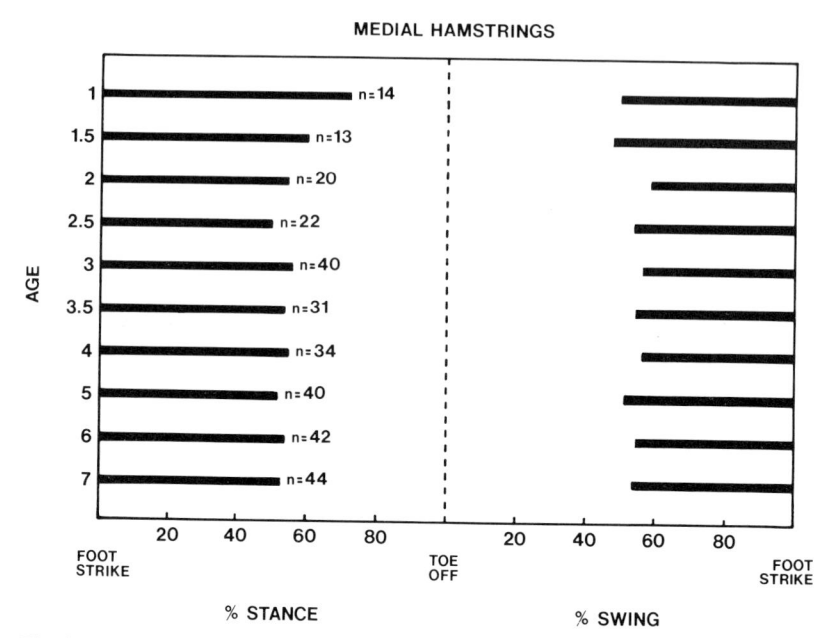

Fig. 8.4. Mean times of onset and cessation of EMG activity in the medial hamstrings.

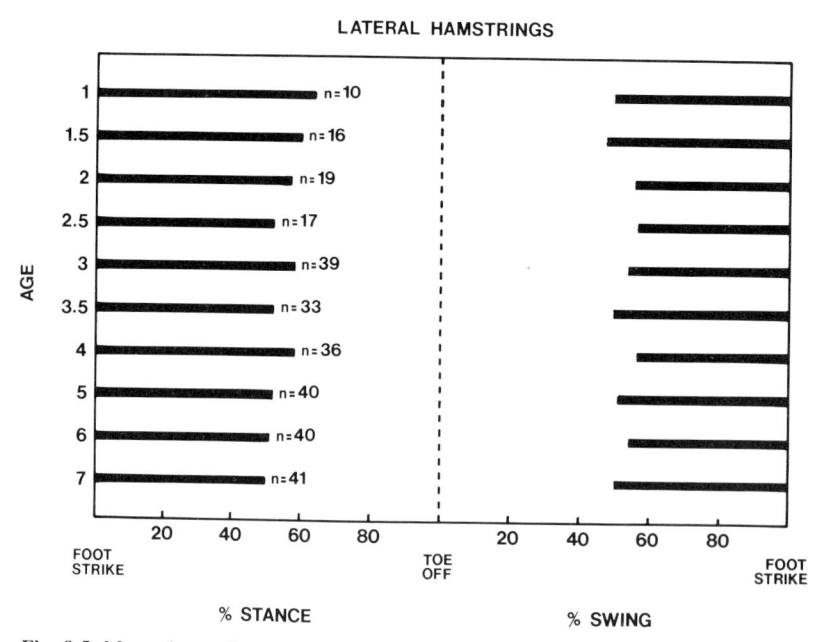

Fig. 8.5. Mean times of onset and cessation of EMG activity in the lateral hamstrings.

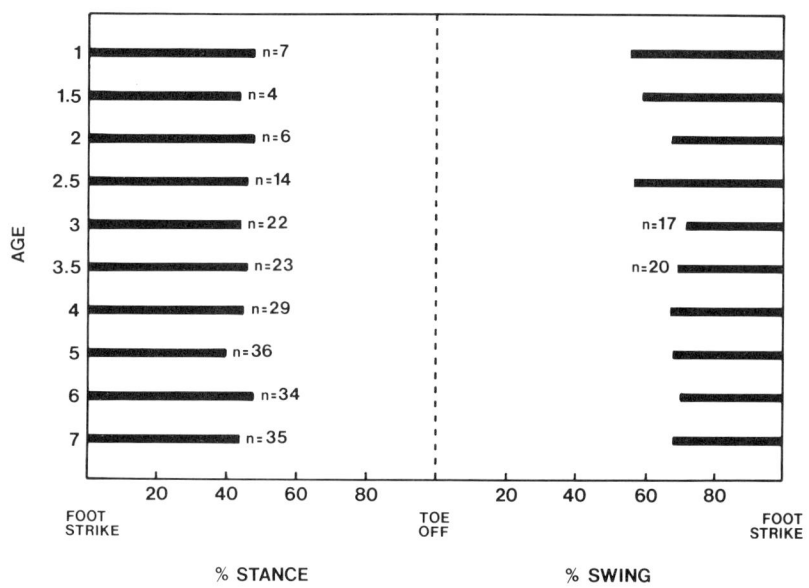

Fig. 8.6. Mean times of onset and cessation of EMG activity in the gluteus maximus. (As indicated, no swing-phase activity was recorded in five 3-year-olds and three 3½-year-olds.)

Gluteus maximus

A description of the function of the gluteus maximus in level walking can be deduced by correlating hip movement, dynamic EMG and joint torque. The gluteus maximus acts concentrically in swing phase to reduce hip flexion prior to foot-strike. It continues to act concentrically in early stance; however, the majority of hip extension in stance phase occurs after this muscle activity has ceased. How does the hip continue to extend while the gluteus maximus is inactive? Hip flexion torque changes to extension torque at 28 per cent of the gait cycle, both in normal children (unpublished data from our laboratory) and in normal adults (Skinner *et al.* 1985). When the force line passes behind the hip joint, no further action of the gluteus maximus is necessary to complete hip extension. The gluteus maximus stops firing also very close to 28 per cent of the cycle (the slightly higher figures reported in Figure 8.6 are, of course, due to calculation of percentage of stance phase rather than of gait cycle). This is an example of the close agreement between muscle activity and extrinsic joint torque.

All age-groups showed similar stance-phase activity in the gluteus maximus. In the 1-, 1½- and 2½-year-olds swing-phase activity was slightly more prolonged than in the 2 years and 3 years and over age-groups, but these differences were minor. A fully mature pattern was evident by 3 years, with onset of activity at about 65 per cent of swing, continuing to around 50 per cent of stance.

Gastroc-soleus
The function of the gastrocnemius-soleus (triceps surae) in mature, level walking is to decelerate the tibia during the first portion of single-limb stance (eccentric action), arrest dorsiflexion and then accelerate the ankle joint before opposite foot-strike (concentric action). This accelerative phase of ankle action coincides with the second peak of the vertical-force curve (see Sutherland et al. 1980b, Winter 1983).

Striking differences were found when the dynamic phasic activity of the gastroc-soleus in our pediatric population was contrasted with that in a normal adult control group (Inman et al. 1981). Swing-phase activity, not usually present in the adult, was commonly seen in our subjects, particularly in the younger age-groups. We found two patterns that require separate descriptions. The first we term the 'immature' pattern because it showed the greatest differences from that of the normal adult controls. It occurred in a very high percentage of the 1- and 1½-year-olds and in approximately one-quarter of the subjects in the remaining age-groups (Fig. 8.7A). It is a 'wrap-around' pattern, beginning near the middle of swing phase and ending with opposite foot-strike. 67 per cent of the 1-year-olds and 63 per cent of the 1½-year-olds demonstrated this immature pattern. There was a precipitous drop in the proportion of subjects with this pattern at 2 years; however, the finding that at 2 years and older approximately one-quarter of our subjects still demonstrated this immature pattern was quite unexpected.

In the second of these patterns (the 'mature' pattern) activity of the gastroc-soleus is confined to the single-stance portion of stance phase, and therefore resembles the adult pattern (Sutherland 1966, Sutherland et al. 1980b, Inman et al. 1981). The mature pattern was present in approximately one-third of the 1- and 1½-year-olds and in around three-quarters of the older children (Fig. 8.7B).

Discussion
What explanations can be given for the differences observed in the time of development of mature phasic activity in the seven muscles or muscle groups in our study? Three possible causes for slower maturity are offered and briefly discussed: (1) the levels of segmental anterior horn cell representation in the spinal cord differ and lower levels might develop more slowly; (2) the sequence of myelination might favor earlier maturation of some muscles over others; (3) some of the movements are more complex than others, necessitating a longer period of development.

Sharrard (1955) has described the distribution of anterior horn cells in the spinal cord. Those of the gluteus medius are located in the L4 and L5 segments, those of the gluteus maximus in the S1 and S2 segments, and those of the gastroc-soleus in the L5, S1, S2 and S3 segments. The gluteus maximus EMG phasic plots show early maturity with no pattern of change after 2 years of age. The gluteus medius plots show only minor change after 2 years and no change after 4 years. By contrast, the gastroc-soleus shows great delay in maturation, so much so that it is necessary to describe two distinct patterns, a 'mature' and an 'immature'.

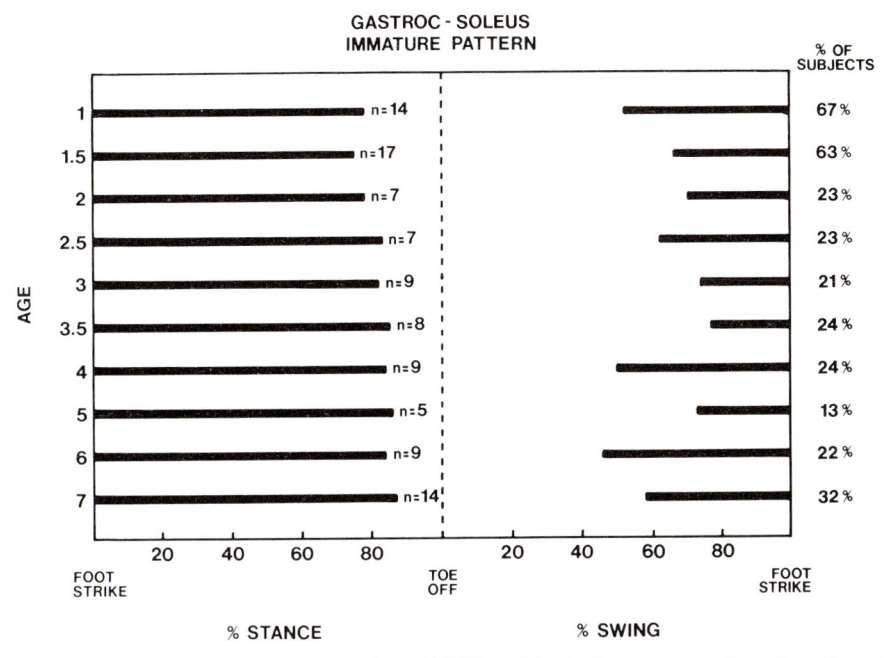

Fig. 8.7A. Mean times of onset and cessation of EMG activity in the gastrocnemius-soleus (immature pattern).

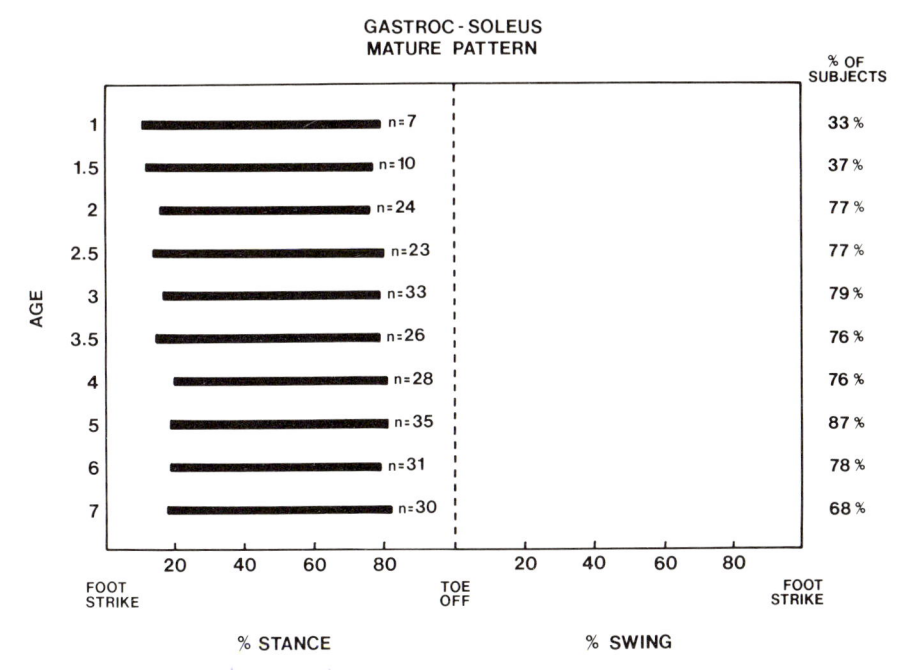

Fig. 8.7B. Mean times of onset and cessation of EMG activity in the gastrocnemius-soleus (mature pattern).

161

Anterior horn cells of the medial and lateral hamstrings are found in the L4, L5, S1 and S2 segments of the spinal cord. The tibialis anterior is unique in this group of muscles in that its anterior horn cells are found in a single spinal segment, L4. The tibialis anterior and both groups of hamstring muscles show a mature pattern of phasic muscle action by 2 years of age.

The quadriceps femoris has anterior horn cells in the L2, L3 and L4 segments of the spinal cord. The primary differences in phasic action are seen in the 1 and 1½ year age-groups, with minor changes from 2 to 3 years and no change thereafter.

The impression is gained that the level of motor innervation in the spinal cord has little to do with the pattern of maturation. Otherwise, how can the very early maturation of gluteus maximus phasic activity be reconciled with the very late maturation of the gastroc-soleus? Both muscles have very nearly the same anterior horn cell representation in the spinal cord. Does the cephalocaudal progress of maturation have any bearing on the question? The answer is probably yes, but the dorsal roots and sensory nerves—not the anterior roots—are most involved in the process. The anterior roots myelinate before the posterior roots, and the lumbar dorsal roots are the last to myelinate (Rafalowska 1979). Motor nerves and anterior roots mature before dorsal nerve roots and sensory nerves. Therefore, myelination cannot be excluded as a component in the maturation process. Conduction delays due to incomplete myelination and the greater distance of the sensory component of the reflex arc are likely significant factors in causing the maturation delay in gastroc-soleus function.

Complexity of movement must also be included in the discussion of maturation. Movement complexity increases progressively from proximal to distal. Hip flexion/extension is the simplest of the lower-extremity motions in walking. Knee flexion/extension is somewhat more complex and ankle motion is the most complicated of the three. This is confirmed by the progressively larger number of Fourier coefficients required to define knee flexion/extension and ankle plantar flexion/dorsiflexion in comparison to hip flexion/extension (Sutherland *et al.* 1980*a*, Olshen *et al.* 1988). Intuitively it seems that complex movements should be slower to mature than simpler ones.

9
FORCE-PLATE VALUES BY AGE

Force data are gathered by means of the force plate, which has been described in Chapter 2 (pp. 5–6) and illustrated in Figure 2.6 (p. 15). These data are useful in describing the development of mature walking, and also in the evaluation of gait for patients with neurological deficits such as spastic diplegia. Simon (1977) has emphasized that both movement measurements and ground-reaction force data are needed, in addition to electromyographic studies, to detect differences between abnormal pathological conditions and compensatory mechanisms.

Before embarking on a description of our analyses of the data, we should first define the basic parameters. *Vertical force* is the vertical ground-reaction force, as measured by the force plate. Further parameters such as vertical acceleration are readily derived from the vertical-force measures. *Fore/aft shear* is the ground-reaction force acting horizontally in the line of progression of the child's walk. We usually refer to shear from the subject's point of view—hence, fore (forward) shear occurs when the foot is pushing ahead. *Medial/lateral shear* is the ground-reaction force acting horizontally, perpendicular to the line of progression of the child's walk. All these force measures are normalized by conversion to percentage of body weight. Again, further parameters (such as joint torque, described below) can be derived from these measurements of shear. The *ground-reaction force vector* is the resultant of the vertical-force, fore/aft shear and medial/lateral shear vectors. The point of application of the ground-reaction force is termed the *center of pressure*. The moment which the subject's foot exerts in the plane of the floor about the center of pressure is referred to as *torque*; this is measured in newton-meters.

Although there are certain problems in measuring lever arms (that is, the perpendicular distance from line of action to point of pivot), joint torques can be evaluated from force vectors. Each such torque value is the product of the force acting on the joint and the length of the lever arm. Just as force measurements are normalized by body weight, so with joint torque the length of the lever arm is normalized by relation to body height. The resulting product is then scaled by being multiplied by 100. Thus, normalized torque is 100 times the product of normalized force and normalized lever arm. For an application of sagittal-plane joint-torque measurements to the study of normal walking, see Sutherland *et al.* (1980*b*). Applications of joint-torque measurements to the study of crouch gait in spastic diplegia are described by Sutherland and Cooper (1978). Hip, knee and ankle torques may be of special interest in specific applications.

Analysis

The statistical analyses of the force data, like those of the motion data, depend on having adequate means of describing both their average values at the different points in the gait cycle and their variability. In considering motion data, we took the angles as measured during the gait cycle and 'fitted' a Fourier series to them. This Fourier series could be used to calculate the angle at any stated point in the gait cycle. A basic difference between motion and force is that while motion is very smooth (that is, the movement during one phase of the cycle flows into the next in an orderly fashion), force is not. Force values can be collected only while the subject's foot is on the floor, but stance phase forms only part of the gait cycle. Thus, although force curves may be qualitatively very similar from step to step, they have a distinct beginning at foot-strike and end at toe-off. Also, there is randomness in the fraction of the cycle during which the foot is in contact with the force plate. These aspects of the data add a new wrinkle of difficulty to our analyses.

'Cubic splines' are one way of describing curves such as those that arise from force data. As applied here, a 'spline' consists of a group of smoothly joined curves, each of which describes a particular portion of the gait cycle. The process of fitting involves choosing the points in the cycle which correspond to the end-points of the intervals to be approximated. (These end-points are known as 'knots'.) The data are approximated between the knots using a cubic (third degree polynomial equation). To do this, we rely on an approach that is in the same 'linear' spirit as the previous Fourier fits, in that the fitted values are certain weighted averages of all the observed values. As before, the weights are determined by the method of least squares. [Software used for this process is from the International Mathematics and Statistics Library routine ICSFKU (I.M.S.L. 1983). Interested readers are directed to the important treatise by de Boor (1978).]

The points at which the knots are placed are necessarily among those for which we have force data from virtually every child. We chose: 0, 3, 7, 12, 20, 32, 40 and 50 per cent. The last, of course, corresponds approximately to opposite foot-strike and exactly to the end of the intervals that we report. The concentration of knots at the beginning of the cycle reflects particular difficulty modeling near the point at which the foot strikes the force plate. As mentioned, the spline is computed so that it is smooth across each knot. (The function and its first two derivatives are required to be continuous.)

The advantage to our approach is that data gathered during each interval tend to influence the fit for that interval. Thus, the early portion of the force curve, where load is being applied rapidly, is approximated by an equation that is specific to that portion of the cycle, and the smooth-flowing portions of the curve in mid-stance are approximated using equations specific to that area. Each interval contributes the equivalent of one 'degree of freedom' to the fit. For technical reasons there are an additional three degrees of freedom so that, with our choice of knots, 10 degrees of freedom are used. This is analogous to using an overall constant, the first four sine and cosine harmonics, and either of the two fifth-order harmonics in the context of motion. However, since we have only 16 to 33 digitized data points for a typical rotation, but typically 150 to 200 data points for each force curve, we are using a much smaller fraction of available degrees of freedom to model force than we used with the motion data. Visually, the fits appear to be good; multiple correlation coefficients are roughly 0.65, that is, 65 per cent. We observe that the transient changes in force just after foot-strike are responsible for the consistently lower multiple correlations observed with force than with motion. Were we to use a higher fraction of available degrees of freedom, it is certain that we could improve the values.

In many respects, our analyses of force are to be viewed as more preliminary than our studies of motion. More work on understanding force will be undertaken in our laboratory in the future. The cited multiple correlations may be poor indicators of how useful spline-fitted force curves are in clinical practice. We feel the correlations are being diminished by small 'phase' shifts of fitted curves near foot-strike. The method of least squares looks at vertical distances between data and fit. It is easy to visualize two rapidly changing curves whose perpendicular distance is very small but which are, in vertical distance, quite far apart.

The bootstrap process described in Chapter 3 is, in principle, applicable to forming prediction regions for force. We have done some initial computations on prediction regions based on polynomial rather than spline models. As of this writing we do not feel that we have a definitive technique for analysis of the variability in force data.

Although we have not analyzed force as completely as motion, two issues which have arisen are worthy of note. (1) Vertical forces cannot be negative, that is, the subject cannot pull up on the force plate. This complicates the definition of a prediction region, since it will be forced to have zero width at foot-strike. (2) Both the length of the stance phase of the cycle and the time of opposite foot-strike are random. This means simply that one must find some way to account for subjects with variable lengths of stance phase. In addition, children whose step length is shorter than the length of the force plate will have data only up until opposite foot-strike. (The force data obtained with both feet on the plate are such that the forces on each foot individually cannot be determined.) The combination of these effects causes the estimated width of the prediction regions from opposite foot-strike to toe-off to be much wider than during the earlier portions of the cycle.

Faced with these problems we have chosen to present only the mean curves for each age-group, and to limit these to the period from foot-strike to 50 per cent of the cycle (approximately, opposite foot-strike). The mean curves within groups were found by simple averaging across subjects. We eliminated consideration of the 1- and 1½-year-olds, as force data were obtained for a combined total of only 11 limbs at these ages, compared with at least 10 limbs in each of the remaining age-groups. Data were collected from many more children than are included in the final analysis due to the complexity of the data and data-handling problems.

Vertical force
The normal adult's vertical-force curve during free-speed walking consists of two peaks connected by a trough—the shape resembles a cursive 'm'. The first peak occurs between about 12 and 16 per cent of the gait cycle. The curve from foot-strike to this first peak is called the loading portion. The first peak exceeds 100 per cent of body weight, usually by no more than 20 per cent. The force then drops below body weight, with the trough occurring around 30 per cent of the cycle. This

portion of the curve is called the mid-stance trough. The unweighting phenomenon that produces the trough occurs when the center of mass of the body is at its highest point in the cycle and when it is positioned vertically over the supporting foot. At this instant, potential energy is very high and kinetic energy is low (Inman *et al.* 1981). The second peak occurs between 40 and 50 per cent of the cycle; it is produced by the fall of the center of mass, resisted by the action of the ankle plantar flexors acting concentrically to diminish ankle dorsiflexion. This phase of the curve is known as the push-off portion; however, there is controversy concerning this term. The work of Perry (1974) and Simon *et al.* (1978) casts doubt on the existence of push-off. Sutherland *et al.* (1980*b*) reported an initial eccentric action of the plantar flexors in stance phase, followed by an accelerative phase (concentric action), peaking just before opposite foot-strike. Investigations by Winter (1983) also support the existence of an accelerative phase of action of the ankle plantar flexors. Vertical force declines rapidly with the beginning of second double support, at about 50 per cent of the cycle, as weight is transferred from one leg to the other.

The fitted vertical-force curves for the 2 to 7 year age-groups are presented in Figure 9.1 (pp. 168–169). As indicated, they end at 50 per cent of the gait cycle; while incomplete, they show the loading portion, the mid-stance trough and most but not all of the second peak. The decline in force that occurs during second double support is missing.

A common finding in all age-groups was the time of the mid-stance trough. This occurred regularly at 30 per cent of the gait cycle. The trough appears to be less well developed in the younger age-groups than in the more mature children. The depths of the fitted troughs, measured from the top of the first peak, were from 17 to 24 per cent of body weight in the 2, 2½ and 3 year age-groups, increasing to 30 per cent at 3½, 4 and 5 years, and to about 40 per cent at 6 and 7 years. Mean vertical force at 50 per cent of the gait cycle was consistently less than peak force in the loading phase in all age-groups, though by 5 years the difference was small.

Fore/aft shear
Forward shear begins at foot-strike and ends when the center of mass passes in front of the supporting foot. It increases rapidly during initial double support and recedes after opposite toe-off. The time of transition from forward to aft shear occurs shortly after 30 per cent of the gait cycle in normal adults, generally matching the trough for vertical force. Aft shear peaks at about the time of opposite foot-strike. The dynamic aspects of fore/aft shear can be illustrated by imagining walking on an extremely slippery surface. A step onto such a surface can produce a backward fall, while a loss of footing occurring after the center of mass of the body has passed in front of the point of support produces a forward fall. We are dependent upon friction between the foot and the supporting surface to carry out the alternate processes of deceleration and acceleration essential to human walking. If we are deprived of the necessary conditions for safe walking—for example, when walking on ice with a thin layer of water on top—we instinctively take very small steps and keep the body and limbs very upright. Under normal

conditions, the timing, quality and magnitude of forward and aft shear give important information about the speed and efficiency of walking. Both forward and aft shear are exaggerated by faster walking. Gait abnormalities which interfere with loading are reflected in decreased forward shear, while deficiencies affecting single-limb stance, such as paralysis of the plantar flexors, reduce aft shear (Sutherland *et al.* 1980*b*).

The fitted fore/aft shear curves for our 2- to 7-year-old subjects are presented in Figure 9.2 (pp. 170–171). The times of direction change are remarkably constant across all eight age-groups. The peak of forward shear occurs at, or shortly before, 10 per cent of the gait cycle at all ages. The time of reversal of fore/aft shear occurs after 30 per cent of the cycle in all age-groups; however, there is a slight increase with increasing maturity. Overall, the differences in fore/aft shear from ages 2 to 7 are not very great, and the pattern is very similar to that of adults.

Medial/lateral shear
A very small medial-shear force is produced by foot-strike. This peaks quickly, receding to zero by approximately 5 per cent of the cycle. Through the remainder of initial double support and throughout single-limb stance, lateral shear is produced. How is this explained? Intuitively, the center of mass is lateral to the center of pressure for a brief instant after foot-strike, producing a medial-shear force; the center of mass then moves medial to the center of pressure, producing lateral shear until opposite foot-strike. This is a tidy explanation; however, it is probably incorrect. It should be remembered that both lower extremities bear some of the body weight during initial double support, and inspection of the force curves for only one limb is not sufficient for a complete analysis of the double-support phase. We believe the correct explanation is that the lower extremity is adducting at the hip at the moment of foot-strike (see Chapter 7, p. 66), producing a transient medial-shear force. The lateral shear is produced by the medial placement of the body's center of mass over the center of pressure.

The fitted medial/lateral shear curves for ages 2 to 7 years are presented in Figure 9.3 (pp. 172–173). There are very few differences across these age-groups. In general, the lateral-shear force peaks at around 20 per cent of the gait cycle, as was the finding in the adults studied by Cunningham (1950). Lateral-shear forces were higher among our 2½-year-old subjects; we have no explanation for this finding.

Lateral shear cannot be generated effectively with instability of the foot (Sutherland 1984). The presence of well-defined lateral shear in the eight age-groups studied indicates that stable weight-bearing is achieved early. We are not able to define any maturational changes in medial/lateral shear in the children in this study.

Torque
The graph for torque in normal adults is a sinusoidal curve with one peak and one trough. The peak, representing internal torque, occurs after foot-strike at around

(Continued on page 176)

VERTICAL FORCE

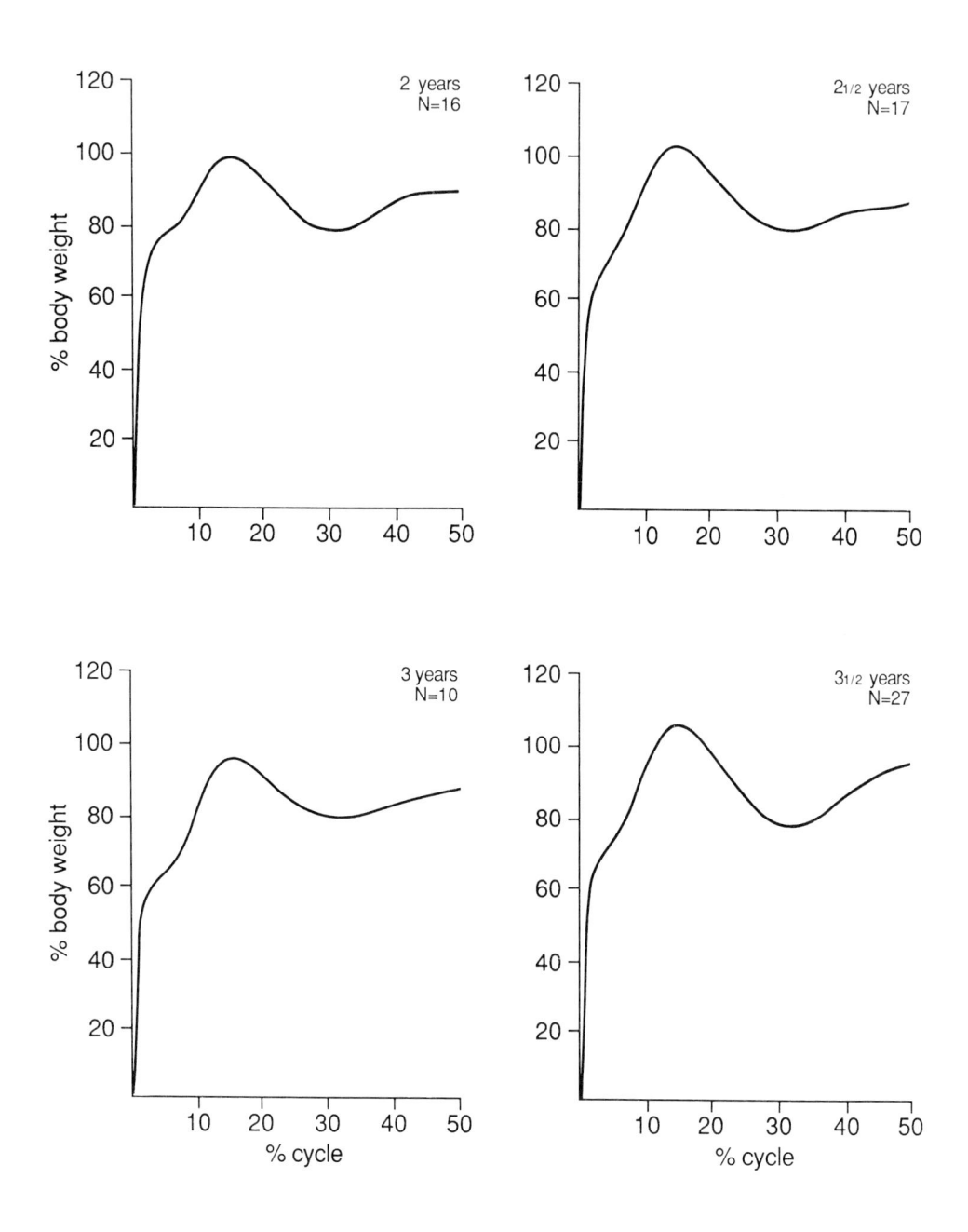

Fig. 9.1A. Fitted vertical-force curves in 2 to 3½ year age-groups.

VERTICAL FORCE

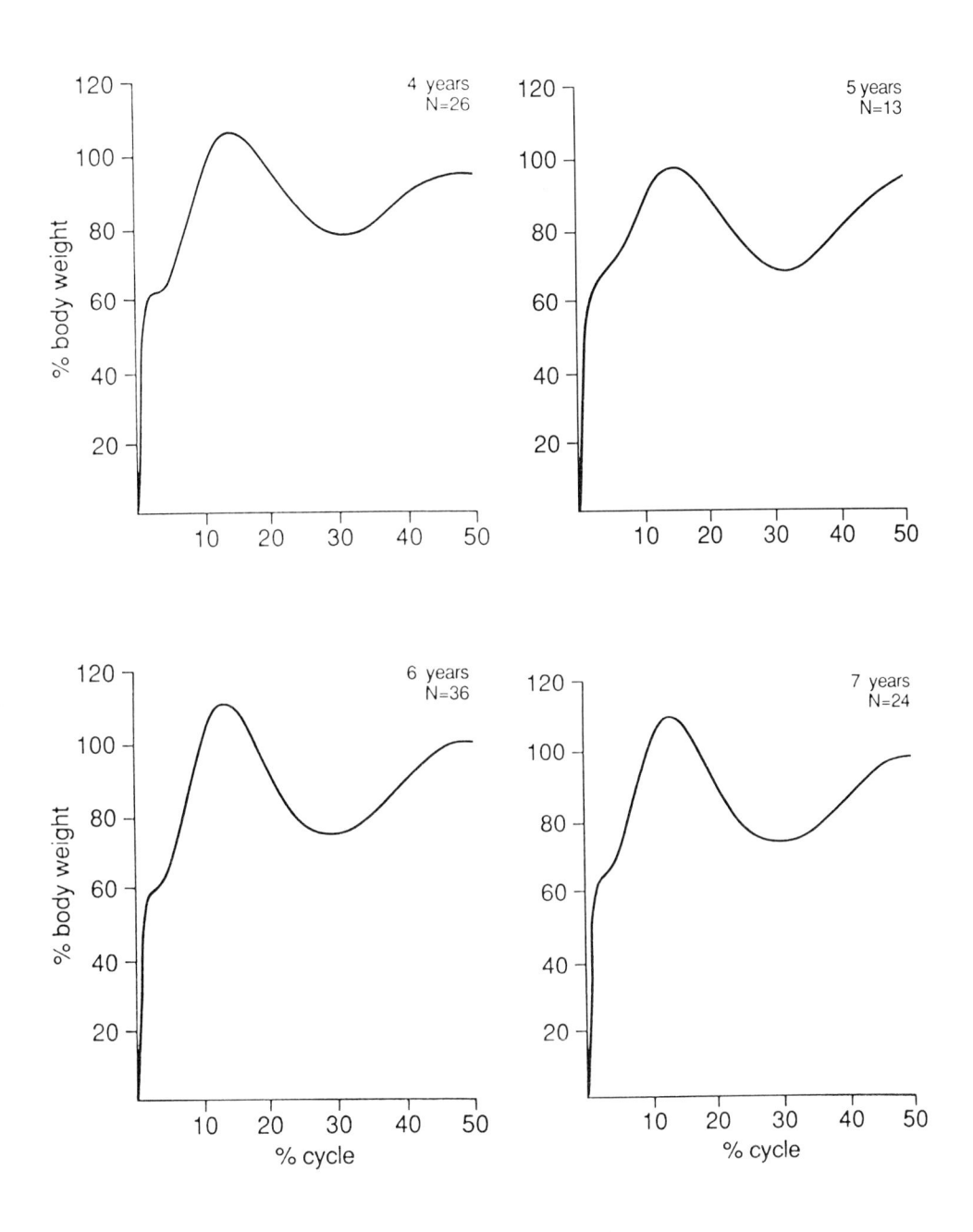

Fig. 9.1B. Fitted vertical-force curves in 4 to 7 year age-groups.

FORE/AFT SHEAR

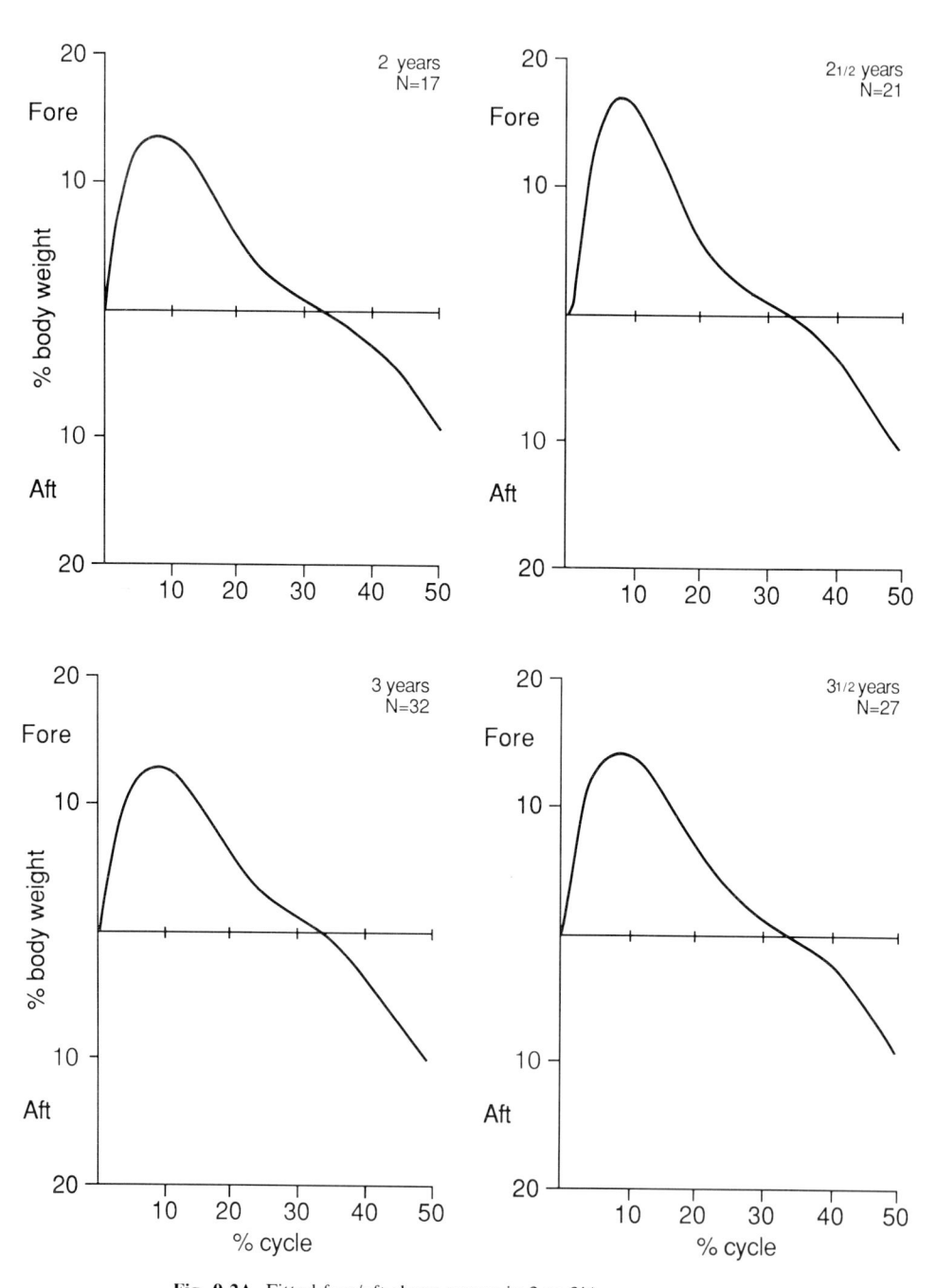

Fig. 9.2A. Fitted fore/aft shear curves in 2 to 3½ year age-groups.

FORE/AFT SHEAR

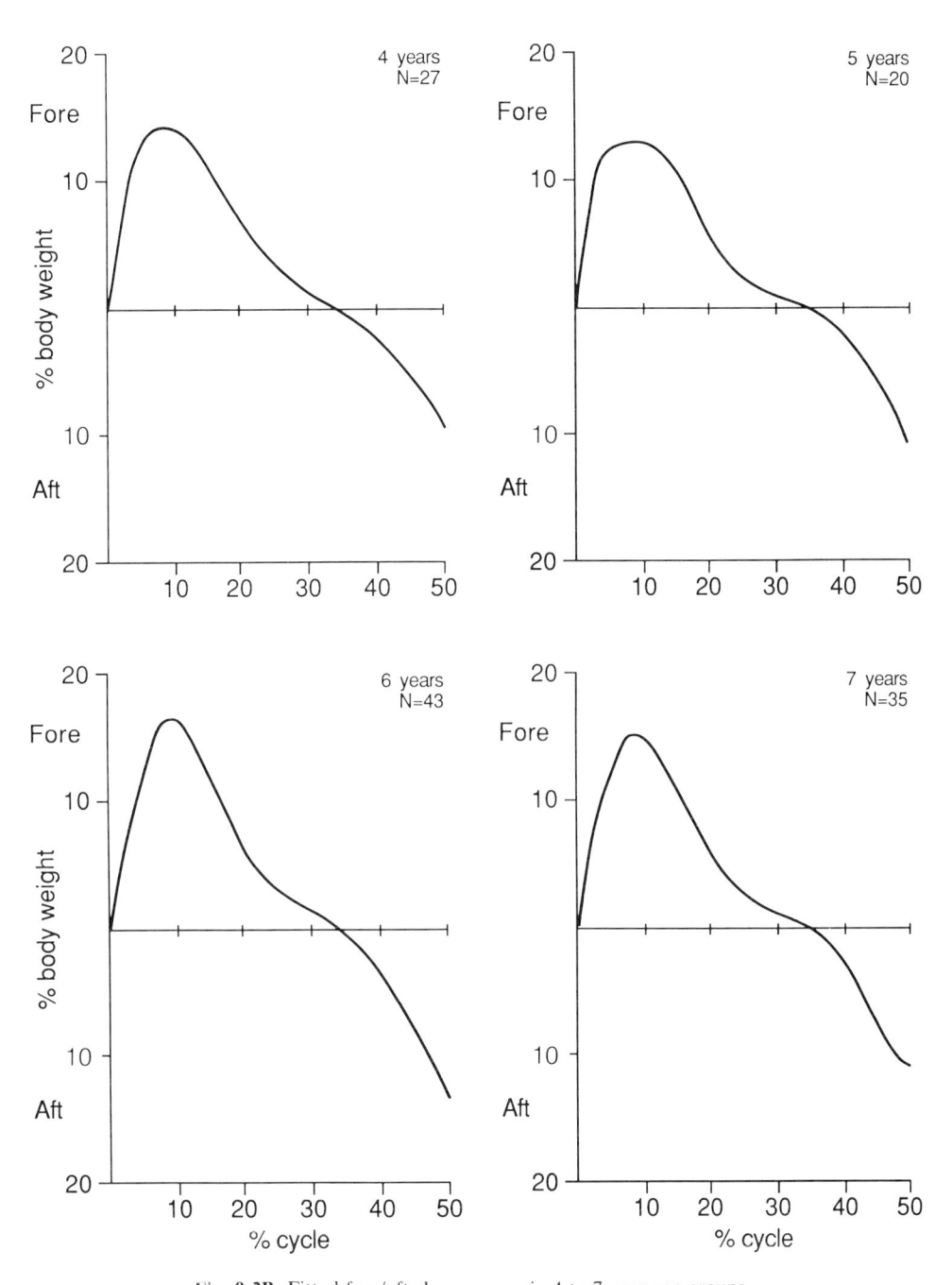

Fig. 9.2B. Fitted fore/aft shear curves in 4 to 7 year age-groups.

MEDIAL/LATERAL SHEAR

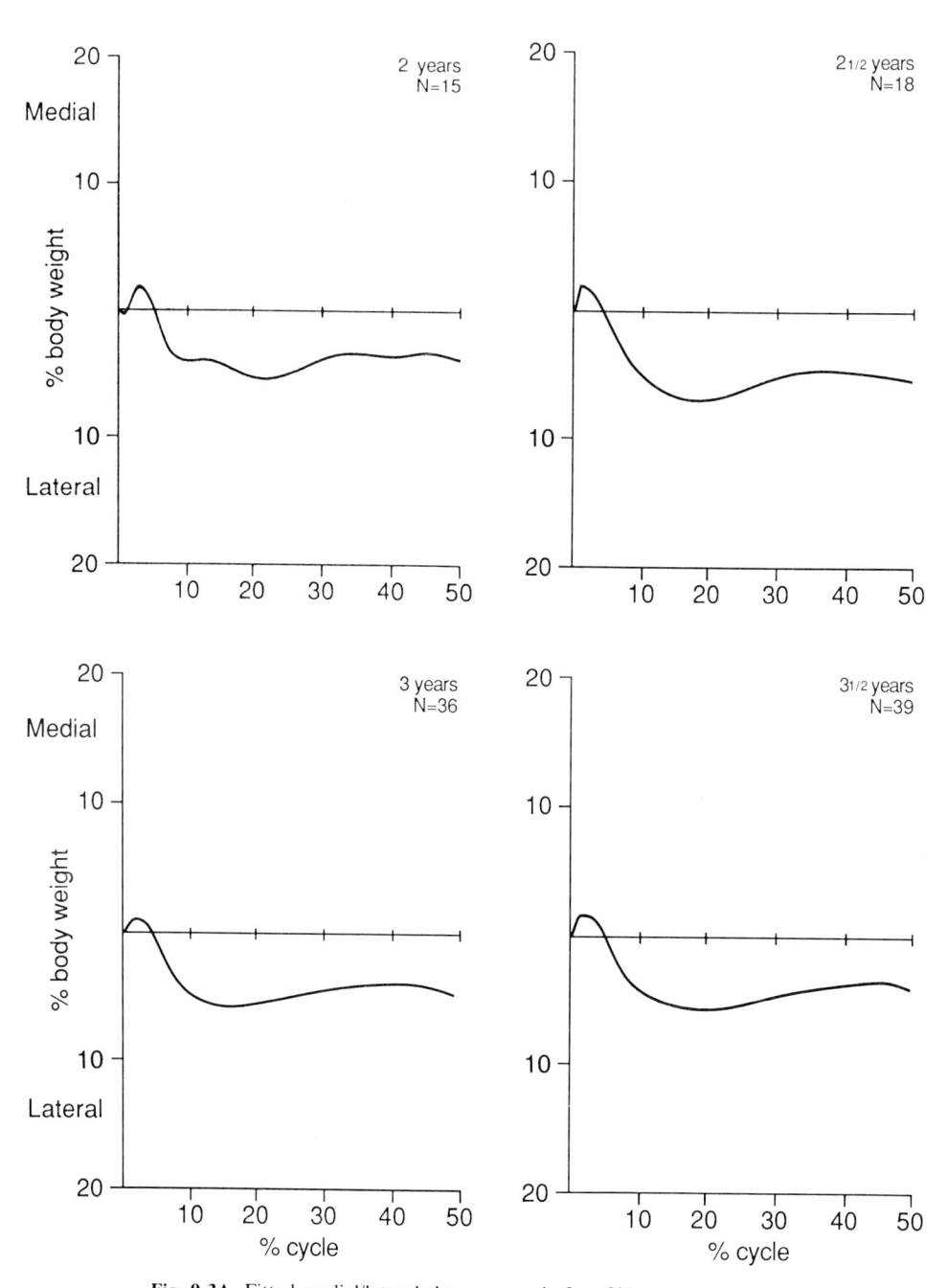

Fig. 9.3A. Fitted medial/lateral shear curves in 2 to 3½ year age-groups.

MEDIAL/LATERAL SHEAR

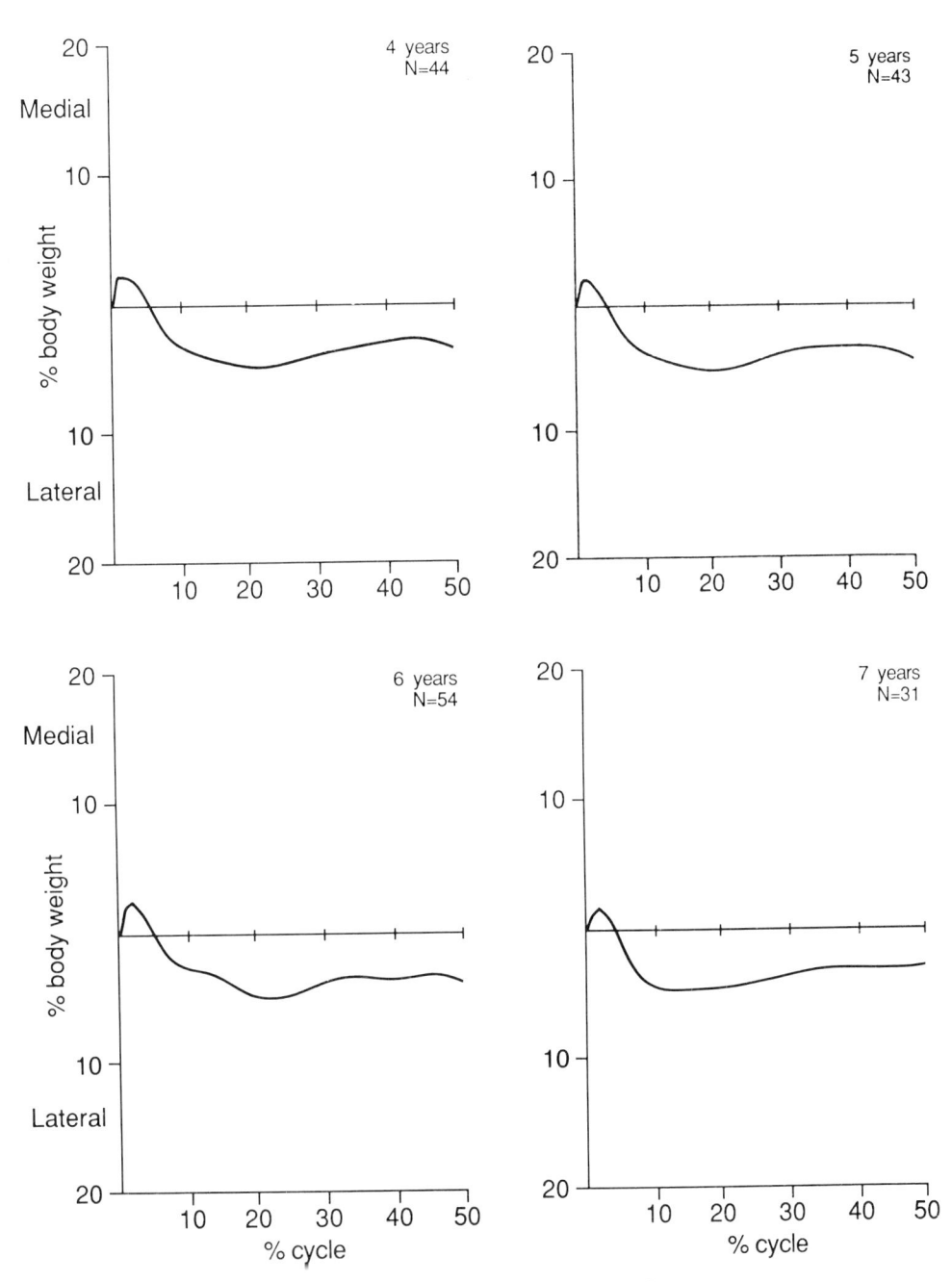

Fig. 9.3B. Fitted medial/lateral shear curves in 4 to 7 year age-groups.

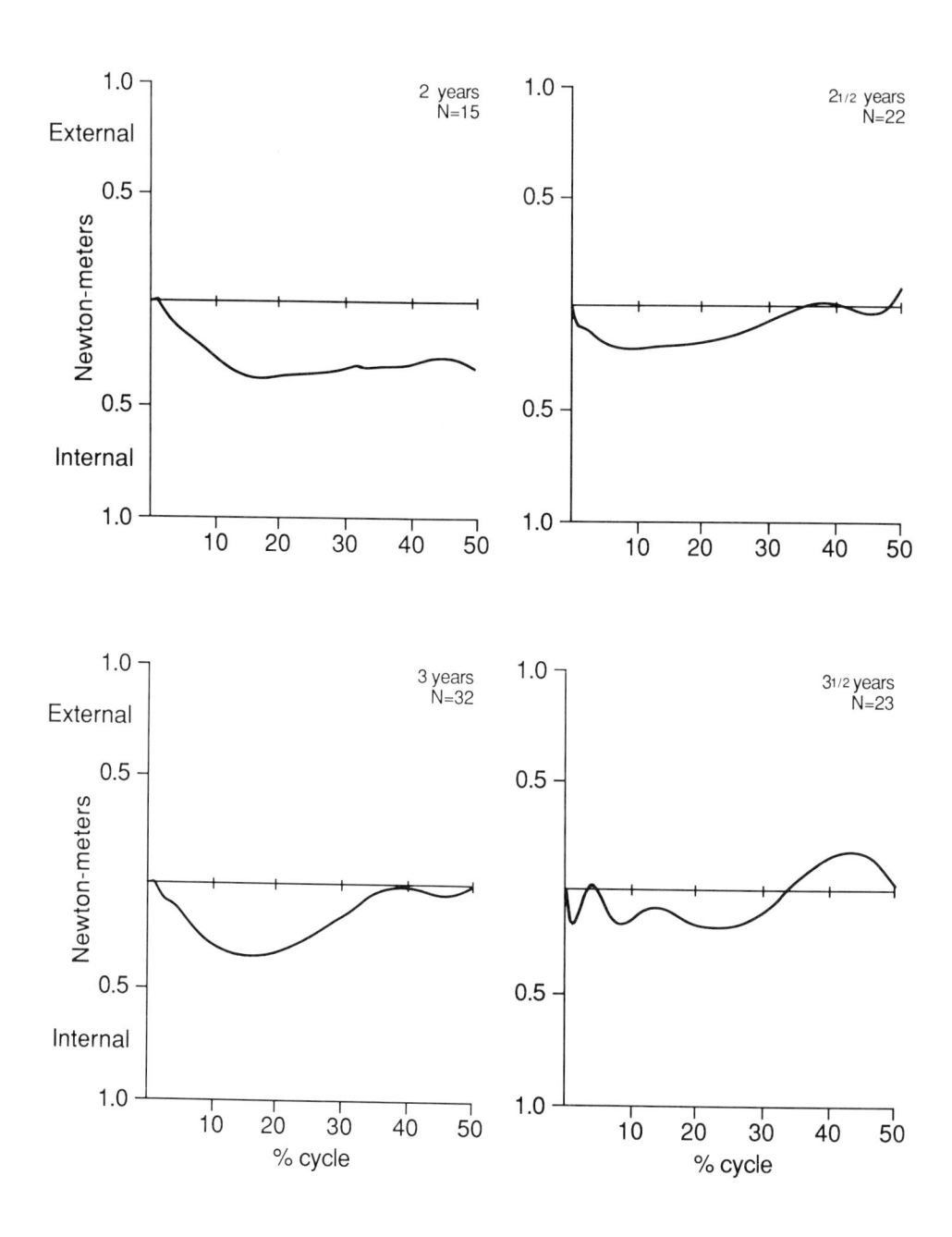

Fig. 9.4A. Fitted torque curves in 2 to 3½ year age-groups.

TORQUE

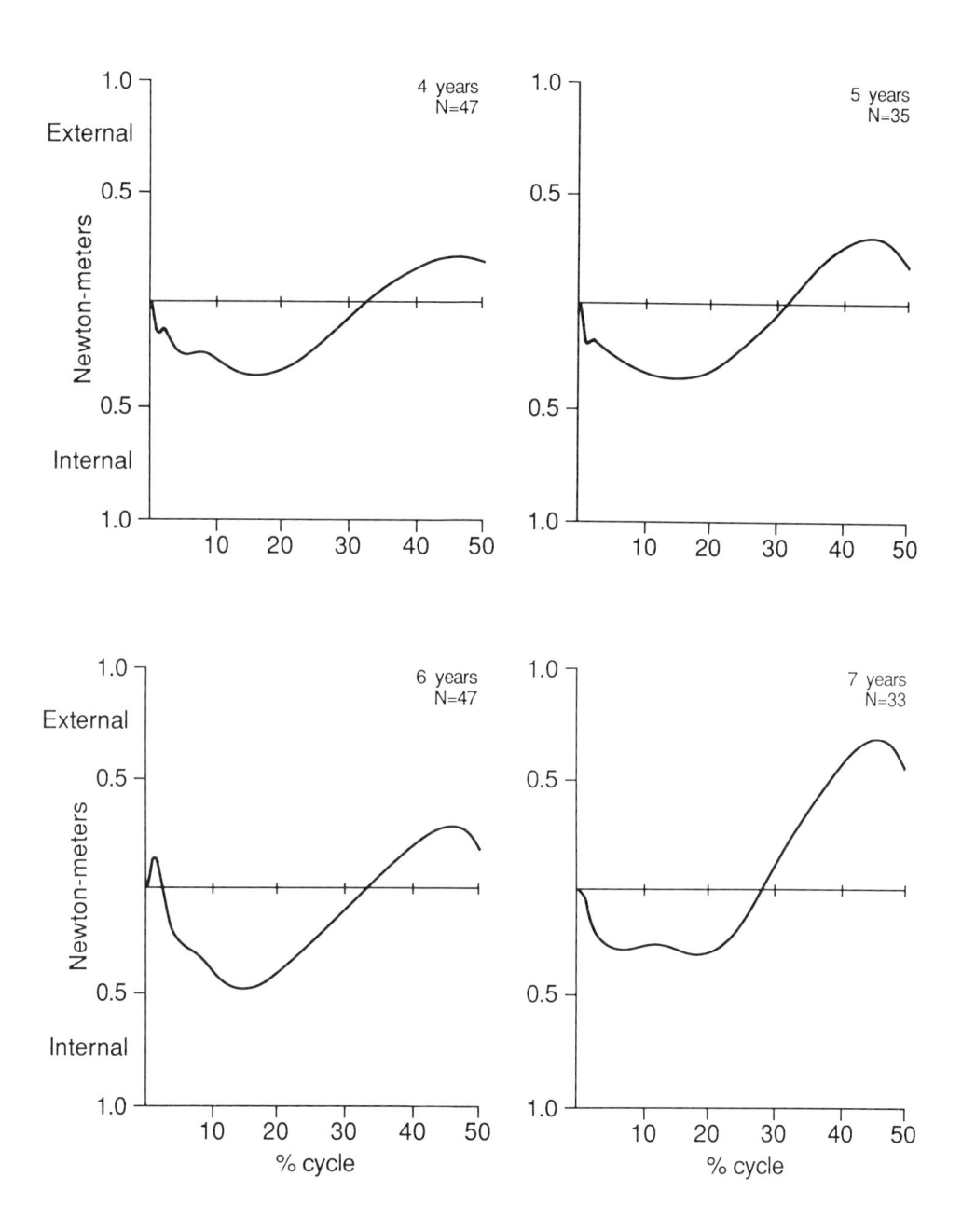

Fig. 9.4B. Fitted torque curves in 4 to 7 year age-groups.

10 per cent of the gait cycle. The transition from internal to external torque is at around 30 per cent of the cycle, matching both the transition point for fore/aft shear and the mid-stance trough in the vertical-force curve. The trough representing maximum external torque occurs at approximately 40 per cent of the gait cycle.

The fitted torque curves for our 2- to 7-year-old subjects are presented in Figure 9.4. Those for children up to age 3 years show no external torque. The five remaining age-groups from 3½ to 7 years all have well-developed external as well as internal torque. The transition from internal to external torque occurs slightly later than in normal adults, varying from approximately 31 to 33 per cent.

In mature gait, internal torque accompanies loading of the limb, pronation of the foot, and internal rotation of the pelvis, femur and tibia. External torque, later in the cycle, accompanies movement of the center of mass of the body in front of the point of support, and external rotation of the pelvis, femur and tibia. The timing of events suggests a relationship with subtalar motion. Pronation of the foot begins at foot-strike and peaks at 20 per cent of the cycle. The transition to supination occurs just before 40 per cent of the cycle, with the peak occurring at about 50 per cent (Inman *et al.* 1981).

We have had substantial difficulties in understanding fitted torque curves, particularly during the first 30 per cent of the gait cycle (which is 60 per cent of the portion of the cycle under consideration). The difficulties may be attributable to at least three causes. (1) Errors of measurement of the center of pressure in these data are unknown (and by now are unknowable since the laboratory no longer has the particular force plate from which the data were gathered). (2) The 'signal-to-noise' ratio tends to be much smaller for torque than for any of the other components of force. (3) If the variability across children is primarily in phase and not functional shape, then combining fits by averaging fitted spline coefficients may be inappropriate. Indeed, perhaps some sort of knot placement that varies with each child, with rescaling before combining, should be attempted.

Discussion
Force data comprise an important part of the data we gather for clinical studies. However, they are generally used less in clinical interpretation of gait than are motion or electromyographic results. This study demonstrated how difficult it is to gather data on very young subjects. Children under the age of 2 years have been described as having 'maximum will with minimum judgement', and as such present a challenge to any investigator. In addition, the design and positioning of our force plate made it difficult to achieve clean foot-strikes with the smaller children. However, we were able to carry out a substantial number of studies on children between the ages of 2 and 7 years. As we have not been able to find studies with comparable numbers in the literature, we feel that this presentation has value despite its limitations.

The authors whose work comprise baselines for comparison are Cunningham (1950) and Endo and Kimura (1972). Endo and Kimura designed a static-gauge force transducer and collected data on six children between the ages of 19 months and 8 years. They compared graphical output for vertical force, fore/aft shear and medial/lateral shear with that of normal adult subjects studied in the same fashion, normalizing the results by relation to body weight. They concluded that the children had force curves which were qualitatively similar to those of the adults, but with exaggerated peaks. They suggested that differences in cadence might explain the differences. Cunningham studied a group of normal adults as well as subjects wearing prostheses. The results for the normal subjects were similar to those for the adults in the study by Endo and Kimura.

Our results are somewhat at odds with both these studies, since we found that the average peak forces were lower in our subjects than those observed in adults. Also, cadence decreases as walking matures, and decreased cadence usually leads to decreased mid-stance troughs in the vertical-force curves. We suggest that the increasing definition of the force curves with maturation is controlled by improved balance and higher velocity.

Our data reflect free-speed walking. We found fewer differences than we had anticipated between the force curves of our children and those of adults. Below we summarize the results for the data collected.

Fore/aft shear shows even less evidence of change with age than vertical force. Reversal of fore/aft shear occurs after 30 per cent of the cycle in all of the eight age-groups considered, although there was a trend toward progressive increase in time of transition. From 4 years on, our subjects displayed transition times and peak levels at the same points in the cycle as the adults studied by Cunningham.

The primary evidence of gait maturation found in our vertical-force data was the increasing definition of the mid-stance trough. We attribute the maturational changes in vertical force to increasing single-limb stance, stride length and walking velocity. The mean loading peaks observed in our study were around 110 per cent of body weight in all groups. These are lower than the 119 to 130 per cent loads measured by Cunningham in his study of normal adults.

Medial/lateral shear showed no maturational changes in the children in our study. Their pattern of medial/lateral shear does not seem to differ from that of adults.

Torque shows a distinct pattern of maturation, with no external torque being observed before the age of 3½ years. From 3½ to 7 years torque becomes progressively more adult in its pattern.

Force data form an interesting component of the information collected under the umbrella of gait analysis. We feel, on a clinical basis, that they provide a useful adjunct to motion and electromyographic data. Care must be used in interpretation, as the data for force at the foot reflect the dynamics of the body above, and it is easy to be led astray if the motions and muscle actions contributing to that force are not considered.

10
AGE AND GAIT

In this chapter we deal with the problem of determining a child's age from measurements that are not necessarily related to his or her physical size. Average hip rotation, for example, is such a variable, while leg length is not. These measurements are termed 'non-age-specific'. A related focus of the chapter is the determination of what constitutes mature walking. An interesting product of this study is a 'binary decision tree' (with accompanying explanations), intended for use in assessing the gait of a possibly neurologically impaired child, by inferring for that child a 'fitted' age. Thus a 5-year-old whose gait most resembles, say, that of a normal 2-year-old, might thereby have his/her deficit quantified in a useful way.

Both parametric and nonparametric statistical techniques were applied to the problem, though only the most easily interpretable is reported here. This is the CART* method of Breiman *et al.* (1984). It was applied to 421 sets of gait data from our study.

Over the last 20 or so years, binary-tree structured methods have been studied theoretically, by simulation, and in applications for various problems of statistics and pattern recognition. The most important area has been that of what is termed 'discrimination' or 'classification'. A classification problem arises when a subject falls naturally into one of a finite number of identifiable groups, or 'classes'. Class membership is determined, at least in part, by certain variables, or 'predictors'. We have a study group for whom both predictors and class membership are known. On the basis of this sample an algorithm, or rule, is derived so that future subjects, for whom predictors are known but class membership is not, can be assigned a class on the basis of these predictors. Here, the 10 age-groups are our classes, while non-age-specific gait measurements are our predictors.

In the customary set-up for studying such classification problems, there are specified parameters termed 'prior probabilities' and 'misclassification costs'. The prior probabilities give respective chances of class membership for all subjects computed without regard to the additional information conveyed by the predictors. The misclassification costs define values for the placing, or 'fitting', of a subject belonging to one class into a different class. In our application, the prior probabilities are equal (at 0.1, there being 10 classes), while the misclassification costs are defined as the square root of the difference in class. (For instance, consider the 6-year-old given a 'fitted' age of 3 years. The classes go: 6, 5, 4, 3½, 3; thus the true age and the fitted age are four classes apart. The 'cost' of this fit is the root of four, that is, two.)

In the CART approach, the range of the predictors (*i.e.* the study-group data) is successively partitioned into 'boxes' by a sequence of linear inequalities.

*CART is a trademark of California Statistical Software, Inc.

(Unordered, discrete predictors, if we had them, could also be used.) The process of partitioning results in a binary decision tree, of which the root node comprises the study-group data, and which leads to a series of terminal nodes, each of which corresponds to an estimate of class membership (*i.e.* a 'fitted' age).

Through these techniques, which are sometimes described as 'recursive partitioning', sequences of simple, optimally chosen questions regarding predictors 'purify' successive nodes. That is, we try to render the subjects who fall into the respective 'daughter' nodes as homogeneous in age as is possible by their answers to simple yes/no questions regarding single predictors. While the technology involves optimal splitting criteria, at least equally important are criteria for pruning large trees on the basis of cross-validatory estimates of risk, applicable if each of a nested sequence of trees were used prospectively for the cited diagnostic purpose. Other salutary aspects of the algorithms are the handling of missing data (which are inevitable in clinical studies), ranking the importance of the predictors to the problem at hand, and the ease with which faulty data (outliers) are detected.

The binary tree displayed in Figure 10.1 was produced by an approach in which the 10 age-groups in our study were considered as 10 classes. Subjects in terminal node A are those with: walking velocity <89.5cm/sec., average hip rotation <−13.2°, and pelvic-span/ankle-spread (P/A) ratio <1.6 – that is, these children walk slowly, cannot rotate their hips internally as they walk, and walk with a broad base of support. Now, referring to Table 10.I, it can be seen that of the 421 children in our study, 34 fell into terminal node A, of whom 33 were 1-year-olds and the other a 1½-year-old. Subjects falling into terminal node B differed from those in A only in that their P/A ratio was greater (*i.e.* their base of support was narrower). It stands to reason that these children should be similar in age, but slightly older; Table 10.I bears this out, indicating an assigned age of 1½ years. Readers are encouraged to study Figure 10.1 and Table 10.I to see what the requirements were for membership in each of the 16 terminal nodes of the tree, and to consider the respective distributions of ages and assigned ages.

Note that variables such as Tib $\hat{\beta}_2$ and Hip $\hat{\beta}_1$ refer to measured values of parameters in the model (**1**) (see Chapter 3, p. 24). 'Tib' refers to tibial rotation and 'Hip' to hip rotation. While it is not easy to develop an intuition as to the clinical implications of these numbers, it should at least be pointed out that the subscripts (2 in the first example and 1 in the second) refer to the harmonic (j) in question—thus Tib $\hat{\beta}_2$ refers to an aspect of tibial motion that occurs twice per cycle. Also, 'Ave' refers to measured values of the α_0 term in the cited model, that is, to average values across the gait cycle.

Ideally, the range of the predictors, which number 18 after extensive screening, is subdivided by the algorithm so that children in each region are exactly, or nearly, the same age. In view of our findings, as shown in Table 10.I, we believe that we did reasonably well.

The fitted age in each terminal node is constant, and is the result of a so-called Bayes classification rule applied to the children at that node. Generally, even if the joint probability distribution of classes and predictors is known, it is not possible to do a perfect job of classifying test subjects. A Bayes classification

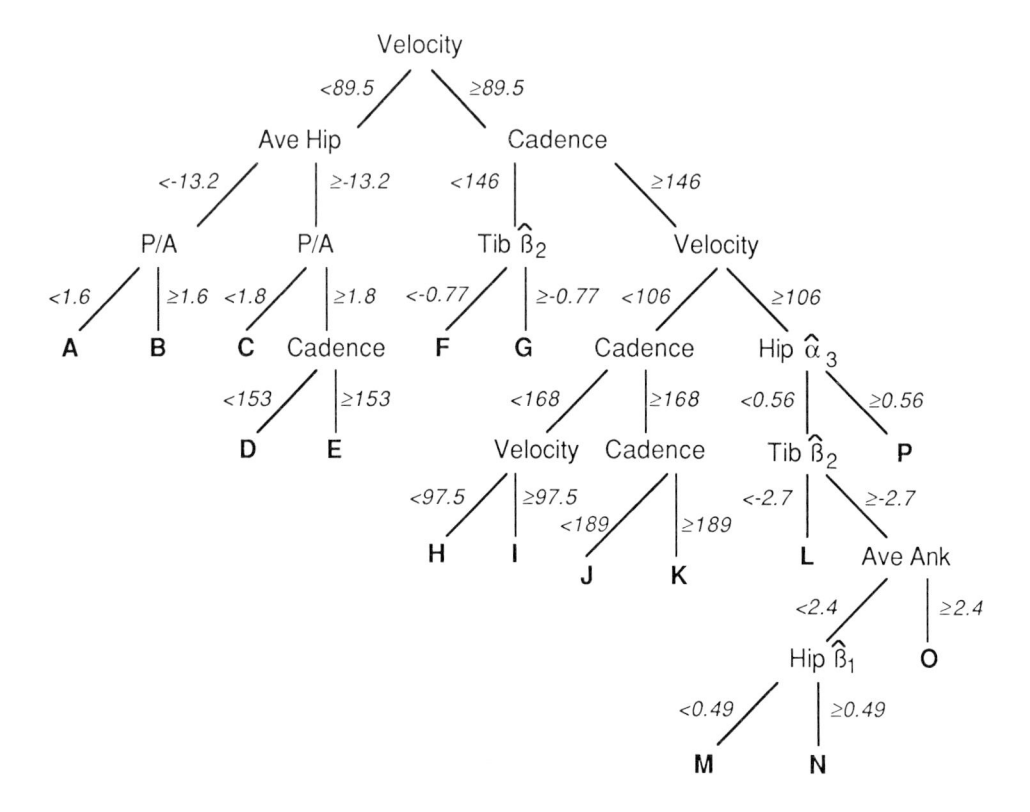

Fig. 10.1. Binary tree for predicting age from gait measurements.
This tree and its accompanying Table 10.I are a device for assigning an age to a test subject based on gait measurements that are not age-specific. At each juncture (node), an optimally chosen question is asked. At the top, for instance, the question is, 'Is walking velocity less than 89.5cm/sec.?' If yes, proceed to the left where the subsequent question is, 'Is hip rotation, averaged across the gait cycle, less than $-13.2°$?' If no, proceed to the right, where the next question concerns cadence. Eventually, the test subject proceeds to one of 16 'terminal nodes' (denoted by the letters A to P). Each of these terminal nodes corresponds to an age which has been assigned on the basis of the ages of the subjects in our study who ended up there. These are listed in Table 10.I. Thus if the test subject, on the basis of seven questions asked in sequence, falls in terminal node M, his/her assigned age is 7 years. Most of the variables about which questions are asked at the various nodes should be obvious to the reader. However, note that 'Ave Ank' refers to values of ankle rotation averaged across the cycle; the Fourier coefficient 'Tib $\hat{\beta}_2$' refers to an aspect of tibial rotation that occurs twice per cycle (see text); 'Hip $\hat{\beta}_1$' likewise refers to an aspect of hip rotation that occurs once per cycle; and 'P/A' refers to the pelvic-span/ankle-spread ratio, higher values of which denote greater maturation.

rule is one that in terms of the prior probabilities and misclassification costs does, on average, the best job possible. In some situations there is a unique Bayes rule; in others there may be infinitely many. What they all have in common is the same overall long-term average misclassification cost. Experience has borne out that our approach successfully approximates a Bayes rule (see Breiman *et al.* 1984).

TABLE 10.I*
Terminal node contents and assigned ages (see Figure 10.1)

Terminal node	Assigned age	1	1½	2	2½	3	3½	4	5	6	7	Total
A	1	33	1	—	—	—	—	—	—	—	—	34
B	1½	12	24	9	4	—	—	—	—	—	—	49
C	2	2	7	13	3	—	—	1	—	—	—	26
D	3	—	—	3	9	18	6	10	3	3	—	52
E	2	1	5	13	10	9	1	1	—	—	1	41
F	6	—	—	—	—	—	—	—	—	15	8	23
G	7	—	—	—	—	1	1	2	4	6	16	30
H	3½	—	—	—	4	8	17	3	4	1	—	37
I	4	—	—	—	—	4	3	8	5	2	—	22
J	2½	—	—	3	5	4	—	2	—	—	—	14
K	1½	2	3	2	—	—	—	—	—	—	—	7
L	4	—	—	1	—	—	4	5	2	—	—	12
M	7	—	—	—	—	—	1	2	5	5	19	32
N	5	—	—	—	1	—	1	—	4	—	—	6
O	5	—	—	—	—	1	1	2	7	1	—	12
P	6	—	—	—	—	1	5	2	4	11	1	24
Total		50	40	44	36	46	40	38	38	44	45	421

*Adapted by permission from Breiman et al. (1984).

TABLE 10.II*
True age vs. fitted age for the 421 study-group subjects

Fitted age	1	1½	2	2½	3	3½	4	5	6	7	Total
1	33	1	—	—	—	—	—	—	—	—	34
1½	14	27	11	4	—	—	—	—	—	—	56
2	3	12	26	13	9	1	2	—	—	—	66
2½	—	—	3	5	4	—	2	—	—	—	14
3	—	—	3	9	18	6	10	3	3	1	53
3½	—	—	—	4	8	17	3	4	1	—	37
4	—	—	1	—	4	7	13	7	2	—	34
5	—	—	—	1	1	2	2	11	1	—	18
6	—	—	—	—	1	5	2	4	26	9	47
7	—	—	—	—	1	2	4	9	11	35	62
Total	50	40	44	36	46	40	38	38	44	45	421

*Adapted by permission from Breiman et al. (1984).

Table 10.II summarizes how well the assigned, or fitted, ages corresponded to the true ages of the subjects in our study group. Of course, one would not do so well were the tree to be applied prospectively to a new group of 421 children; however, cross-validation indicated that it would do quite well, and no worse than could be expected of other more complicated techniques we tried.

As stated, the CART methodology comes equipped with its own technique for assessing the importance of the predictors to the fitting process. The results quoted in Table 10.III are derived from a more sophisticated process of selection than were

TABLE 10.III

Relative variable importance* (for growing the tree of Figure 10.1)

Walking velocity	100
Average hip rotation	64
Right single stance %	56
Pelvic-span/ankle-spread ratio	52
Hip $\hat{\alpha}_2$	44
Cadence	40
Hip abduction/adduction $\hat{\beta}_2$	36
Hip $\hat{\beta}_1$	36
Average tibial rotation	36
Hip $\hat{\alpha}_4$	32
Average ankle rotation	28
Foot $\hat{\alpha}_1$	28
Hip abduction/adduction $\hat{\beta}_1$	28
Tib $\hat{\beta}_2$	28
Hip $\hat{\alpha}_3$	24
Tib $\hat{\beta}_1$	24
Hip $\hat{\beta}_4$	24
Dominance	16

*In order to rank predictors as to their importance, there are at least two extremely different criteria one might consider. A feature could be 'important' if good prediction can be achieved when it is the only one available. Alternatively, one might call a feature 'important' if, when all the features are used, node purification is most degraded by deletion of that single feature. The CART methodology that we employed takes an approach that is a compromise of these two criteria, and involves asking how well a feature does in imitating the 'best' split at each node. Thus a feature which has a high relative importance may never actually be chosen for a 'best' question anywhere in the decision tree.

related results reported by Sutherland *et al.* (1980*a*); nevertheless, it is clear that the two lists are similar in that all non-age-specific measurements deemed important in the earlier study are still found to be so here. Note that not one piece of sagittal-plane information made the list of variables retained for this run, let alone was deemed 'important' for classification. This result stands in marked contrast to our previous determinations of important measurements in classifying children with Duchenne muscular dystrophy (Sutherland *et al.* 1981).

11
RELATIONSHIP OF NEURAL DEVELOPMENT AND WALKING

Introduction
It is a curious fact that the newborn human infant is totally dependent, and that the development of mobility occurs more slowly than in the majority of animal species. What are the reasons for the usual 12-month interval between human birth and independent walking and for the additional 2 years required for gait maturation? Intuitively, bipedal gait with its demand for single-limb support is more difficult than quadrupedal gait. Does it take more time to learn to cope with gravity on two feet rather than four, or does the answer lie in the slower development of the motor control system in the human species, as suggested by Robinson and Tizard (1966) and Norton (1981)? Alternatively, it may be that both maturation of the motor control system and learning are needed.

The human motor control system has been studied extensively, but many questions regarding its function remain unanswered. One such question is, what are the relative roles of the voluntary supraspinal centers and reflexes mediated through spinal centers in controlling walking? It is commonly believed that only the command to walk or to modify walking speed or direction are voluntary supraspinal activities. The timing of muscle action and the intensity of muscle contractions are handled through spinal centers and peripheral nerves. In the mature normal human, peripheral receptors in the skin, muscles and joints provide afferent stimuli which are automatically processed through spinal centers to modify muscle action in walking (Grillner 1975). This physiological fact explains the lack of conscious effort required to sustain walking and it helps us to understand how it is possible to walk across a darkened room with little difficulty (at least until an unexpected obstacle is encountered). In normal walking, visual stimuli are of less importance than kinesthetic stimuli in judging limb position, although they do provide information about terrain and other moving objects. If you are skeptical, note that on your way from office to automobile you commonly see terrain, other individuals and vehicles but seldom, if ever, your lower limbs. Sensory input from the vestibular system derived from sway-related linear and angular accelerations of the head may also contribute to balance and walking; however, it seems to play a secondary role to kinesthetic and visual sensory input except when the support surface is disrupted, or when visual stimuli are lost or impaired (Begbie 1967, Nashner *et al.* 1982). An efficient conduction system is required to link peripheral receptors with the central nervous system centers where motor commands originate. Intuitively, cortical control, an efficient conduction system and well-developed interneuron connections are all needed to achieve mature gait, but independent walking can begin before the system reaches maturity.

Pre-walking development
What about spontaneous kicking in infants and reflexive stepping? How do they fit into the complexities of gait maturation? Thelen and associates have presented evidence that both these features may be forerunners of mature locomotion (Thelen *et al.* 1981, Thelen and Fisher 1982). They found that the patterns of movement are identical, although some modification occurs when weight is placed on the soles in the stepping reflex. They demonstrated by a combination of kinematic, electromyographic and motivational comparisons that newborn stepping was the same stereotyped movement as spontaneous kicking seen in newborns in the supine position, and that both movements were probably a muscle synergism later incorporated into erect locomotion. They concluded that step-like movements were not specifically triggered by the upright position, as is generally believed, but, like kicking, are reactivated by tonic increases in generalized behavioral arousal. Reflexive stepping usually disappears at around 2 months of age, but spontaneous kicking persists and, according to Thelen and Fisher (1982), may represent a basic component of locomotion.

The maturation process which leads to independent human locomotion is complex. Learning, emergence of cortical control, sensory integration and myelination are taking place simultaneously, making it difficult to identify a single responsible element. According to Byers (1941), all the neuronal cells are present by 7½ months from conception. No mitotic figures are detectable in neurons after this age (Rabinowitz 1964). If this information is correct, the long postnatal period required for walking in man cannot be due to lack of neuronal development. The subsequent fourfold growth of the brain is mainly due to deposition of myelin and to a vast elaboration of dendritic processes, although there is also a considerable increase in vascular tissues (Rabinowitz 1964). While the brain of a fullterm newborn infant is already a quarter of the weight of the adult brain, the other organs of the body are only approximately one twentieth of their final adult weight, indicating that the brain is proportionately more mature at birth than are the other organs (Rabinowitz 1964). It is not known if myelin development is crucial, or if the dendrite/soma relationships which develop during the same period of postnatal growth are the major factors in the development of upright walking.

Function of myelin in the nervous system
The benefits of myelination include: lower energy requirements for nerve conduction; rapid conduction; and marked reduction in space required (Morell and Norton 1980). Myelin has been described as an electrical insulator that speeds conduction with a relatively small nerve fiber, thus allowing a large number of nerve fibers in a small space. A much reduced flow of sodium ions is required for nerve conduction with myelin present, and the conduction signal leaps from node to node of Ranvier (saltatory conduction). Without myelin, the entire axonal membrane must depolarize and then repolarize.

If myelin were lacking, the control system would be slow and energy requirements high, as in multiple sclerosis. Otherwise, the size of the fibers would have to be greatly increased until the central nervous system occupied a disproportionate share of body space (Morell and Norton 1980).

Composition of myelin
Both lipids and proteins develop from the cell-surface membranes of the Schwann cells. The lipid layers alternate with the protein layers. The lipids include cholesterol, phospholipid and glycolipid. The concentration of lipid is high, and thus it excludes water and water-soluble ions including sodium and potassium. The glycolipid, cerebroside, which is found primarily in the myelin sheaths, represents 20 per cent of the total dry weight of the myelin. Myelin basic protein and proteolipoid protein comprise the protein layers which alternate with the lipid layers (Morell and Norton 1980).

Sequence of myelin formation in man
Biochemical studies reveal that myelination is primarily a postnatal process in humans. The most rapid rate of myelination occurs between 32 weeks gestational age and 6 months after birth (Martinez and Ballabriga 1978). With some exceptions, the process moves cephalocaudally and from proximal to distal (Rafalowska 1979). The spinal roots myelinate earlier than the central tracts of the cord. The anterior roots of segments C8 to T1 are the first to myelinate, followed by the posterior roots of C8 to T1 and the anterior roots of L5 to S1, and finally the dorsal roots of the lumbar segment (Rafalowska 1979). According to Matthews (1968), the increase in axon diameter stimulates myelination. The thinnest mature myelinated fibers in the peripheral nervous system are about 1μm in diameter, while in the central nervous system even thinner myelinated fibers are present.

Myelin formation in mammals
Norton (1981) has noted that the central nervous systems of rats and other nest-building animals myelinate postnatally for the most part, and these animals are helpless at birth. In contrast, grazing animals with considerable myelin in the central nervous system at birth are active from the moment they are born. Man is a 'mother-clinging animal', helpless at birth much as the nest animals (Robinson and Tizard 1966).

Functional assessment of myelination
The best functional assessment of myelination comes from sensory and motor conduction velocity studies. Studies of normal children reveal maturation, as evidenced by adult conduction velocities, at between 2 and 5 years of age, depending on the nerves sampled (Gamstorp 1963, Baer and Johnson 1965). Conduction velocities in the infant are less than half of those in older children, and these low velocities have been shown to correlate with the incomplete myelination of the nerves. Motor nerves and anterior roots mature before dorsal nerve roots and sensory nerves. This differential is helpful in explaining at least one aspect of delayed maturation of the control system. Motor action takes place before there is adequate modification through sensory feedback.

Correlation of myelination with development of walking
The striato-acoustic system has completed myelination before birth (Meyersburg and Post 1979). The motor roots are developed by the first month of life. The optic

radiations and tracts have achieved maturity by 4 months, the sensory roots by 6 months, and the sensory tracts by 12 months. The pyramidal tracts and striatum also are largely complete by the age of 1 year. The cerebellar peduncles, limbic system and acoustic radiations are complete by 5 years (Meyersburg and Post 1979). The child stands alone by 10 or 11 months, and usually walks by 12 months.

Walking impairment in demyelinating diseases

There are a number of experimental and natural diseases in which demyelination is a common finding, and all of these diseases are characterized by disturbed gait.

The experimental model for demyelination in *multiple sclerosis* is allergic encephalomyelitis, produced in monkeys by repeated injection of cerebral tissue (Rivers and Schwentker 1935). Paresis, ataxia, nystagmus and blindness can also be induced in monkeys by this method (Wolf *et al.* 1947). While multiple sclerosis is rare in infants and children, disturbed gait and impaired vision are the most common presenting complaints in children with this disease (Low and Carter 1956, Gall *et al.* 1958, Menkes 1985).

Acute infectious polyneuritis (Landry-Guillain-Barre syndrome), also a demyelinating disease, begins in the lower extremities and ascends, with paralysis presenting in around 50 per cent of patients, and recovery, often complete, in a period of from 2 to 18 months (Menkes 1985). Both motor and sensory impairments occur, and in paralytic cases the clinical presentation can vary from minor involvement to total quadriplegia and respiratory paralysis.

Charcot-Marie-Tooth disease produces atrophy and weakness of the distal musculature of the lower extremities and, to a lesser extent, of the upper extremities (Charcot and Marie 1886, Tooth 1896, Menkes 1985). In the Dejerine-Sottas variety, distal sensory impairment is usual, with impairment of vibratory sensation (Dejerine and Sottas 1893, Menkes 1985). The *Lévy-Roussy syndrome* adds tremor of the hands to the clumsy gait, areflexia and deformity of the feet found in Charcot-Marie-Tooth disease (Roussy and Lévy 1926, Menkes 1985).

Friedreich's ataxia is a heterodegenerative condition producing cavus deformities of the feet, kyphoscoliosis and severe ataxia. In addition to demyelination, there is axonal degeneration and compensatory gliosis, particularly involving the cerebellar afferents in the spinal cord and the dorsal-ventral roots (Menkes 1985).

Discussion

The timetables for human myelination and for the development of complex motor functions, including walking, are roughly parallel. It is logical to assume that rapid transmission of neural impulses from both central and peripheral receptors is necessary for gait modification, and that myelination is required to speed neural transmission. Furthermore, demyelinating diseases do seriously impair or prevent walking. In spite of this circumstantial evidence suggesting a crucial role for myelination, it is important to remember that other processes of maturation are proceeding simultaneously. It may be that too heavy an emphasis has been placed upon myelination because it can be identified with relative ease, in comparison with the establishment of synaptic connections which are not readily measured (Dobbing and Sands 1973). Be that as it may, it is safe to say that maturation of the motor control system is the key factor in both the landmark event of independent walking and in the process of transformation of the shaky, staccato movements of the toddler into the smooth, energy-efficient pattern which we recognize as mature walking.

Does learning play a significant role in early walking? Perhaps, although it seems unlikely that the onset of walking can be accelerated in advance of a critical level of central nervous system maturation. Any parent who has tried to coax a child to take first steps will attest to the futility of attempting to speed the process. The child, usually but not always, goes through stages of creeping, crawling, pulling to stand, cruising (see footnote, p. 50) and finally independent walking, *when the time is right*. The process seems to be instinctive rather than cognitive and maturation is the determining factor. The transformation of immature to mature walking also follows an orderly pattern which is best explained by progressive maturation (Grillner *et al.* 1985).

We are confident that the insights gained from the research presented herein provide a scientific description of the early changes in human gait. Current and future research in the neurosciences will clarify the roles of the various components of the maturation process.

12
RELEVANCE TO CLINICAL PRACTICE

Introduction
As shown in the preceding chapters, the walking patterns of young children differ substantially from those of adults. Knowledge of these age-related changes provides the foundation for studies of children with suspected pathological gait. The observer who lacks an understanding of the changes that occur with growth and development may exaggerate the significance of movement alterations which are part of normal development, or may miss clinically important deviations from normal. For those who do not have access to a gait laboratory, a data base comprising measurements of time/distance parameters, joint angles, muscle phasic activity and ground-reaction forces in a normal population, together with tracings from cine film, are substantial aids in improving skills in observation and in understanding gait. For those with a gait lab, such aids are indispensable. Obviously it is futile to consider pathological gait without normal measurements for comparison.

But why perform gait studies at all? The first reason is to provide a description of the subject. Gait is a sensitive measure of neuromuscular development or impairment, and a sound descriptive model is useful in defining normal versus abnormal gait, giving some clues as to the underlying cause of abnormality. Secondly, by following children through a treatment program it bcomes possible to predict what is likely to happen in future cases.

Gait analysis has been used extensively in the evaluation of patients with cerebral palsy. In our own medical center we rely on objective gait measurements supplemented by careful clinical examination to prepare treatment plans and to assess the outcome of treatment. This level of care prevails in a growing number of medical centers. What are some of the contributions of gait studies to the understanding of gait abnormalities in cerebral palsy, and has treatment changed as a consequence of them? We can look to the medical literature for examples of their positive influence, and we can anticipate the development of gait systems which will make results such as those reported in this book widely available to clinicians.

In this chapter, then, we look first at examples of gait analysis from the literature, followed by two cases from our own laboratory.

Gait analysis in the literature
Mann *et al.* (1975) used an optical system of movement measurement to demonstrate the unfavourable effects upon pelvic alignment and hip extension of proximal hamstring release. They concluded that while the operation achieved the desired improvements in knee extension and step length, the unfavorable side-effects of increased anterior pelvic tilt and diminished hip extension made this particular procedure a poor choice for the treatment of hamstring contractures in ambulatory patients.

Sutherland *et al.* (1975) used movement measurements to show the improvement in early swing-phase flexion following rectus femoris release in patients with stiff-knee gait associated with rectus femoris spasticity.

Simon *et al.* (1977) used force vectors and measurements from cine film to devise 'stick' figures to demonstrate the effect of below-knee orthosis in reducing early stance-phase genu recurvatum.

Sutherland and Cooper (1978) described the pathomechanics of progressive crouch gait in spastic diplegia, using force-plate and joint-torque measurements. These revealed excessive stance-phase knee-flexion torque, which was illustrated by superimposing the force vector on sequential film tracings.

Studies of cerebral-palsied children's energy consumption while walking have shown it to be considerably greater than in normal children (Campbell and Ball 1978). This is evidenced by a higher heart rate (the best clinical indicator) and a greater consumption of oxygen during walking, and explains why these children become fatigued easily and need frequent rest. Findings from studies such as these have important implications for parents, doctors and therapists in setting realistic treatment goals, and suggest that many children should be given mobility aids at an earlier age to enable them to keep up with their peers.

Baumann *et al.* (1980) reported pre- and postoperative gait studies of 34 patients with cerebral palsy who had distal lengthenings of the hamstring muscles to overcome excessive knee flexion. The dynamic joint angles of hip, knee and ankle were plotted before and after surgery in 20 patients. A large reduction in knee flexion in stance was achieved, although this improvement was also accompanied by a moderate loss of flexion in swing phase.

Perry *et al.* (1974) used electromyography to investigate the validity of the Silverskiold test. The positive test is this: when there is a contracture in the gastrocnemius but not in the soleus muscle, the foot will remain in equinus deformity despite forcible dorsiflexion when the knee is extended, but not when it is flexed. 17 patients with persistent equinus gait were studied in the sitting position, with slow and then rapid stretching of the heel cord; gait EMGs were also performed. Perry and her associates concluded that the presence of a primitive synergy of the extensors, with increased tone in both muscles when the knee is extended, invalidates the Silverskiold test. To be meaningful, the test must be carried out with the patient anesthetized—this eliminates the primitive extensor reflex, and the presence of selective contracture of the gastrocnemius or soleus can then be determined.

The same authors carried out clinical stretch tests about the hip while monitoring individual muscles with indwelling electrodes, and found that these tests are non-specific and cannot be relied upon to separate the gracilis from the hamstring muscles, nor the adductors from the iliopsoas (Perry *et al.* 1976). Similar observations about the rectus test were made by Roosth (1971) and Sutherland *et al.* (1975). If the traditional passive stretch testing cannot separate muscle activities, it would appear highly desirable to obtain EMGs of individual muscles in normal, level walking as an essential part of preoperative planning (Sutherland *et al.* 1969, Hoffer *et al.* 1974, Perry *et al.* 1976, Perry and Hoffer 1977, Simon 1977).

Postoperative electromyography was used by Gritzka *et al.* (1972) to evaluate posterior tibial transfer through the interosseous membrane to correct equinovarus deformity in cerebral palsy. Nearly all the muscles failed to contract during the swing phase, but seven of the 10 ambulatory limbs were converted from equinovarus gait to heel-strike gait. Gritzka and colleagues attributed the improvement to a 'check-rein' effect: they postulated that the presence of swing-phase activity in the tibialis posterior would act as a dorsiflexor, and that if it were not present the tension of the muscle complex would maintain better swing-phase alignment.

Hoffer *et al.* (1974) used electromyography in planning the treatment of children with spastic varus hind foot. When the EMG revealed spasticity in the tibialis anterior, a split anterior tibial transfer was performed. The report covers 21 such transfers.

Perry and Hoffer (1977) used electromyography in planning tendon transfers in 24 children with cerebral palsy. 16 of these children were treated for flexible hind-foot deformities and four for internally rotated lower limbs. The remaining four children were treated for flexion deformities of the forearm and wrist. When deforming muscles acted exclusively in one portion of either the gait cycle or the movement of an upper extremity, appropriate tendon transfers were performed; but when continuous muscle activity was noted, tendon lengthening was carried out. Varus posture of the hind foot was treated by posterior transfer or split anterior tibial transfer, depending on the EMG pattern. Valgus hind foot was treated by peroneus brevis transfer, internal rotation of the lower limb by hamstring transfer, and pronated forearm and flexed elbow and wrist during grasp and release by flexor carpi ulnaris transfer. 'Only when the timing of muscle activity is known can a rational operative plan be made' (Perry and Hoffer 1977).

Electromyography and movement measurements have been used to evaluate the effects of rectus femoris release (Sutherland *et al.* 1975). Preoperative EMG revealed an increase in early swing-phase activity in patients with rectus spasticity which interfered with the initiation of knee flexion. EMGs were found useful in selecting patients for rectus release surgery by excluding those who demonstrated swing-phase activity of the entire quadriceps muscle, as it was thought that the procedure would be useless in the presence of total quadriceps spasticity.

As Simon (1977) has pointed out, both movement measurements and ground-reaction data are needed, in addition to electromyography, to detect the difference between abnormal and compensatory mechanisms. EMG activity which is out of phase may be truly pathological or may indicate a compensatory mechanism, and if the activity is in normal phase it can still be pathological if there is either increased or decreased muscle tension. This is illustrated by the study of 10 patients with genu-recurvatum gait reported by Simon *et al.* (1977). In these patients an abrupt halt in tibial motion was noted early in stance phase if the calf muscles were overworking, and late in stance phase if the calf muscles were weak. Forward tibial motion was absent in all 10 patients before and during the occurrence of recurvatum, as a result of abnormal calf-muscle activity. Recurvatum occurred when the femur and tibia were in a direct line, and the principal causative factor was the position of the trunk and femur in relation to the tibia/foot complex at the time of the tibia's halt. Below-knee orthosis prevented recurvatum by locking the ankle, but did not change walking ability as measured by velocity, cadence and stride length. This work is valuable in pointing out the complexity of movements in the lower extremities and the need to combine EMG, movement measurements and ground-reaction force studies for full analysis.

Perry (1987) and Gage *et al.* (1987) have applied motion analysis techniques to evaluate a new operation, transfer of the rectus femoris to the sartorius or gracilis to improve swing-phase knee flexion in cerebral palsy. The idea for this procedure came from Perry and it was first performed by Gage. Pre- and postoperative gait studies reported by Gage *et al.* (1987) and similar studies in our own Motion Analysis Laboratory (unpublished) validate the efficacy of this exciting new procedure. It can be carried out alone or in conjunction with distal hamstring lengthenings. The EMG change which characterizes this motion disorder is prolongation of activity in the rectus femoris, extending into swing phase. For the rectus transfer to improve swing-phase knee flexion, the remaining elements of the quadriceps femoris must be silent during the same period.

Case studies

Two examples from our own laboratory have been selected to demonstrate the use of our normal prediction regions, time/distance parameters, dynamic EMG and force measurements to determine whether a child's gait is pathological.

Case 1: Preterm 5-year-old with questionable neuromuscular impairment
Subject #8.506 was born prematurely, with a gestational age of 32 weeks and a birthweight of 1701g. His Apgar score was 9 at 1 minute and again at 5 minutes. At 6½ hours of age, he was transported from an outlying community hospital to the neonatal intensive care unit because of labored respiration and cyanosis. At the time of transport an umbilical artery catheter was placed via sub-umbilical cut-down because intra-umbilical attempts had been unsuccessful. He remained for 27 days in the neonatal intensive care unit for treatment of mild respiratory distress syndrome (requiring oxygen only). The umbilical artery catheter was removed at 7 days of age, and at 10 days oxygen was stopped. His weight had increased to 2150g at the time of discharge from hospital. His parents say that he sat at 3 months, crawled at 4 months, pulled to stand at 4½ months, walked at 10 months and ran at 10 months. The ages given for the first three developmental milestones cast doubt on the accuracy of recall of the parents!

An examination and gait analysis were performed at 5 years corrected age. His height was 108cm (50th percentile of normal subjects) and he weighed 17.3kg (75th percentile). The passive ranges of motion of lower-extremity joints were within normal limits. No pathological reflexes were found. The time/distance parameters are listed in Table 12.I. Note the asymmetry in right and left single stance (35 *vs.* 40 per cent). Stride length is at the 75th percentile of normal subjects, cadence is below the 25th percentile and walking velocity is at the 27th percentile (see Chapter 6)

TABLE 12.I

Time/distance parameters for subject #8.506 at 5 years corrected age

Parameter measured	Right	Left
Opposite toe-off (% cycle)	14	13
Opposite foot-strike (% cycle)	49	53
Single-limb stance (% cycle)	35	40
Toe-off (% cycle)	62	66
Step length (cm)	43	45
Stride length (cm)	88	
Cycle time (secs.)	0.89	
Cadence (steps/min.)	135	
Walking velocity (cm/sec.)	99	
Walking velocity (m/min.)	59	

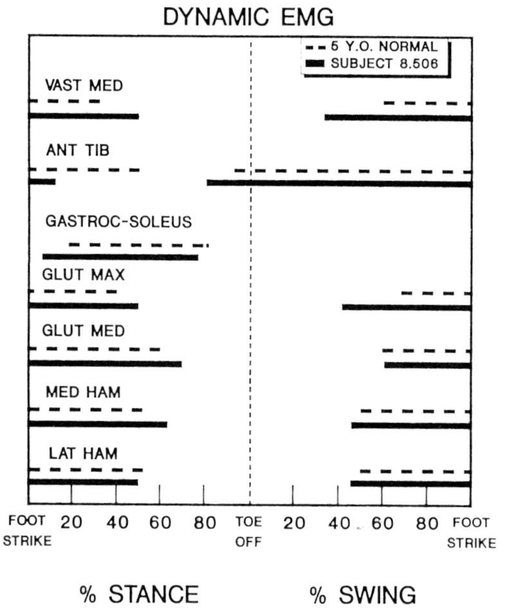

Fig. 12.1. Normalized stance- and swing-phase dynamic EMGs in subject #8.506 compared with mean phasic activity in 5-year-old normal controls.

DYNAMIC ELECTROMYOGRAPHY

EMGs were obtained with surface electrodes from the vastus medialis, anterior tibialis, gastroc/soleus, gluteus maximus, gluteus medius, and medial and lateral hamstrings (Fig. 12.1). Mild abnormalities were noted in vastus medialis, anterior tibialis and gluteus maximus. Activity in the gluteus maximus and vastus medialis began early in swing phase; in the anterior tibialis activity stopped prematurely in stance phase. EMGs of the gluteus medius, medial and lateral hamstrings and gastroc/soleus did not differ significantly from those of normal subjects of the same age (see Chapter 8).

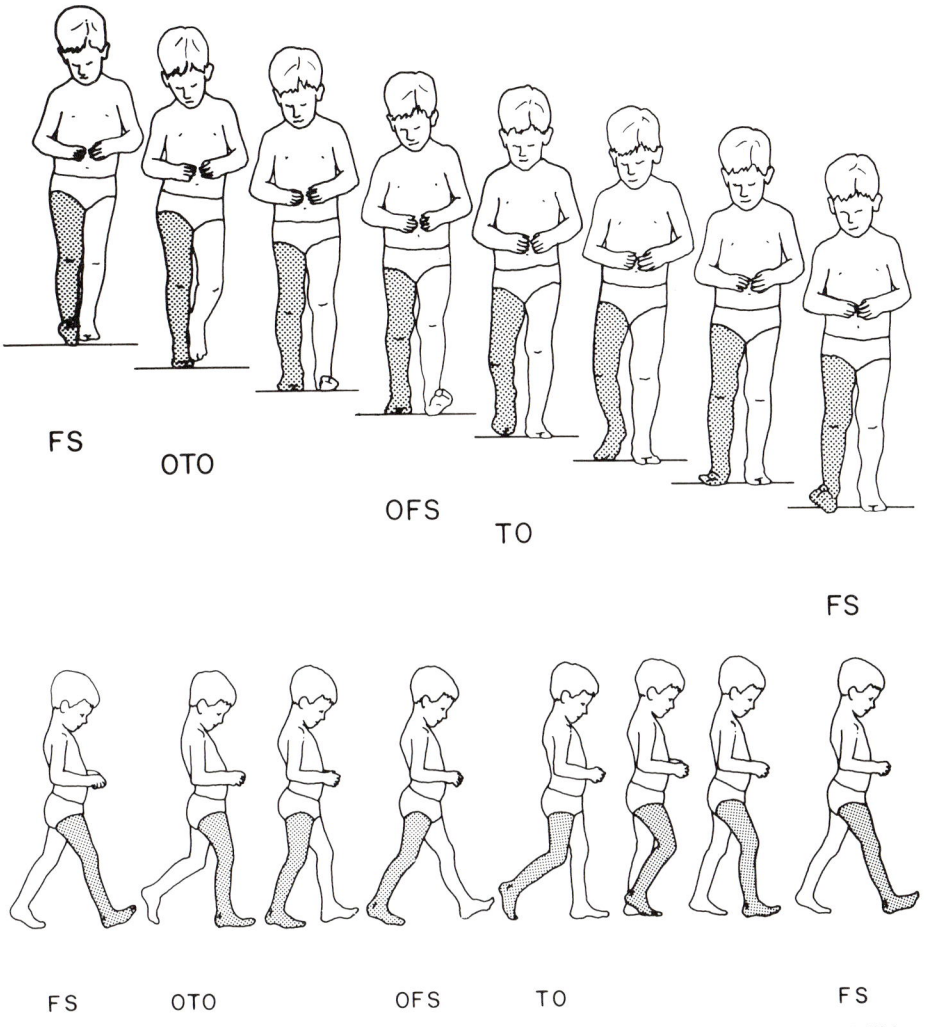

Fig. 12.2. Film tracings from representative gait cycle, side and front views, of subject #8.506.

FILM TRACINGS

Reciprocal arm swing is missing but in other respects his gait appears normal (Fig. 12.2).

JOINT ANGLES

Of 24 joint-angle plots (Figs. 12.3A–X, pp. 194–197), two fell slightly outside the 95 per cent prediction regions: right hip abduction/adduction (Fig. 12.3B) and right foot rotation (Fig. 12.3L). Right heel-strike was absent, as indicated by lack of increasing plantar flexion after foot-strike in the right ankle dorsi-/plantar flexion curve (Fig. 12.3F).

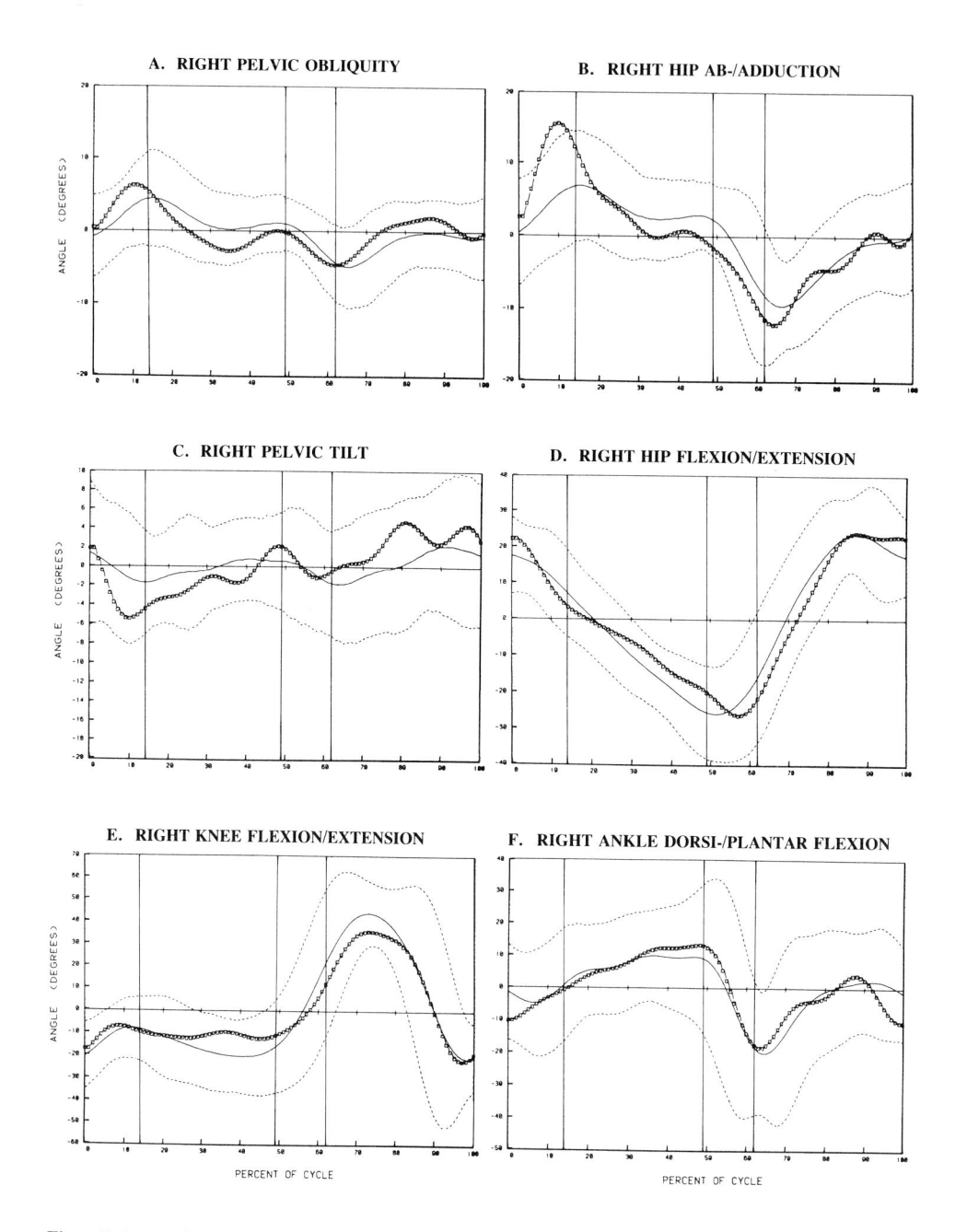

Figs. 12.3A–F. Graphs plotting the sum of harmonic terms (α_0 term removed: see Chapter 3) in the fitting of the right-side joint-angle data from subject #8.506.

In each case the heavy line is from the subject. The upper and lower broken lines are the boundaries of the 95 per cent prediction region. The solid central line represents the population average for 5-year-old normal subjects. The three vertical lines indicate opposite toe-off, opposite foot-strike and toe-off.

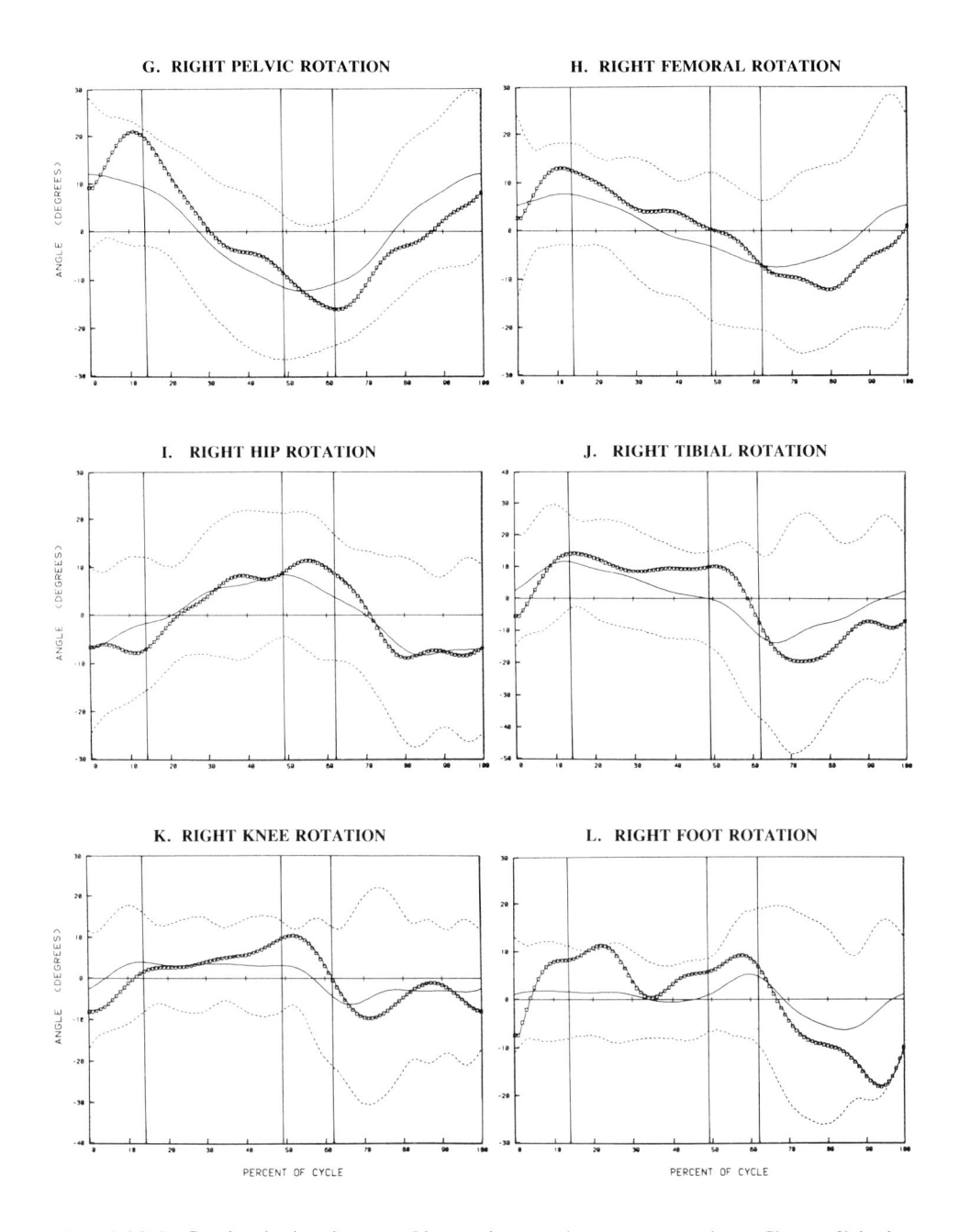

Figs. 12.3G–L. Graphs plotting the sum of harmonic terms (α_0 term removed: see Chapter 3) in the fitting of the right-side joint-angle data from subject #8.506.

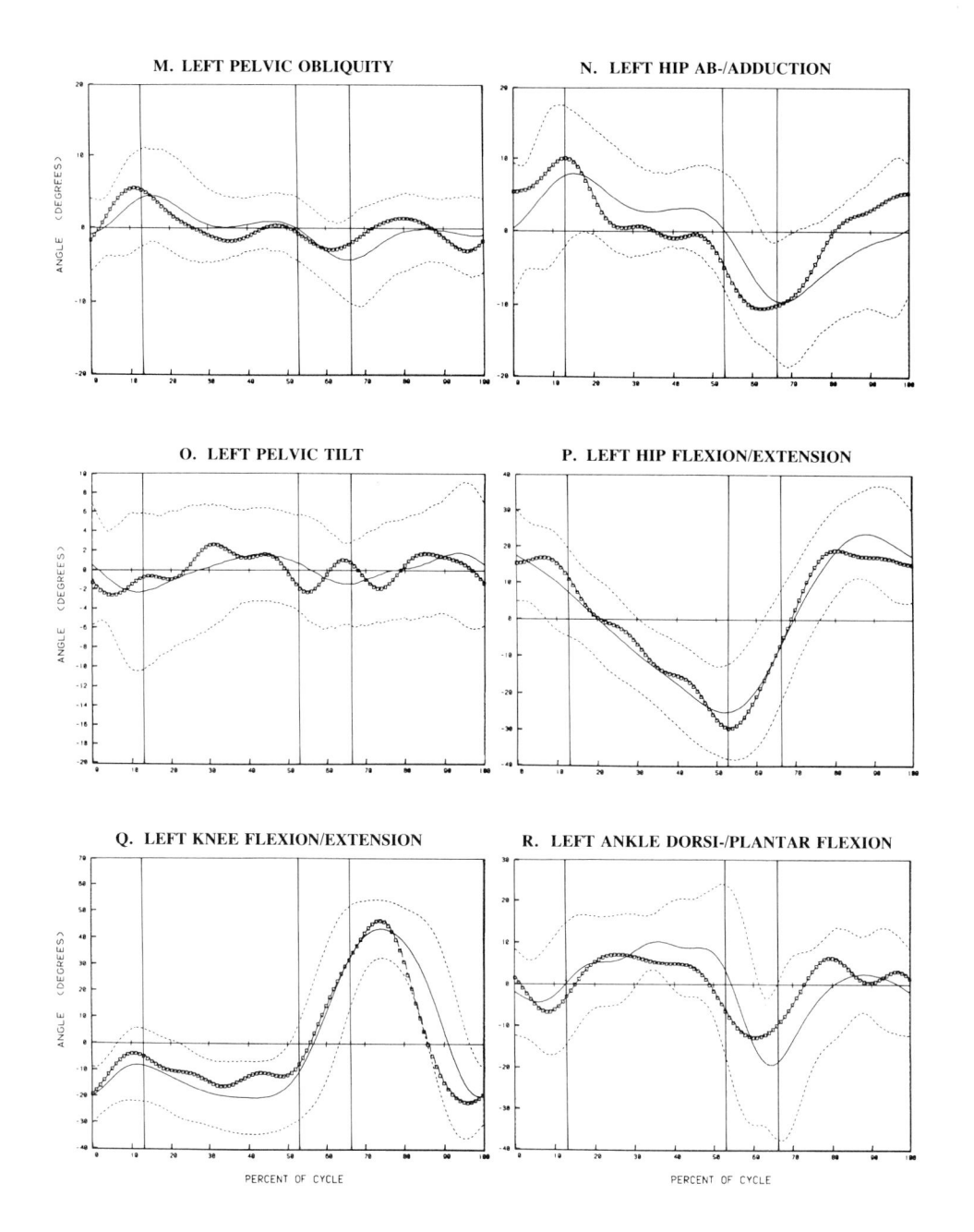

Figs. 12.3M–R. Graphs plotting the sum of harmonic terms (α_0 term removed: see Chapter 3) in the fitting of the left-side joint-angle data from subject #8.506.

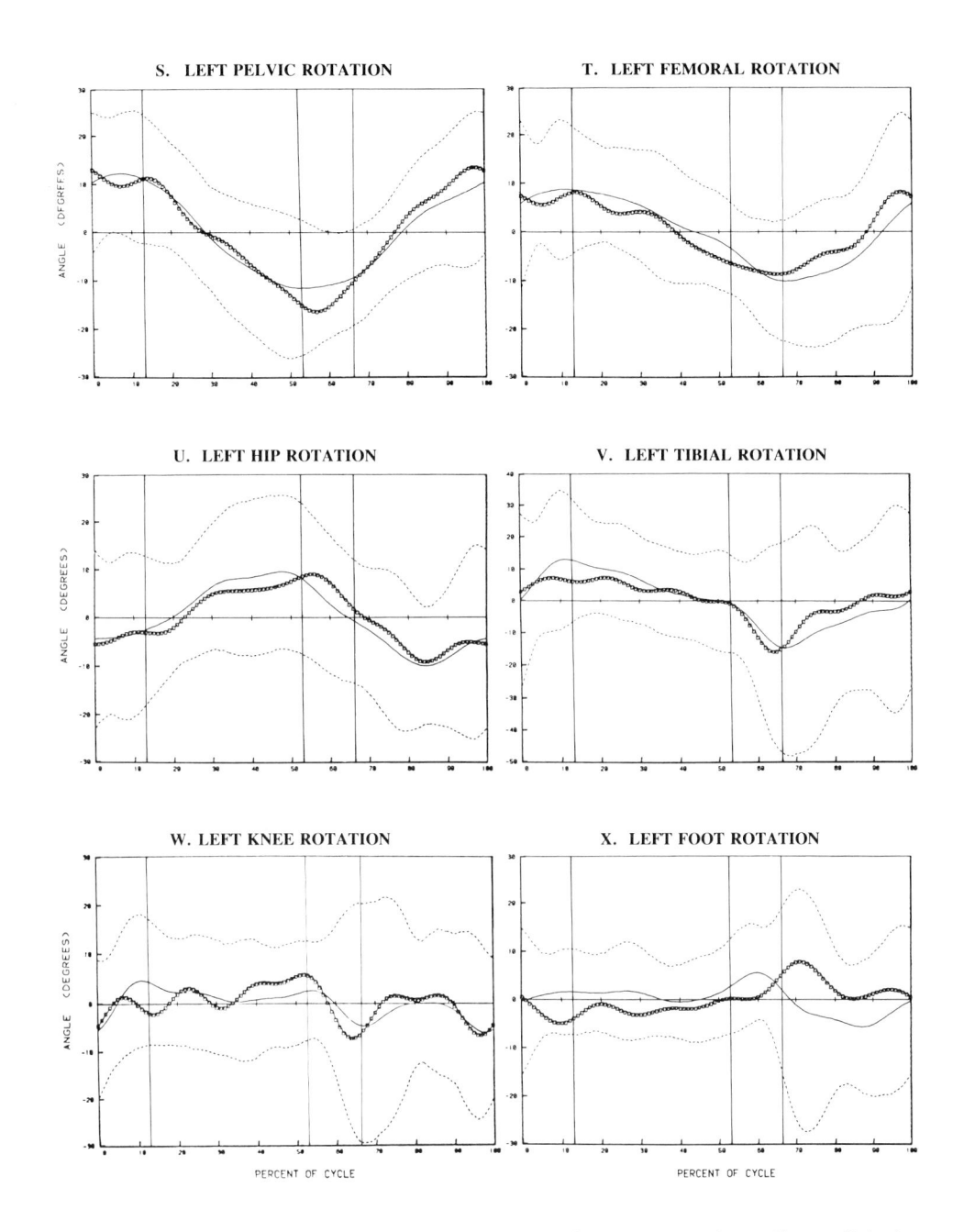

Figs. 12.3S–X. Graphs plotting the sum of harmonic terms (α_0 term removed: see Chapter 3) in the fitting of the left-side joint-angle data from subject #8.506.

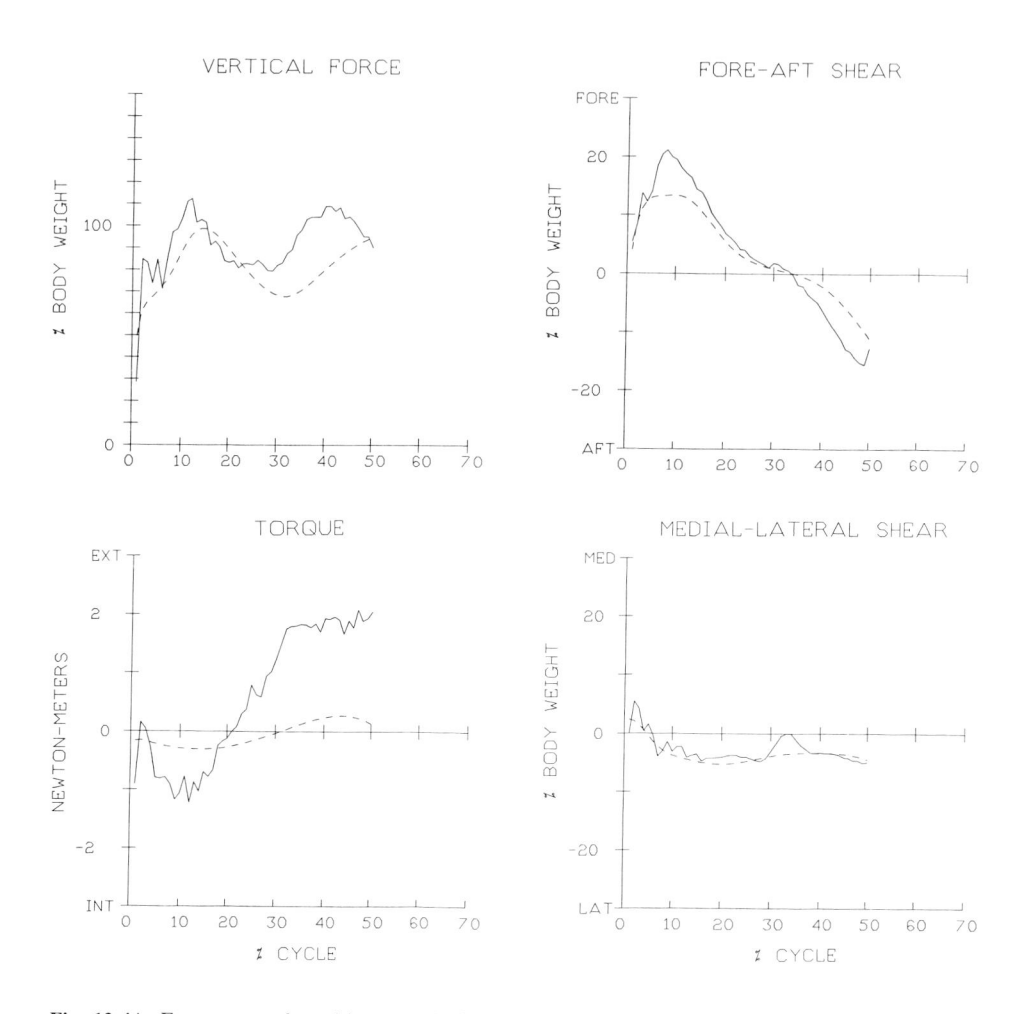

Fig. 12.4A. Force curves for subject #8.506 (right foot). The broken lines indicate normal 5-year-old force curves.

FORCE-PLATE MEASUREMENTS
The force measurements for the right foot appear normal with the exception of torque. Internal and external torque are exaggerated (Fig. 12.4A). Measurements for the left foot show exaggerated loading, increased forward shear, absent initial medial shear, increased lateral shear, diminished internal torque and absent lateral torque (Fig. 12.4B).

AGE-PREDICTION TREE
The subject was studied according to the classification tree of Chapter 10 (p. 180), in which children are assigned to age on the basis of measured gait parameters. His data put him in terminal node G, indicating that he walks like a 7-year-old.

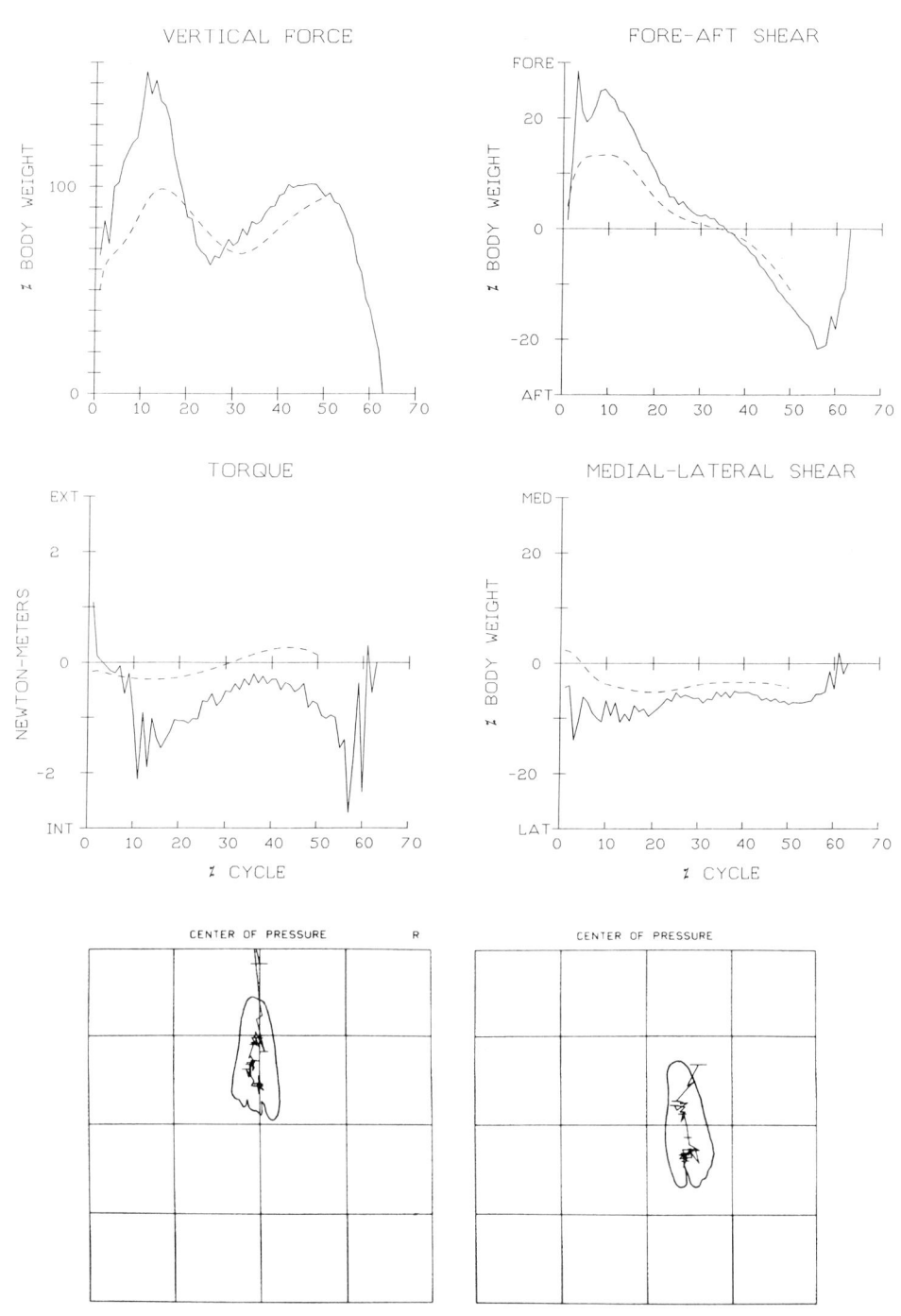

Fig. 12.4B. Force curves for subject #8.506 (left foot). The broken lines indicate normal 5-year-old force curves. Also reproduced are pressure plots for right and left feet.

CONCLUSIONS
In spite of the history of prematurity, the absence of reciprocal arm swing, and the fact that the hip abduction/adduction and foot rotation curves both have points lying outside the 95 per cent prediction regions, this subject's walking pattern does not demonstrate neurological impairment. The minor gait deviations shown might be due to self-consciousness, producing 'doctor visit walking', or to distractibility. The age-prediction tree was particularly helpful in this case as the authors had differing views about possible neurological impairment until the tree data classification was completed. We then agreed that he is unimpaired with respect to walking. This conclusion is the expected one from the early history. There were no serious risk factors in the neonatal intensive care record. Also, his pediatrician's office records confirm 'well child' status at age 10 years.

Case 2: Preterm 5-year-old with cerebral palsy
Subject #8.519 was born prematurely at home to a gravida 1, para 0, 26-year-old caucasian female. His gestational age was 30 weeks and his birthweight was 1300g. Apgar scores are not available because of the home birth. He was taken to a community hospital, placed in oxygen, and the Children's Hospital transport team was called. Upon their arrival, intubation was performed and an umbilical catheter was inserted. He was given sodium bicarbonate plus 25 per cent salt-poor albumin and 25 per cent dextrose in water. He was transported in 100 per cent oxygen, arriving at the neonatal intensive care unit in fair condition 4 hours after birth. His hospital course was prolonged (76 days). Discharge diagnoses were as follows:

1. Prematurity, 30 weeks gestation, weight appropriate for gestational age.
2. Idiopathic respiratory distress syndrome severe, requiring assisted ventilation for 9 days.
3. Pulmonary interstitial emphysema severe.
4. Patent ductus arteriosus severe.
5. Renal tubular defect, resolving.
6. Anemia of prematurity.

Two operations were performed: ligation of patent ductus arteriosus and selective intubation of the right main-stem bronchus. His weight on discharge was 2354g.
  The developmental milestones were delayed. He pulled to stand at 14 months, crawled at 19 months, and began to walk with a walker at 3 years. At 5 years he was still dependent on a walker for support in ambulation and had not undergone any orthopaedic surgical procedures.
  His height was 99cm (1st percentile of normal). The crown-to-pubis length, measured supine, was 56.5cm (50th percentile). The pubis-to-toe length was 47cm right and 47.5cm left: these measures are less than the minimum values in normal children. His arm span was 103.3cm (slightly below 50th percentile). His weight was 15kg (slightly below 25th percentile). (Normal anthropometric measurements are given in Chapter 5.)
  Passive range of motion tests revealed restricted extension of both knees and restricted abduction of the left hip. The deep tendon reflexes at the knee and ankle

TABLE 12.II
Time/distance parameters for subject #8.519 at 5 years corrected age

Parameter measured	Right	Left
Opposite toe-off (% cycle)	29	20
Opposite foot-strike (% cycle)	55	40
Single stance (% cycle)	26	20
Toe-off (% cycle)	76	76
Step length (cm)	8	21
Stride length (cm)	29	
Cycle time (secs.)	1.09	
Cadence (steps/min.)	110	
Walking velocity (cm/sec.)	27	
Walking velocity (m/min.)	16	

were hyperactive in both legs. The asymmetric tonic neck reflex was retained. He could walk independently with a walker but was unable to heel-walk, stand on one leg, squat or run.

The time/distance parameters are listed in Table 12.II. All the measurements are outside the minimal or maximal values of normal 5-year-old children (see Chapter 6). Left opposite foot-strike, right and left step length, right and left single stance, stride length, cadence and walking velocity are below the minimal values; right and left opposite toe-off, right opposite foot-strike, right and left toe-off, and cycle time are higher than the maximal values.

JOINT ANGLES
Twelve joint-angle graphs show deviation outside the 95 per cent prediction regions (Figs. 12.5A–L). This is overwhelming evidence of pathological motion.

FILM TRACINGS
The flexion posture and gait pattern of this child is very familiar to experienced observers (Fig. 12.6). He *looks* as if he has cerebral palsy.

DYNAMIC ELECTROMYOGRAPHY
Electromyograms were obtained with surface electrodes (Fig. 12.7). Only one of the seven muscles studied, the tibialis anterior, had clearly normal phasic activity. The activity of the gastroc/soleus resembled the immature pattern found in a small number of normal 5-year-olds (see Fig. 8.7A, p. 161). the gluteus maximus, vastus medialis, and medial and lateral hamstrings all began activity prematurely in swing phase and were active overlong in stance phase. The gluteus medius was delayed in onset and activity was prolonged. Alterations in phasic activity such as these are common in cerebral palsy.

AGE-PREDICTION TREE
The subject was studied according to the age-prediction tree of Chapter 10 (p. 180). Even supported, his gait data put him in terminal node C, and so our best estimate is that he walks like a 2-year-old.

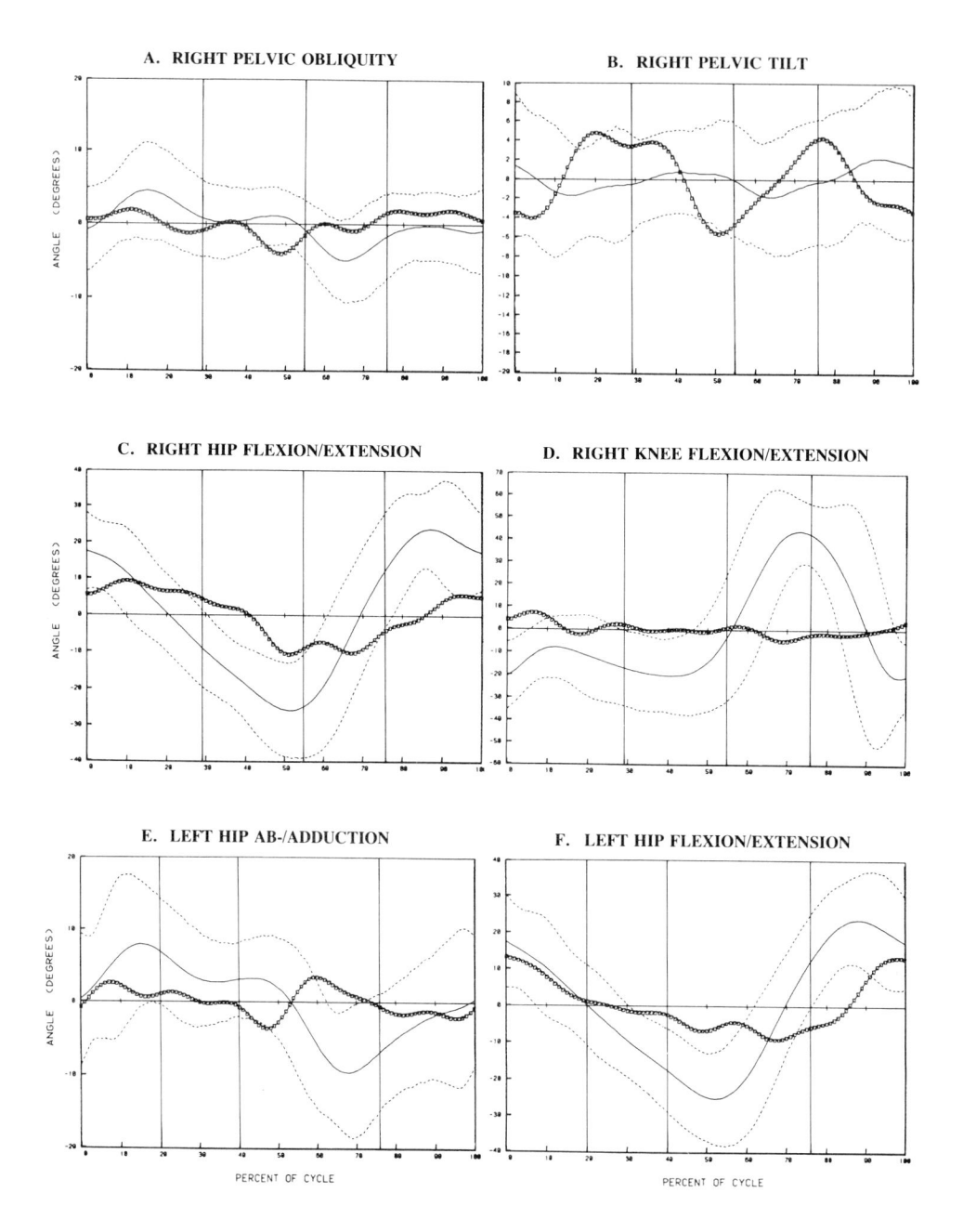

Figs. 12.5A–F. Graphs plotting the sum of the harmonics (α_0 term removed: see Chapter 3) in the fitting of the joint-angle data from subject #8.519.

In each case the heavy line is from the subject. The upper and lower broken lines are the boundaries of the 95 per cent prediction region. The solid central line represents the population average for 5-year-old normal subjects. The three vertical lines indicate opposite toe-off, opposite foot-strike and toe-off.

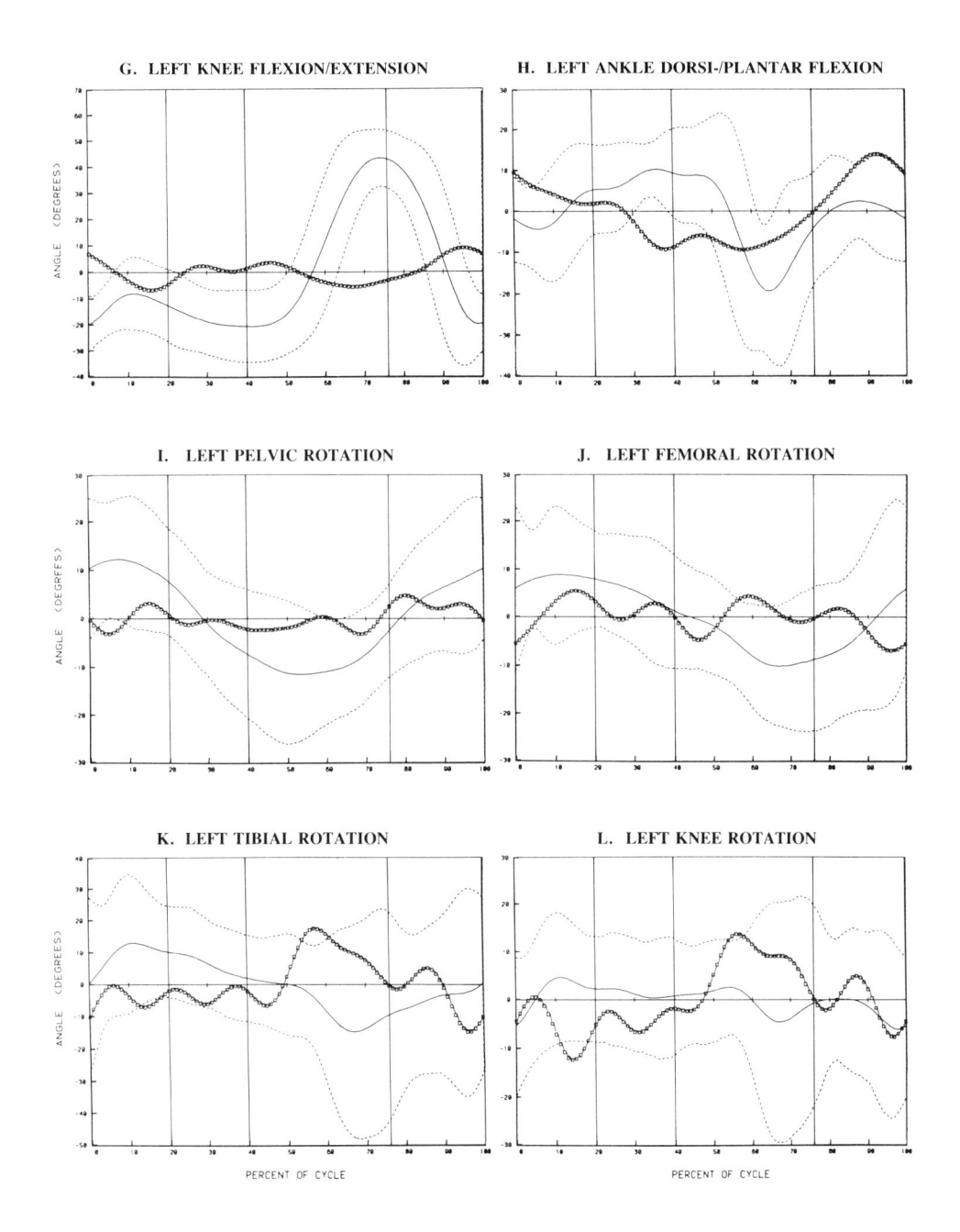

Figs. 12.5G–L. Graphs plotting the sum of the harmonics (α_0 term removed: see Chapter 3) in the fitting of the joint-angle data from subject #8.519.

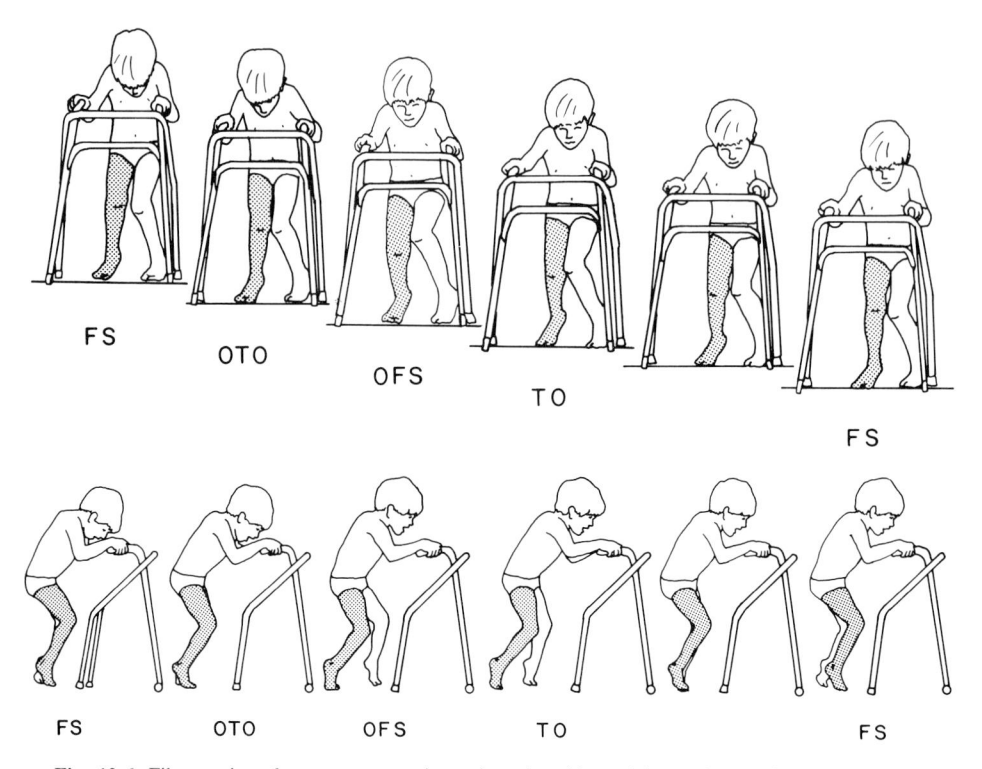

Fig. 12.6. Film tracings from representative gait cycle, side and front views, of subject #8.519.

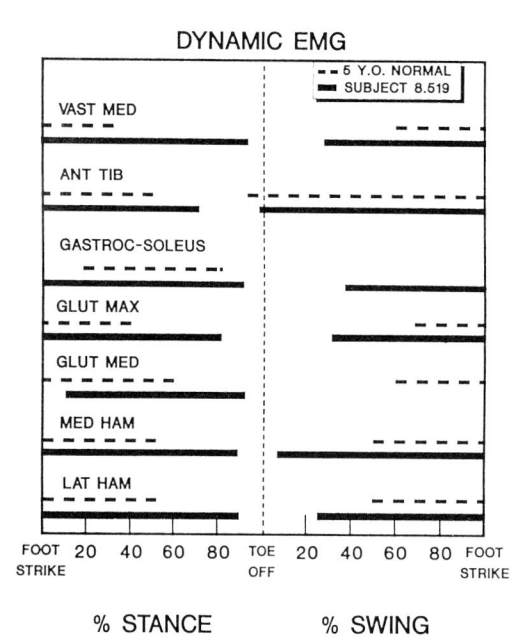

Fig. 12.7. Normalized stance- and swing-phase EMGs in subject #8.519 compared with mean phasic activity in 5-year-old normal controls.

CONCLUSIONS

The time/distance parameters, dynamic EMG plots, joint angles, and fitted age according to the classification tree are all consistent with neuromuscular impairment. This child has cerebral palsy of the spastic diplegic type. Recognizing the cerebral palsy is not difficult; however, the discipline of arriving at this conclusion through specific gait measurements could be important in part for preparation of treatment plans and assessment of outcome. Also, studies such as these will lay the groundwork for future computer-assisted decision making and expert systems in motion analysis.

13
FUTURE DIRECTIONS

This book summarizes over a decade of data collection, reduction and interpretation. The data presented range from simple measures of height and weight to complex analyses of movement. In this final chapter we describe a vision of the future in which these data represent but a building block.

History
Locomotion is an integral part of our daily lives. Interest in the how and why of walking, as well as in ways to compensate for disability, has no doubt existed since prehistoric times. The ability to compare the gait of different individuals or the gait of the same person at different times depends upon an ability to quantify the actions. Gait happens very quickly—a typical gait cycle in an adult takes less than a second—and it is difficult to observe the many things that happen simultaneously. Two very important components of gait—muscle activity and the force exerted—are invisible to the eye. The questions become: (1) how does one record those events which happen very quickly or are invisible? and (2) how does one interpret the resultant data?

As technology has advanced, the field of gait analysis has been quick to incorporate developments. Around the turn of the century, Muybridge and others began to use stop-action photography to record gait (see Muybridge 1979). This allowed motions to be studied at leisure and in slow motion, a process which has remained very useful as better cine cameras and now video systems have been developed. With improvements in electronic instrumentation, electrogoniometry and electromyography have become easier to perform. Electrogoniometry still suffers in that even the lightest system affects the gait of small children, and so we have persisted in using remote photographic or other means of recording motion. Force plates, uncommon in the late 1960s, now are standard equipment and are available from several vendors. Transducers have also become simpler, lighter and cheaper as the electronics revolution has progressed. Perhaps the most dramatic change in this area is the availability of relatively inexpensive digital computers which can both gather data from the outside world and be used to process them. Indeed, gait analysis as we practise it resembles some areas of modern radiology in that it simply could not exist without high-speed computation equipment.

Despite the growing availability of technology, gait analysis has not yet become a very common tool for the physician. Gait laboratories have developed around individuals or groups willing to make the investment in time, effort and money to assemble and operate systems. They have flourished best where a combination of physician input and referral was coupled with day-to-day clinical expertise in the form of physical therapists or other health-care specialists and with technical expertise in the form of engineers and other technical staff.

Because systems have developed one by one, there has been little standardization. Each laboratory tends to have chosen those technologies which solved the problems they found of interest, and most labs contain a variety of equipment unique to themselves. Despite a few 'clones' where labs have been duplicated, the situation has been very much one of every lab for itself.

With laboratories working in isolation, and with most clinical applications being local in nature, there was little in the way of cross-comparison between data collected in different labs. Each lab also tended to have its measurement system evolve in a way distinct from that of any other, making comparisons still less easy. Processing the data has generally required a lot of labor-intensive work, especially for movement data acquired using cine film. Moreover, an even more critical aspect has been the relative unfamiliarity of physicians in general, and even of orthopaedists, with physics. Although familiar with biological procedures and heavily trained in anatomy, many physicians find themselves at a loss when faced with typical gait data. The triumph of devices such as CT scanners in part reflects the fact that the data presented are well known and easy to understand. Gait data, on the other hand, concern much that is inaccessible to the naked eye. Whereas one can dissect a cadaver and know the basics of how the body is assembled, there is no such simple way to acquire an understanding of gait.

Changes to this basic pattern began in the late 1970s and '80s. First came the emergence of imaging systems that could watch a subject and communicate his or her movements and other data as recorded by transducers to digital computers. Such commercial systems meant that more than one lab could now have similar equipment, and the incentive to share data became greater as the mechanics became easier. With imaging systems, the promise of eliminating much of the manual labor associated with cine film moved closer to reality and more labs appeared. This increased interest in gait has not yet produced as active a field as one might hope, since many of the early systems were oversold and under-supported. However, the technology was there.

The Present

As we write this in 1988, several commercial gait systems are on the market or planned for the near future. The field is much more mature than it was 5 years ago, and the design of systems is much more targeted on gait. As our own laboratory has progressed, we have begun the process of moving from the cine system with which the data in this book were collected to one based on video cameras linked directly to our computer. The major hurdle of 'automation' has been to design a system which is as accurate, reliable and easy to use as our old cine system, but which at the same time reduces the data processing time and hence the cost of performing the service. We presently operate a five-camera VICON system for data collection, with our own locally developed software for producing clinically useful output.

The VICON system works as follows. Each camera has a strobe light set around the lens. This emits an infra-red signal, which strikes reflective markers attached to the subject. The reflected signals are fed directly from the camera to a computer, and this automatically determines the positions of the markers in space to build up a continuous 3D picture of the subject's motion. Simultaneously, the system allows collection of data from two force plates. We continue to collect EMGs apart from the motion studies, but now this function too is computer based. This system, which we have had in use since 1985, has allowed us to cut our turn-around time for a study from the 4 to 6 weeks typical in the past to around 10 days for routine studies and as little as a few hours for urgent cases.

While we have changed our system, we have still incorporated an array of color video cameras and recorders to provide high quality clinical pictures of the patients walking. We feel that being able to look at the whole person and to compare clinical impressions with the hard data in a timely fashion is *very* important.

Increased interest in gait and in 'automated' measurement systems has touched us in another way as well. We are in the midst of a study which will combine the results of studies from five widely separated labs, each running different systems. Initial comparisons between their movement data and those presented here indicate that the harmonic components of the curves are comparable for the sagittal plane and for movements of the pelvis, hip and foot. The major differences lie in the transverse-plane rotations, which suffer from disagreement on the definitions of the motions as well as on their actual measures. The compatibility of such systems suggests that gait data have the potential to be as universally applicable as are radiographic and other common diagnostic test data.

This book describes some of the statistics used to analyze gait. These provide an objective way of assessing patient progress and the efficacy of surgery or other treatment. They, together with the high-speed data processing available with new systems, are the foundations upon which the next generation of gait analysis will rise.

The Future
The keys to the future of gait analysis lie in the ability of new systems to process data much more quickly than was possible before, in the development of better descriptive methods to characterize gait, and in the ability to 'simplify' gait analysis to make it accessible to a wider audience.

Consider changes due to faster processing times. In the past it was impracticable to apply many gait analysis techniques because of the time it took to process the data, a good example being the monitoring of progress in stroke or head-injury patients during rehabilitation programs. Such patients change steadily over the course of their rehabilitation, making even a 2-week turn-around of data little short of useless. On the other hand, quantitative analysis of the efficacy of such programs is possible and practical if data can be processed and returned to the treatment units in 1 or 2 days.

In the past, gait analysis has been used for subjects with relatively static disorders, where the planning of treatment encompassed a long period of time. With shorter turn-around, the latent interest in quantitative measures of gait for stroke and head-injury patients, for amputees, and in other areas of movement problems where changes occur quickly, is likely to expand and become a major part of the business.

Increased speed in analysis is likely to lower significantly the cost of providing the service, as the staff involved will be able to be more productive.

Moving for a moment out of the strictly medical field, the ability to analyze gait quickly also opens doors in the area of sports and other recreational activities.

The second issue, that of improved descriptive methods, is important in that, if methods can be derived which will work for any gait facility, then the ability to analyze data will be less dependent on individual expertise and more of a science. Techniques mentioned in this book, for instance, allow gait measurements to be expressed as percentiles of normal values and are applicable in any setting using the same measurement system, and indeed appear to be applicable to most measurements even if they are made under quite different circumstances.

The future holds the promise of such descriptive techniques being used routinely to assess the efficacy of treatment or to categorize subjects as having particular disorders, or particular subsets of some disorder. Ultimately such techniques may be used to match certain disorders with appropriate treatments by using the same criteria that the clinician uses but in an automated way. The advances would be aided by further analyses quantifying the relationship between motions, electromyographic and force data.

This leads to the third point, that of making gait analysis accessible to more physicians. So-called 'expert systems' now used in some scientific and commercial applications to apply decision-making rules based on previously defined criteria almost certainly have application in gait analysis. Such systems tend to be computer intensive, but, as stated, gait systems also are becoming more and more dependent on computers. The systems are becoming both more powerful and less expensive, and it is likely that soon some form of 'expert system' will be used to interpret gait. We believe that the data and graphics presented in this book could be fundamental ingredients of any expert system for gait analysis in children.

The ability to set up rules based on the way experts in the field make decisions means that the inexperienced practitioner has at his or her disposal an 'expert in a box' which can aid in decision making, but which can be over-ruled if clinical experience so dictates. The existence of a system which can gather and process data and also assist with interpretation is the change which may make gait analysis a real winner.

It is likely that in the next few years gait analysis will consolidate. The manufacturers of gait analysis systems will settle into their niches in the field, and the procedures and practices will become much more standard. Simply having many centers with common equipment will have the effect of streamlining the collaborative process.

We feel very positive about gait analysis in our center. It has been used well with many patients having benefited. We see no reason why that should be anything but improved upon by the changes which are upon us.

APPENDICES

A. HEALTH SCREENING QUESTIONNAIRE

Health history form for children having motion studies (to be completed by parent)

Subject #

Identifying information

Name ....
            last   first   initial(s)

Address ....
        number   street   city   zip

Date of birth ....

Phone ....

Parent's name ....

Past history

                                      (* Circle appropriate answer)

Born: At term / Premature *

Sex: M / F *

Birthweight ....

Caesarean section?   Yes / No *

Breech birth: Yes / No *

Difficult breathing at birth?   Yes / No *

Any chronic medical conditions?   Yes / No *
    If yes, please describe ....
....

Wears glasses? Yes / No *

Handedness/footedness:
    Prefers to use which hand to:
        Eat? Right / Left *
        Write? Right / Left *
        Throw? Right / Left *
    Prefers to kick with which foot? Right / Left *

Any family history of:
    1. Congenital dislocation of hip? Yes / No *
    2. Club foot? Yes / No *
    3. Rotational problems of lower limbs? Yes / No *
    4. Severe bow legs? Yes / No *
    5. Severe knock knees? Yes / No *

Any major injury or illness requiring hospitalization? Yes / No *
    If yes, please describe ....

Any fracture, dislocation, or other bone or joint problem? Yes / No *
    If yes, please describe ....

Developmental milestones

At which age did s/he first:
    Sit?   (months)
    Crawl?   (months)
    Pull to stand?   (months)
    Walk alone?   (months)
    Run?   (months)

Present health status

Any illness at present (including minor problems, *e.g.* cold, etc.)? Yes / No *
    If yes, please describe ....

Any problems with vision? Yes / No *
    If yes, please describe ....

B. CONSENT FORM

Consent to act as human subject

Subject's name ....

Date ....

I do hereby give my consent for the inclusion of my daughter/son .... as a subject in the research proposal entitled 'Gait Study of Normal Children in their Growing Years'. I understand that there are no benefits to be gained directly by my child as a result of this study. Benefits to be gained will be to other children with abnormal walking patterns produced by a variety of diseases. I understand that the movies taken and the measurements recorded will be used for scientific purposes. I consent to the use of the movies and the various measurements for scientific purposes at the discretion of the principal investigator and his colleagues on the study.

....
    Parent or parent's agent   Witness

C. FORM FOR RECORDING ANTHROPOMETRIC AND DEVELOPMENTAL EVALUATIONS

Name ....
Birth date ....
Age .... yrs. .... mos.

1st Evaluation Date			2nd Evaluation Date	
		Heights (cm) Standing Crown-to-pubic (supine) Pubic-to-toe (ankle neutral) Sitting Weight (kg, g) (lbs., oz.) Arm span (cm)		
Right	*Left*	Range of motion Hip .. Flexion .. Extension .. Abduction .. Adduction .. Internal rotation (prone) .. External rotation (prone) Knee .. Flexion .. Extension Ankle .. Dorsiflexion Tibial torsion	*Right*	*Left*
Lying	*Standing*	Lower-extremity alignment (cm) Valgus (intermalleolar distance) Varus (intercondylar distance)	*Lying*	*Standing*
Right	*Left*	Muscle strength Upper extremity .. Normal Lower extremity .. Normal Joint laxity .. Fingers .. Wrists .. Elbows	*Right*	*Left*

	1st Evaluation				2nd Evaluation	

	Right	Left	Joint laxity .. Knees
			.. Ankles
			Deep tendon reflexes
			   Elbow .. Normal
			          .. Hyper
			          .. Hypo
			   Knee .. Normal
			         .. Hyper
			         .. Hypo
			   Ankle .. Normal
			          .. Hyper
			          .. Hypo
					Right	Left

Yes	No	N/A	Mobility
			  Walking independently
			  Walking on toes
			  Walking on heels
			  Standing on one leg
			  Hopping
			  Squatting
			  Getting up off floor
			  Walking on balance beam
			  Tandem-walking on balance beam
			  Running
			  Reflexes .. Retained neonatal
			             .. Protective extension
				Yes	No	N/A

	Right	Left	Foot preference (kicking ball)
			Hand preference (writing or eating)
			Measurements to be converted to
			  degrees of tibial torsion
			    Ankle width (cm)
			    Medial malleolus to heel (cm)
			    Lateral malleolus to heel (cm)
					Right	Left

Comments/Summary

....
Therapist's signature

REFERENCES

Anderson, M., Green, W. T., Messner, M. B. (1963) 'Growth and predictions of growth in the lower extremities.' *Journal of Bone and Joint Surgery*, **45A**, 1–14.
Anderson, T. W. (1971) *The Statistical Analysis of Time Series.* New York: John Wiley.
Baer, R., Johnson, E. W. (1965) 'Motor nerve conduction velocities in normal children.' *Archives of Physical Medicine*, **46**, 698–704.
Basmajian, J. V., DeLuca, C. J. (1985) *Muscles Alive, 5th Edn.* Baltimore: Williams & Wilkins.
Baumann, J. U., Ruetsch, H., Schurmann, K. (1980) 'Distal hamstring lengthening in cerebral palsy. An evaluation by gait analysis.' *International Orthopedics*, **3**, 305–309.
Bayley, N. (1969) *Manual for the Bayley Scales of Infant Development.* New York: Psychological Corporation.
Begbie, G. H. (1967) 'Some problems of postural sway.' *In* de Reuck, A. V. S., Knight, J. (Eds.) *Myotatic, Kinesthetic, and Vestibular Mechanism.* London: Churchill.
Biden, E., Olshen, R., Simon, S., Sutherland, D., Gage, J., Kadaba, M. (1987) 'Comparison of gait data from multiple labs.' *Paper presented at the 23rd Annual Meeting of the Orthopaedic Research Society, San Francisco.*
Breiman, L., Friedman, J. H., Olshen, R. A., Stone, C. J. (1984) *Classification and Regression Trees.* Belmont, CA: Wadsworth International.
Byers, R. K. (1941) 'Evolution of hemiplegias in infancy.' *American Journal of Diseases of Children*, **61**, 915–927.
Campbell, J., Ball, J. (1978) 'Energetics of walking in cerebral palsy.' *Orthopedic Clinics of North America*, **9**, 374–377.
Capozzo, A., Leo, T., Pedotti, A. (1975) 'A general computing method for the analysis of human locomotion.' *Journal of Biomechanics*, **8**, 307–320.
Carter, C., Wilkinson, J. (1964) 'Persistent joint laxity and congenital dislocation of the hip.' *Journal of Bone and Joint Surgery*, **46B**, 40–45.
Charcot, J. M., Marie, P. (1886) 'Sur une forme particulière d'atrophie musculaire progressive: souvent familiale débutant par les pieds et les jambes, et atteignant plus tard les mains.' *Revue de Médecine*, **6**, 97–138.
Cunningham, D. M. (1950) *Components of Floor Reactions During Walking. (Prosthetic Devices Research Project. Series 11, Issue 14.* Berkeley: Institute of Engineering Research, University of California. (Re-issued October 1958).
de Boor, C. (1978) *A Practical Guide to Splines.* New York: Springer-Verlag.
Dejerine, J., Sottas, J. (1983) 'Sur la névrite interstitielle hypertrophique et progressive de l'enfance.' *Société Biologique Comptes Rendus*, **5**, 63–96.
Dobbing, J., Sands, J. (1973) 'Quantitative growth and development of human brain.' *Archives of Disease in Childhood*, **48**, 757–767.
Dubowitz, V. (1968) 'The floppy infant. A practical approach to classification.' *Developmental Medicine and Child Neurology*, **10**, 706–710.
Efron, B. (1979) 'Bootstrap methods: another look at the jackknife.' *Annals of Statistics*, **7**, 1–26.
—— (1982) *The Jackknife, the Bootstrap, and Other Resampling Plans.* Philadelphia: Society for Industrial and Applied Mathematics.
Endo, B., Kimura, T. (1972) 'External force of foot in infant walking.' *Journal of the Faculty of Science, The University of Tokyo*, Sect. V., Vol. IV, Part 2, pp. 103–117.
Frankenberg, W. K., Dodds, J. B. (1967) 'The Denver Developmental Screening Test.' *Journal of Pediatrics*, **71**, 181–191.
—— Fandel, A. W., Sciarillo, W., Burgess, D. (1981) 'The newly abbreviated and revised Denver Developmental Screening Test.' *Journal of Pediatrics*, **99**, 995–999.
Gage, J. R., Perry, J., Hicks, R. R., Koop, S., Werntz, J. R. (1987) 'Rectus femoris transfer to improve knee function of children with cerebral palsy.' *Developmental Medicine and Child Neurology*, **29**, 159–166.
Gall, J. C., Hayles, A. B., Siekert, R. G., Keith, H. M. (1958) 'Multiple sclerosis in children. A clinical study of 40 cases with onset in childhood.' *Pediatrics*, **21**, 703–709.
Gamstorp, I. (1963) 'Normal conduction velocity for ulnar, medial and peroneal nerves in infancy, childhood and adolescence.' *Acta Paediatrica Scandinavica*, Suppl. 146, 68–76.
Grieve, D. W., Gear, R. J. (1966) 'The relationships between length of stride, step frequency, time of swing and speed of walking for children and adults.' *Ergonomics*, **5**, 379–399.

Grillner, S. (1975) 'Locomotion in vertebrates: central mechanisms and reflex interaction.' *Physiological Review*, **55**, 247–303.
—— Stein, P. S. G., Stuart, D. G., Forssberg, H., Herman, R. M. (Eds.) (1985) *Neurobiology of Vertebrate Locomotion. Proceedings of an International Symposium held at The Wenner-Gren Center, Stockholm, June 17th–19th, 1985.* London: Macmillan.
Gritzka, T. L., Staheli, L. T., Duncan, W. R. (1972) 'Posterior tibial transfer through the interossus membrane to correct equinovarus deformity in cerebral palsy.' *Clinical Orthopedics and Related Research*, **89**, 201–206.
Hamill, P. V. V., Drizd, P. A., Johnson, C. L., Reed, R. B., Roche, A. F. (1977) *National Center for Health Statistics (NCHS) Growth Curves for Children, Birth to Eighteen Years.* Washington, D. C.: US Government Printing Office. DHEW pub'n. no. (PHS) 78–1650.
Hart, H., Bax, M., Jenkins, S. (1978) 'The value of a developmental history.' *Developmental Medicine and Child Neurology*, **20**, 442–452.
Hennessy, M. J., Dixon, S. D., Simon, S. R. (1984) 'The development of gait: a study in African children ages one to five.' *Child Development*, **55**, 844–853.
Hoffer, M. M., Reiswig, J. A., Garrett, A. M., Perry, J. (1974) 'The split anterior tibial tendon transfer in the treatment of spastic varus hind foot of childhood.' *Orthopedic Clinics of North America*, **5**, 31–38.
Hupprich, F. L., Sigerseth, P. O. (1950) 'The specificity of flexibility in girls.' *Research Quarterly*, **21**, 25–33.
Inman, V. T. (1973) 'Biceps cineplasty EMG studies and EMG tension length studies.' *Technical report of Biomechanical Group, San Francisco University of California Biomechanics Laboratory*.
—— Ralston, H. J., Todd, F. (1981) *Human Walking.* Baltimore: Williams and Wilkins.
International Mathematics and Statistics Library (1983) *Problem-solving Software System for Mathematical and Statistical FORTRAN Programming. I.M.S.L. User's Manual, Vol. 2.* (Chapter I). Houston: I.M.S.L., Inc.
Johansen, S., Johnstone, I. (1988) 'Hotelling's theorem on the volume of tubes: some illustrations in simultaneous inference and data analysis.' *Annals of Statistics, (in press).*
Kotz, S., Johnson, N. L. (1982) *Encyclopedia of Statistical Sciences, Vol. 2.* New York: John Wiley.
Lasko, P. (1986) 'Kinematic variability and relationships during the walking cycle of children.' *Unpublished PhD thesis, University of Southern California.*
Low, N. L., Carter, S. (1956) 'Multiple sclerosis in children.' *Pediatrics*, **18**, 24–30.
McKusick, V. A. (1972) 'The Ehlers-Danlos syndrome.' *In:* McKusick, V. A. (Ed.) *Heritable Disorders of Connective Tissue, 4th Edn.* St. Louis: C. V. Mosby.
Mann, R. A., Larsen, L. J., Mahoney, M., Hagy, J. L. (1975) 'Proximal hamstring release in children with spastic cerebral palsy.' *Paper presented at meeting of the American Academy for Cerebral Palsy, New Orleans.*
Marshall, J. L., Johanson, N., Wickiewicz, T. L., Tischler, H. M., Koslin, B. L., Zeno, S., Meyers, A. (1980) 'Joint looseness: a function of the person and the joint.' *Medicine and Science in Sports and Exercise*, **12**, 189–194.
Martinez, M., Ballabriga, A. (1978) 'A chemical study on the development of the human forebrain and cerebellum during the brain growth spurt period. 1. Gangliosides and plasmalogens.' *Brain Research*, **159**, 351–362.
Matthews, M. A. (1968) 'An electron microscopic study of the relationship between axon diameter and the initiation of myelin production in the peripheral nervous system.' *Anatomical Record*, **161**, 337–351.
Menkes, J. H. (1985) *Child Neurology, 3rd Edn.* Philadelphia: Lea and Febiger.
Meyersburg, H. A., Post, R. M. (1979) 'An holistic developmental view of neural and psychological processes: a neurobiologic-psychoanalytic integration.' *British Journal of Psychiatry*, **115**, 139–155.
Morell, P., Norton, W. T. (1980) 'Myelin.' *Scientific American*, **242**, (5), 88–117.
Moseley, C. F. (1977) 'A straight line graph for leg-length discrepancies.' *Journal of Bone and Joint Surgery*, **59A**, 174–178.
Muybridge, E. (1979) *Muybridge's Complete Human and Animal Locomotion. All 781 Plates from the 1887 Animal Locomotion.* New York: Dover Publications.
Nashner, L. M., Black, F. O., Wall, C. (1982) 'Adaptation to altered support and visual conditions during stance: patients with vestibular deficits.' *Journal of Neuroscience*, **2**, 536–544.
Norton, W. T. (1981) 'Patterns of myelination.' *In* Siegel, G. J., Albers, R. W., Agranoff, B. W., Katzman, R. (Eds.) *Basic Neurochemistry, 3rd Edn.* Boston: Little, Brown.
Ogg, H. L. (1963) 'Measuring and evaluating the gait patterns of children.' *Journal of the American Physical Therapy Association*, **43**, 717–720.

Olshen, R. A., Biden, E. N., Wyatt, M. P., Sutherland, D. H. (1988) 'Gait analysis and the bootstrap.' *Annals of Statistics, (in press).*

Perry, J. (1974) 'Kinesiology of lower extremity bracing.' *Clinical Orthopedics,* **102,** 18–31.

—— (1987) 'Distal rectus femoris transfer.' *Developmental Medicine and Child Neurology,* **29,** 153–158.

—— Hoffer, M. M. (1977) 'Preoperative and postoperative dynamic electromyography as an aid in planning tendon transfers in children with cerebral palsy.' *Journal of Bone and Joint Surgery,* **59A,** 531–537.

—— —— Giovan, P., Antonelli, D., Greenberg, R. (1974) 'Gait analysis of the triceps surae in cerebral palsy: a preoperative and postoperative clinical and electromyographic study.' *Journal of Bone and Joint Surgery,* **56A,** 511–520.

Powell, M. J. D. (1981) *Approximation Theory and Methods.* Cambridge: Cambridge University Press.

Rabinowicz, T. (1964) 'Cerebral cortex of the premature infant of the 8th month.' *Progress in Brain Research,* **4,** 39–92.

Rafalowska, J. (1979) 'Some problems of development and ageing of the nervous system. II. Myelination of spinal roots in the second half of life and in early infancy.' *Neuropatalogia Polska,* **3,** 407–420.

Ralston, H. J., Inman, V. T., Strait, L. A., Shaffrath, M. D. (1947) 'Mechanics of human isolated voluntary muscle.' *American Journal of Physiology,* **151,** 612–620.

—— Polissar, M. J., Inman, V. T., Close, J. R., Feinstein, B. (1949) 'Dynamic features of human isolated voluntary muscle in isometric and free contractions.' *Journal of Applied Physiology,* **1,** 526–533.

Rao, C. R. (1965) 'The theory of least squares when the parameters are stochastic and its application to the analysis of growth curves.' *Biometrika,* **52,** 447–458.

Rivers, T. M., Schwentker, F. F. (1935) 'Encephalomyelitis accompanied by myelin destruction experimentally produced in monkeys.' *Journal of Experimental Medicine,* **61,** 689–702.

Robinson, R. J., Tizard, J. P. M. (1966) 'The central nervous system in the newborn.' *British Medical Bulletin,* **22,** 49–55.

Roosth, H. P. (1971) 'Flexion deformity of the hip and knee in spastic cerebral palsy: treatment by early release of spastic hip-flexor muscles. Technique and results in thirty-seven cases.' *Journal of Bone and Joint Surgery,* **53A,** 1489–1510.

Roussy, G., Lévy, G. (1926) 'Sept cas d'une maladie familiale particulière. Troubles de la marche, pieds bots, et aréfléxie tendineuse généralisée, avec, accessoirement, légère maladresse des mains.' *Revue de Neurologie,* **33,** 427–450.

Scrutton, D. R. (1969) 'Footprint sequences of normal children under five years old.' *Developmental Medicine and Child Neurology,* **11,** 44–53.

Salenius, P., Vankka, E. (1975) 'The development of the tibiofemoral angle in children.' *Journal of Bone and Joint Surgery,* **57A,** 259–261.

Sharrard, W. J. W. (1955) 'The distribution of the permanent paralysis in the lower limb in poliomyelitis.' *Journal of Bone and Joint Surgery,* **37B,** 540–558.

Shibata, R. (1981) 'An optimal selection of regression variables.' *Biometrika,* **68,** 45–54.

Simon, S. R. (1977) 'Use of gait analysis in cerebral palsy.' *Orthopedic Transactions,* **1,** 76.

—— Deutsch, S. E., Rosenthal, R. K. (1977) 'Genu recurvatum in spastic cerebral palsy: a preliminary report.' *Orthopedic Transactions,* **1,** 75.

—— Mann, R. A., Hagy, J. L., Larsen, L. J. (1978) 'Role of the posterior calf muscles in normal gait.' *Journal of Bone and Joint Surgery,* **60A,** 465–472.

Skinner, S. R., Antonelli, D., Perry, J., Lester, D. K. (1985) 'Functional demands on the stance limb in walking.' *Orthopedics,* **8,** 355–361.

Solomonow, M., Baratta, R., Zhou, B., Shoji, H., d'Ambrosia, R. (1986) 'Historical update and new developments on the EMG-force relationships of skeletal muscles.' *Orthopedics,* **9,** 1541–1543.

Staheli, L., Engel, G. M. (1972) 'Tibial torsion: a method of assessment and a survey of normal children.' *Clinical Orthopedics and Related Research,* **86,** 183–186.

Sutherland, D. H. (1966) 'An electromyographic study of the plantar flexors of the ankle in normal walking on the level.' *Journal of Bone and Joint Surgery,* **48A,** 66–71.

—— (1981a) 'The events of gait.' *Bulletin of Prosthetic Research,* **10–35,** 281–282.

—— (1981b) 'Clinical use of force data.' *Bulletin of Prosthetic Research,* **10–35,** 312–315.

—— (1984) *Gait Disorders in Childhood and Adolescence.* Baltimore: Williams & Wilkins.

—— Bost, F. C., Schottstaedt, E. R. (1960) 'Electromyographic study of transplanted muscles about the knee in poliomyelitis patients.' *Journal of Bone and Joint Surgery,* **42A,** 919–939.

—— —— Larsen, L. J., Ashley, R. K., Callander, J. N., James, P. M. (1969) 'Clinical and electromyographic study of seven spastic children with internal rotation gait.' *Journal of Bone and*

Joint Surgery, **51A,** 1070–1082.
—— Larsen, L. J., Mann, R. (1975) 'Rectus femoris release in selected patients with cerebral palsy: a preliminary report.' *Developmental Medicine and Child Neurology,* **17,** 26–34.
—— Cooper, L. (1977) 'Crouch gait in spastic diplegia.' *Orthopedic Transactions,* **1,** 76.
—— —— (1978) 'The pathomechanics of progessive crouch gait in spastic diplegia.' *Orthopedic Clinics of North America,* **9,** 143–154.
—— Olshen, R., Cooper, L., Woo, S. (1980*a*) 'The development of mature gait.' *Journal of Bone and Joint Surgery,* **62A,** 336–353.
—— Cooper, L., Daniel, D. (1980*b*) 'The role of the ankle plantar flexors in normal walking.' *Journal of Bone and Joint Surgery,* **62A,** 354–363.
—— Olshen, R., Cooper, L., Wyatt, M., Leach, J., Mubarak, S., Schultz, P. (1981) 'The pathomechanics of gait in Duchenne muscular dystrophy.' *Developmental Medicine and Child Neurology,* **23,** 3–22.
Thelen, E., Bradshaw, G., Ward, J. A. (1981) 'Spontaneous kicking in month-old infants: manifestation of a human central locomotor program.' *Behavioral and Neural Biology,* **32,** 45–53.
—— Fisher, D. M. (1982) 'Newborn stepping: an explanation for a "disappearing" reflex.' *Developmental Psychology,* **18,** 760–775.
Tooth, H. H. (1896) *The Peroneal Type of Progressive Muscular Atrophy. Cambridge University Thesis.* London: H. K. Lewis.
Touwen, B. C. L. (1979) *Examination of the Child with Minor Neurological Dysfunction, 2nd Edn. Clinics in Developmental Medicine No. 71.* London: S.I.M.P. with Heinemann; Philadelphia: J. B. Lippincott.
Vaughan, V. C., Litt, I. F. (1987) 'Developmental pediatrics.' *In* Behrman, R. E., Vaughan, V. C. (Eds.) *Nelson Textbook of Pediatrics, 13th Edn.* Philadelphia: W. B. Saunders.
Winter, D. A. (1979) *Biomechanics of Human Movement.* New York: John Wiley.
—— (1980) 'Overall principle of lower limb support during stance phase.' *Biomechanics,* **13,** 923–927.
—— (1983) 'Biomechanical motor patterns in normal walking.' *Journal of Motor Behavior,* **15,** 302–330.
Wolf, A., Kabat, E. A., Bezer, A. E. (1947) 'The pathology of disseminated encephalomyelitis produced experimentally in the Rhesus monkey and its resemblance to human demyelinating disease.' *Journal of Neuropathology and Experimental Neurology,* **6,** 333–357.

ACKNOWLEDGEMENTS

It is customary in research monographs to acknowledge the help of individuals and institutions without whom publication would not have been completed. For us, however, it scarcely seems possible to say in words how indebted we are to a variety of people whose intelligence, hard work and patience contributed to our interdisciplinary, and long-standing, efforts. We shall, nonetheless, attempt to give credit where it is due, and we apologize to those who are not explicitly mentioned but perhaps should have been. It is easy to lay blame for any remaining errors: we are responsible.

Two individuals are due special thanks: Les Cooper and Sherill Marciano. Les was an important participant in writing and work associated with the original grant that paid for our research. He helped recruit subjects, gathered data, designed its original storage, and generally did much to make possible the monograph. Sherill, who joined the team during the data-gathering phase, did major work typing and collating the manuscript. With our material flying in and out of San Diego, London, Fredericton and Stanford, sometimes at a dizzying pace, and none of the authors blessed with special organizational skills, it was imperative that someone take charge of knowing where everything was. Sherill was the person upon whom we relied.

Early in our work Kacy Barlow did much in regard to administration and typing. Later, typing was done by several individuals in the Motion Analysis Laboratory, notably Jennifer Boyd and the late Elizabeth Wright. Additional help was provided by Judi Davis of Stanford University and Joan Pappas of the University of California, San Diego (UCSD).

We would have had nothing to present without the initial screening of our subjects. Physical therapists Jan Taylor and Valerie Thom set up the original protocol for screening and took many of our anthropometric measurements, and Judy Leach screened and measured about half of the children. Yet another physical therapist, Patricia Silva, analyzed some of the anthropometric data in conjunction with work on her Master's degree at San Diego State University.

The technical staff of the Motion Analysis Laboratory were crucial to many aspects of our research. Patty Dedrick provided some of the artwork that is fundamental to our descriptions of walking and of the laboratory. In addition, she helped with studies of subjects and with digitizing data. Craig Brueninger made important technical contributions at the outset of our work, especially with data collection and reduction. The efforts of Patty and Craig were continued and supplemented in many ways by Don Nothdurft, Tracy Grindeland, Shawn Chambers, Lesley Wise, Susan Millard and Joe Rodriguez.

Of course, our work on gait analysis is highly data- and computer-intensive, and much technical help was given us with data management, computation, and graphics. We cite in particular Louise Focht of the Motion Analysis Laboratory, who contributed to data management, and Gary Underhill of the

Manufacturing Technology Centre of the University of New Brunswick (UNB), who prepared data for analysis. Thanks are also owed to Evelyn Richards of UNB, and to Christine Justice and Julie Morris of UCSD. Evelyn prepared data for analysis; Christine helped with computations that are the basis of Chapter 10; and Julie helped with some graphics.

Charles Jablecki of UCSD and Keith Brown of the University of Edinburgh offered valuable criticism of Chapter 11. Savio Woo, also of UCSD, was a participant in the original grant and in our preliminary report on these data. Peggy Lasko's work (in our laboratory) on her University of Southern California Ph.D. dissertation contributed to our present understanding of the reproducibility of motion data.

The bootstrap-based prediction regions that we introduce here for the first time are somewhat novel, particularly in the context of gait analysis. Statistical colleagues gave advice concerning them and other aspects of our work. We benefited especially from the comments of Peter Bickel of the University of California, Berkeley; Morris Eaton of the University of Minnesota; Bradley Efron and Iain Johnstone of Stanford University; Søren Johansen of the University of Copenhagen; Charles McCulloch of Cornell University; and John Rice of UCSD. Johansen and Johnstone have shown in very recent work how to derive analytically (without bootstrapping) prediction regions that are very similar to what we have computed with the bootstrap. They have shared with us some impressive graphics that illustrate the possibilities of their approach. We are pleased to have helped stimulate their research.

Institutional support of the most generous sort was provided us by the Children's Hospital and Health Center, San Diego. We mention in particular administrative help from Donald Krebs, Blair Sadler and Anna Edwards. Several units of both UNB and UCSD were supportive of our efforts. In addition to the Manufacturing Technology Center at UNB, we thank the Department of Mechanical Engineering and the Computing Centre. At UCSD, the Division of Orthopaedics and especially its Chair, Wayne Akeson, were important to our success. The Laboratory for Mathematics and Statistics, very ably administered by Joy Kirsch, and the Department of Mathematics helped support our research and travel.

Duke Johnston made key material contributions to constructing the building that houses the Motion Analysis Laboratory, and to equipping it. Important help was provided subsequently by the Weingart Foundation, the Easter Seals Society of San Diego, Mr and Mrs Frederick W. Schrempf, the San Diego Children of the Church of Jesus Christ of Latter-Day Saints, and Margaret B. Wall (in honor of Luba S. Johnston).

Research that is summarized in part in this monograph was generously aided by support from various grants. In particular, we are grateful for NIH grants 5 RO1 HD08520 and 5 RO1 HD15801 to the Children's Hospital and Health Center, San Diego—the first of which supported the gathering of data on our study group of normal children. Three grants to UCSD supported the statistical work that has been so essential to these efforts: NIH grant 5 RO1 PHS CA41628, and NSF grants DMS 85-05609 and DMS 87-22306. Richard Olsen's work on the monograph that was accomplished during a recent sabbatical was supported in part by the John Simon Guggenheim Memorial Foundation, as well as by a Research Scholar in Cancer Award from the American Cancer Society and by the University of California.

Wadsworth International kindly allowed us to adapt two tables published in *Classification and Regression Trees* (Breiman *et al.* 1984) for use in Chapter 10. We thank them.

We recognize the magnificent help that has been provided us by those at Mac Keith Press. Pat Chappelle was a persistent and demanding, and extremely helpful editor of this volume. Though we did not always see eye to eye on how best to deal with each of his many queries, we acknowledge that the monograph is very much the better for his contributions. We thank Martin Bax not only for his very kind Foreword, but also for his encouraging, threatening, cajoling and other energies expended over too many years in the hopes that he would eventually see this monograph in print. We hope, Martin, that what you see now was worth your efforts—and perhaps even the wait.

Finally, but by no means least, we thank the hundreds of children and their families who gave so generously of their time and energies to participate in our project. If we have substantially improved what is known about the development of mature walking, then the benefits to future children will render everyone's contributions worthwhile.

San Diego, California
July 1988

DAVID H. SUTHERLAND
RICHARD A. OLSHEN
EDMUND N. BIDEN
MARILYNN P. WYATT

INDEX

A
Acute infectious polyneuritis (Landry-Guillain-Barre syndrome) 186
Aft shear *see* Fore/aft shear
Age
  distribution of study group 31 (table), 31–32
  prediction from gait measurements 178–82, 180 (fig.), 181–2 (tables)
  case studies 198, 201
Allergic encephalomyelitis 186
α_0 term *see* Population average
Analysis of data *see* Statistical analysis
Ankle
  center 10
  dorsiflexion
    passive 40, 41 (fig.)
  dorsiflexion/plantar flexion
    abnormal 203 (fig.)
    complexity 162
    description 148–9
    measurement 4–5, 10, 12 (fig.)
    motion curves and prediction regions 93–97 (figs.)
  joint laxity 47
  spread, definition of 15
Anterior horn cells, distribution 160
Anterior tibialis *see* Tibialis anterior
Anthropometric measurements 7, 14, 33–48
  form for recording 213–4
Arm span 14, 34, 36 (fig.)
Arm-swing, reciprocal 129 (fig.), 131 (fig.), 152, 153 (fig.)
Automated gait analysis systems 207–9

B
Balance beam
  tandem-walking on, assessment 53, 54 (fig.)
  walking on, assessment 14, 53, 54 (fig.)
Bayes classification rule 179–80
Binary decision tree for age prediction 178–82, 180 (fig.), 181–2 (tables)
Blount's disease 43
Body weight 14, 34, 36 (fig.)
Bootstrap 17, 27–29, 65, 165, 220

C
Cadence 1, 14, 15, 151, 177
  and age 62, 63 (fig.), 64, 129–47 (tables)
  and cycle time 64
  definition of 16
Cameras 3, 10, 22–23 (tables)
  see also VICON video system
CART binary-tree method for age prediction 178–82
Case studies 191–205
Center of mass 166, 167, 176

Center of pressure 5, 6, 15 (fig.)
  case study, plots 199 (fig.)
  definition of 17, 163
  measurement errors 176
  x,y coordinates 14, 15 (fig.)
Cerebral palsy
  benefits of gait analysis 188–91
  case study 200–5
    EMGs 201, 204 (fig.)
    film tracings 201, 204 (fig.)
    joint angles, abnormal 201, 202–3 (figs.)
Charcot-Marie-Tooth disease 186
Computer systems 6–7, 22–23 (tables), 206
Conduction velocity studies, and myelination 185
Consent form 31, 212
Coronal (frontal) plane
  definition of 65, 67 (fig.)
  movement in, 65–67
Crouch gait in spastic diplegia 163
Crown-pubis height 14, 34, 35 (fig.)
Cruising 50, 50 (footnote), 187
Cubic splines 164
Cycle time 14, 15
  and age 55, 62, 63 (fig.), 129–47 (tables)
  and cadence 64

D
Data handling (collection and reduction) *see* Force measurements; Motion data
Demyelination, and impaired gait 186
Dendritic processes, gait maturation and 184
Developmental screening 7, 14, 48–54
  form for recording 213–4
Diapers 153
Digitization 4–5, 5 (fig.), 7, 9 (fig.), 17–21
  aberrant values, replacement of 25–26
  human *vs.* automatic 21
  inter-observer differences 17–21, 20 (figs.)
  timing errors 18–19
Dominance
  foot 14, 49–50, 50 (table)
  hand 14, 49–50, 50 (table)
  mixed 50, 50 (table)
Double-limb support 14
  initial 16, 17 (fig.), 55, 64
  second 16, 17 (fig.), 55, 64
Duchenne muscular dystrophy 182
Dynamic electromyography *see* Electromyography

E
Efron, Bradley 27
Ehlers-Danlos syndrome 45
Elbows, joint laxity 45, 46 (fig.)
Electrogoniometry 205

Electromyography 6, 7–9, 14, 154–61
  case studies 192, 192 (fig.), 201, 204 (fig.)
  equipment used 7–9, 22 (table)
  numbers of completed studies 31 (table)
  test procedure 7–9
  see also Muscle activity
Equipment 21, 207–8, 209
  in present lab 23 (table), 207–8
  used in study 3–21 *passim*, 22 (table)
Ethnic composition of sample 32
Eulerian movement 65, 65 (footnote)

F
Femoral rotation
  abnormal 203 (fig.)
  description 149
  measurement 4–5, 11, 13 (fig.)
  motion curves and prediction regions 103–7 (figs.)
Femoral/tibial angle 14, 43, 44 (fig.)
Femoral/tibial alignment *see* varus/valgus alignment
Film
  analysis 4–5
  cameras 3, 10, 22 (table)
  editing 3–4
  frame errors 18–19, 21
  processing 3
  tracings 1, 65, 66, 129–47 (figs.)
    case studies 193 (fig.), 204 (fig.)
Fingers, joint laxity 45, 46 (fig.)
Finite moment 25 (footnote)
Floor, getting up from, assessment 14, 50
Foot
  dominance 14, 49–50, 50 (table)
  rotation
    abnormal 193, 195 (fig.)
    description 150–1
    measurement 4–5, 11, 13 (fig.)
    motion curves and prediction regions 123–7 (figs.)
Foot-strike 6, 7, 15, 16, 17 (fig.), 55
  flat 129 (fig.), 149
  see also Opposite foot-strike
Footswitches 6, 7, 22 (table)
Force measurements 5–6, 14, 15 (fig.)
  analysis 163–5
    limitations of 165
    modeling 164–5
    splines 164
    variability and prediction regions 165
  by age 163–7
  case study 198, 198–9 (figs.)
  clinical usefulness 176
  components 14, 15 (fig.)
  data reduction 14
  number of studies 31 (table)
  as percentage of body weight 14, 103
  previous studies 176–7

  see also Fore/aft shear; Medial/lateral shear; Torque; Vertical Force
Force plate 3, 4 (fig.), 5–6, 7, 15 (fig.), 22–23 (tables), 206
Fore/aft shear
  definition of 16, 163
  description 166
  maturation 167, 170–1 (figs.), 177
  mean values by age 167, 170–1 (figs.)
  measurement 5, 14, 15 (fig.)
  reversal 16, 17 (fig.)
  vector 15 (fig.), 16
  see also Force measurements
Fourier analysis 5, 17, 19, 24–27, 65
Fourier coefficients 17, 24–25, 26, 162
Frame errors 18–19, 21
Friedreich's ataxia 186

G
Gait analysis
  accessibility 209
  case studies 191–205
  clinical benefits 188–205
    future developments 208–9
    literature 188–91
  commercial systems 207–8
  current development 1, 207–8
  future of 208–9
  history of 202–7
  in sport and recreational activities 209
  study objectives 1
  study plan 30–32
  test procedure 7–10
Gait cycle 15, 17 (fig.)
  definition of 15, 55
  digitization 15
  film tracings 129–47 (figs.)
    case studies 193 (fig.), 204 (fig.)
    of normal 7-year-old girl, 17 (fig.)
  subdivisions 16, 17 (fig.), 55
Gait impairment, and demyelination 186
Gait laboratories
  collaboration 208, 209
  development of 206–7
Gait maturation, indicators of 151–3
Gait problems *see* Pathological gait
Gastrocnemius-soleus (triceps surae)
  EMG activity 14, 160
    immature pattern 160, 161 (fig.)
      case study 201, 204 (fig.)
    mature pattern 160, 161 (fig.)
  flexibility and age 40
  function 160
  maturation 160–2
Gaussian distribution 26
Gluteus maximus
  EMG activity 14, 159, 159 (fig.)
    abnormal 192, 192 (fig.), 201, 204 (fig.)
  function 159

223

maturation 159, 160, 162
Gluteus medius
  EMG activity 156, 157 (fig.)
    abnormal 201, 204 (fig.)
  function 156
  maturation 156, 160, 162
Graf-Pen sonic digitizer 4, 9 (fig.), 22 (table)
Gross manual muscle test, 14, 45
Ground-reaction force 6, 16–17
  definition of 16
  line of application 15 (fig.), 148
  location on foot 6
  vector 163
Growth velocity, and time/distance parameters 56, 64

H

Hamstrings
  EMG activity 14
    abnormal 201, 204 (fig.)
    lateral 156, 158 (fig.)
    medial 156, 158 (fig.)
  flexibility and age 36, 40
  function 156
  and hip abduction 39
  maturation 156, 162
Hand dominance 14, 49–50, 50 (table)
Harmonics 17, 24, 26
  and degrees of freedom 26
  variance of the sum of 27
Health screening questionnaire 30, 210–1
Heel-strike 15, 16, 17 (fig.), 149
  absent 193
  as indicator of gait maturity 133 (fig.), 151, 152
Heel-walking, assessment 14, 51, 52 (fig.)
Height
  crown-to-pubis 14, 33, 35 (fig.)
  pubis-to-toe 14, 33, 35 (fig.)
  ratio of upper-body to lower-body, change with age 34
  sitting 14, 34, 35 (fig.)
  standing 14, 33, 34, 35 (fig.)
  and step length 56, 57 (fig.)
Hip
  abduction/adduction
    abnormal 193, 194 (fig.), 202 (fig.)
    description 66
    measurement 4–5, 11, 13 (fig.)
    motion curves and prediction regions 73–77
    adduction, increase at age 2 years 133 (fig.)
  center 10
  extension, muscle action and joint torque 159
  flexion/extension
    abnormal 202 (fig.)
    complexity 162
    description 148
    measurement 4–5, 10, 12 (fig.)
    motion curves and prediction regions 83–87 (figs.)
  passive range of motion 14
    abduction 38–39, 41
    adduction 39
    extension 36, 37 (fig.), 41
    flexion with knee extended (straight-leg raising) 36, 37 (fig.), 41
    rotation 37–38, 41, 150
  rotation
    calculation 14
    description 149–50
    external, decreased at age 2 133 (fig.)
    motion curves and prediction regions 108–112 (figs.)
Hopping, assessment 14, 51–52, 53 (fig.)
Hypermobility 45–48

I

Initial double-limb support 16, 17 (fig.), 55
Initial swing 16, 17 (fig.), 55
Intercondylar distance 43
Intermalleolar distance 43

J

Joint angles
  case studies 193, 194–7 (figs.), 201, 202–3 (figs.)
  composite 128–46 (figs.)
  coronal (frontal) plane 4–5, 66–67
  as evidence of pathological gait 201
  gait events and changes in 151
  measurement 4–5, 10–14, 12–13 (figs.), 19–21, 66
  motion curves and prediction regions 128–46 (figs.)
    case studies 193, 194–7 (figs.), 201, 202–3 (figs.)
  parallax correction 4–5, 10
  prediction regions 17, 25, 26–29, 65, 128–46 (figs.), 193, 201, 220
  sagittal plane 4, 67, 148–9
  transverse plane 4–5, 149–51
  see also Motion data; and under individual joint rotations

K

Kicking, spontaneous 184
Knee
  center 10
  flexion/extension
    abnormal 202–3 (figs.)
    complexity 162
    description 148
    and gait maturity 133 (fig.), 151, 152, 152 (fig.)
    measurement 4–5, 10, 12 (fig.)
    motion curves and prediction regions 88–92 (figs.)
  hyperextension 40
  joint laxity 45, 47 (fig.)
  passive extension 14, 40

rotation
  abnormal 203 (fig.)
  calculation 14
  description 150
  motion curves and prediction regions 118–122
Knots 164

L

Landry-Guillain-Barre syndrome (acute infectious polyneuritis), 186
Lateral hamstrings *see* Hamstrings
Learning, and gait development 183, 184, 187
Leg length
  and age 56, 57 (fig.)
  and step length 56, 57 (fig.)
Lévy-Roussy syndrome 185
Loading peaks 165–6, 168–9 (figs.), 177
  exaggerated 198, 199 (fig.)
Loading portion 165
Lower-extremity dominance 14, 49–50, 50 (table)

M

Markers and marker sticks
  in measuring joint angles 10–11, 12–13 (figs.), 15–16
  positioning 7, 8 (fig.), 9 (fig.), 21
  errors 18–19
  x,y coordinates 4, 5 (fig.)
Medial hamstrings *see* Hamstrings
Medial/lateral shear
  definition of 16, 163
  description 167
  maturation 167, 177
  mean values by age 167, 172–3 (figs.)
  measurement 5, 14, 15 (fig.)
  see also Force measurements
Mid-stance 16, 17 (fig.), 55
  trough 166, 177
Mid-swing 16, 17 (fig.), 55
Modeling *see* Statistical analysis
Motion, developmental screening of passive 34–41
Motion Analysis Laboratory, Children's Hospital, San Diego 1, 3–7, 207
  see also Equipment
Motion analyzer 4–5, 5 (fig.), 14–16, 22 (table)
Motion curves *see* Joint angles
Motion data
  aberrant, correction of 25–26
  collection 3–5, 14–15
  elimination 31
  handling 6–7, 14–16
  normal variation 21
  reduction (digitization) 15–16
  reproducibility 17–21, 20 (figs.)
  sex differences 32
  statistical analysis 3, 7, 17, 24 29, 65
  see also Movement measurements

Motor control system, gait and maturation of 55, 61, 160, 162, 183–7
Movement measurements
  description 3–5, 7
  equipment used
    in present laboratory 21, 23 (table)
    in study 21, 22 (table)
  numbers of completed studies 31 (table)
  using chalk dust, ink or talc 1, 63
  see also Digitization; Gait analysis; Joint angles; Motion analyzer; Motion data; Time/distance parameters
Multiple sclerosis 184, 186
Muscle activity 154–62
  abnormal 201, 204 (fig.)
  case studies 192, 192 (fig.), 201, 204 (fig.)
  conclusions 160–2
  intensity 154
  maturation of 160, 162
  numbers of completed studies 31 (table)
  'on/off' times
    differentiation 7–9
    as percentage of gait cycle 6, 14, 154–5
    variation in 14
  phasic, definition of 17
  test procedure 8–9
  see also Electromyography; and under individual muscles
Muscle resistance to gait events 151
Muscle strength (gross manual muscle test) 14, 45
Muybridge, Eadweard 206
Myelination, and gait maturation 160, 162, 184–7

N

Neonatal reflexes 54, 184
Nervous system, gait and development of 183–7
Non-age-specific gait measurements 178
Null hypothesis, definition of 153 (footnote)

O

Opposite foot-strike 14, 15, 16, 17 (fig.), 55, 151
  by age 58–59, 59 (table), 60 (fig.), 129–47 (tables)
Opposite toe-off 14, 15, 16, 17 (fig.), 55, 151
  by age 58, 59 (table), 60 (fig.), 129–47 (tables)
  and single-limb stance 61, 61 (fig.)
Oscillograph 6, 7, 22 (table)
Oscilloscope 6, 7, 22 (table)

P

Passive range of motion 34–41
Pathological gait 1, 16
  case study 200–5
Pelvic belt 7, 8 (fig.), 9 (fig.), 11, 12 (fig.), 13 (fig.)
Pelvic obliquity
  abnormal 202 (fig.)
  description 149

225

measurement 4–5, 11, 13 (fig.)
motion curves and prediction regions 68–72 (figs.)
Pelvic rotation
abnormal 203 (fig.)
description 149
measurement 4–5, 11, 13 (fig.)
motion curves and prediction regions 98–102 (figs.)
Pelvic span, definition of 152
Pelvic-span/ankle-spread ratio 14, 67, 151–3, 153 (fig.)
Pelvic tilt
abnormal 202 (fig.)
description 67
measurement 4–5, 10, 12 (fig.)
motion curves and prediction regions 78–82 (figs.)
Phasic muscle activity *see* Muscle activity
Physical therapy examinations 9, 30, 31 (table), 33, 45
Planes of movement 65–66, 67 (fig.)
see also Coronal (frontal) plane; Medial plane; Transverse plane
Population average (α_0 term) 21, 24–27, 65
Prediction interval 29
Prediction regions 17, 25, 26–29, 65, 128–46 (figs.), 220
case-study comparisons 193, 194–7 (figs.), 201, 202–3 (figs.)
for force data 165
Preference *see* Dominance
Pre-walking development 184
Protective extension reflex 14, 54
Pubis-toe length 14, 34, 35 (fig.)
Push-off 166

Q
Quadriceps femoris *see* Vastus medialis

R
Radiography 43
Range of motion *see* Passive range of motion
Reciprocal arm-swing 129 (fig.), 131 (fig.), 152, 153 (fig.)
Reflexes
protective extension 54
retained neonatal 54
stepping 184
Reproducibility of data 17–21, 20 (fig.)
Right/left comparisons 36, 45, 51, 53, 58–59
Running, assessment 14, 51, 52 (fig.), 64

S
Sagittal plane
definition of 65, 67 (fig.)
movement in 65, 67, 148–9
Second double-limb support 16, 17 (fig.), 55
Selection of subjects 30–31

Sex
differences 32–34
distribution of study group 31–32, 32 (table)
Single-limb stance 14, 15, 16, 17 (fig.), 51, 55, 151, 177
and ability to stand on one leg 51
and age 59–60, 64, 129–47 (tables)
duration 16
force on foot, measurement 6
and toe-off 61
Sitting height 14, 34, 35 (fig.)
Spastic diplegia 163, 211
Squatting, assessment 14, 50
Stance phase 16, 17 (fig.)
muscle activity as percentage of 154–5
Standing height 14, 33, 34, 35 (fig.)
relationship to arm span 34
Standing on one leg, assessment 14, 51, 52 (fig.)
Standing up unassisted, assessment 14, 50
Statistical analysis
of force data 163–5
of motion data 5, 7, 17, 24–29
Step length 1, 14, 15, 151
and age 56, 57 (fig.), 64, 129–47 (tables)
definition of 16
and height 56, 57 (fig.)
and leg length 56, 57 (fig.)
Stepping reflex 184
Straight-leg raising, passive 36, 37 (fig.), 41
Stride length 1, 14, 16, 55
and age 56 (fig.), 58, 129–47 (tables), 177
definition of 16
Study plan 30–32
Subjects
age distribution 31, 32 (table)
racial composition 32
recruitment criteria 30
selection 30–31
sex distribution 32, 32 (table)
Support base, width of 67
Swing phase 16, 17 (fig.), 55, 64
EMG activity as percentage of 154–5

T
Tandem-walking on balance beam, assessment 53, 54 (fig.)
Terminal stance 16, 17 (fig.), 55
Test procedure 7–10
Tibial rotation
abnormal 203 (fig.)
description 150
measurement 4–5, 11, 13 (fig.), 18
motion curves and prediction regions 113–7 (figs.)
Tibial torsion (transmalleolar axis) 14, 41–42, 42 (fig.), 43 (fig.)
Tibialis anterior
EMG activity 14, 155, 155 (fig.)
abnormal 192, 192 (fig.)

function 155
maturation 155, 162
Time/distance parameters 4, 14, 55–64
  discussion 62–64
  mean values by age 129–47 (tables)
  measurement 4
  numbers of completed studies 31 (table)
  previous studies 63–64
  see also individual parameters
Toe-off 15, 16, 17 (fig.), 55, 151
  and age 59, 60 (fig.), 129–47 (tables)
  and single-limb stance 61, 61 (fig.)
  see also Opposite toe-off
Toe-walking, assessment 51, 52 (fig.)
Torque
  description 167–76
  exaggerated, in cerebral palsy 198, 198–9 (figs.)
  maturation 174–5 (figs.), 176, 177
  mean values by age 174–5 (figs.), 176
  measurement 5, 14, 163
  see also Force measurements
Transducers 5, 15 (fig.), 206
Transmalleolar axis (tibial torsion), 14, 41–42, 42 (fig.), 43 (fig.)
Transverse plane
  definition of 65, 67 (fig.)
  movement in 65, 67, 149–51
Triceps surae *see* Gastrocnemius-soleus

U
Upper limb
  dominance 14, 49–50, 50 (table)
  protective extension reflex 14, 54

V
Varus/valgus alignment 14, 42–43, 44 (fig.)
Vastus medialis (quadriceps femoris)
  EMG activity 14, 156, 157 (fig.)

abnormal 192, 192 (fig.)
function 156
maturation 156, 162
Vertical acceleration 163
Vertical force
  definition of 16, 163
  description 165–6
  maturation 166, 168–9 (figs.), 177
  mean values by age 166, 168–9 (figs.)
  measurement 5, 14, 15 (fig.)
  vector 15 (fig.), 16
  see also Force measurements
VICON video system 3, 21, 23 (table), 207–8

W
Walking
  assessment
    on balance beam 14, 53, 54 (fig.)
    on heels 14, 51, 52 (fig.)
    on tiptoes 14, 51, 52 (fig.)
  independent, age of 48, 49 (table)
  symmetry of 64
  see also Gait analysis
Walking velocity 1, 14, 55, 151, 167, 177
  and age 62, 63 (fig.), 64, 129–47 (tables)
  control over 64
  definition of 16
  and stride length 64
Walkway, in Gait Analysis Laboratory 3, 6, 7, 8 (fig.), 9
Weight *see* Body weight
Weight-bearing 167
Wrists, joint laxity 45, 46 (fig.)

X
X-ray examination 43
x,y coordinates
  of body markers 4, 5 (fig.), 9 (fig.)
  of center of pressure 14